Informed Consent in Medical Research

Informed Consent in Medical Research

Edited by

Len Doyal

Professor of Medical Ethics, St Bartholomew's and the Royal London School of Medicine and Dentistry, Queen Mary, University of London *and* Honorary Consultant, Bart's and The London NHS Trust, UK

and

Jeffrey S Tobias

Consultant in Clinical Oncology, Meyerstein Institute of Oncology, Middlesex Hospital, London, UK and Chair, Education Committee, Cancer Research Campaign, London, UK

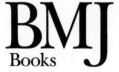

First published in 2001
by BMJ Books, BMA House, Tavistock Square,
London WC1H 9JR

www.bmjbooks.com

British Library Cataloguing in Publication Data
A catalogue record for this book is available from the British Library

ISBN 0-7279-1486-3

Cover design by Landmark Design, Croydon, Surrey
Typeset by Gray Publishing, Tunbridge Wells, Kent
Printed and bound by MPG Books Ltd, Bodmin, Cornwall

Contents

Contributors

SM Louise Abrams
St Bartholomew's and the Royal London School of
Medicine and Dentistry, Queen Mary, University of
London, London, UK

David Benatar
Lecturer, Department of Philosophy and Bioethics
Centre, University of Cape Town, South Africa

Solomon R Benatar
Professor of Medicine, and Director, Bioethics
Centre, Department of Medicine, University of
Cape Town, South Africa

Rebecca Bennett
Lecturer in Bioethics, Institute of Law, Medicine
and Bioethics, University of Manchester, UK

Satish Bhagwanjee
Faculty of Medicine, University of Natal, Durban,
South Africa

Baruch A Brody
Leon Jaworksi Professor of Biomedical Ethics,
Baylor College of Medicine, Houston, Texas, USA

GA Browning
Solicitor, London, UK

John P Bunker
Emeritus Professor of Anaesthesia, Stanford
University, USA; Visiting Professor, Department of
Epidemiology and Public Health, University
College London, UK

Ruth Chadwick
Professor of Bioethics, Philosophy Department,
Lancaster University, UK

Iain Chalmers
Director, UK Cochrane Centre, Oxford, UK

Martin Dennis
Department of Clinical Neurosciences, University
of Edinburgh, Western General Hospital,
Edinburgh, UK

Heather Draper
Senior Lecturer, Centre for Biomedical Ethics, The
Medical School, University of Birmingham, UK

Paul J Edelson
Columbia University College of Physicians and
Surgeons, New York, USA

Bobbie Farsides
Senior Lecturer in Medical Ethics, Centre of
Medical Law and Ethics, Kings College London,
UK

Phil Fennell
Reader in Law, Department of Law, University of
Cardiff, UK

CM Foster
Assistant Secretary, Science, Medicine, Technology
and Environmental Issues, Board for Social
Responsibility, Church of England, UK

Raanan Gillon
Emeritus Professor of Medical Ethics, Imperial
College Ethics Unit, Department of Primary Care,
Imperial College, London, UK

Heather Goodare
Personal Counsellor, Horsham, UK

Angela Hall
Senior Lecturer in Communication Skills, St
George's Hospital Medical School, London, UK

John Harris
Sir David Alliance Professor of Bioethics, Institute
of Medicine, Law and Bioethics, University of
Manchester, UK

Brian Hurwitz
Head, Department of Primary Health Care and
General Practice, Imperial College School of
Medicine, London, UK

Prakash M Jeena
Faculty of Medicine, University of Natal, Durban,
South Africa

Alan G Johnson
Professor of Surgery, the University of Sheffield, UK

Rajendra Kale
Neurologist, Pune, India

Laxmi-Kunj
Neurologist, Pune, India

Richard I Lindley
Consultant Physician and Geriatrician, Lothian University Hospitals NHS Trust, Part-time Senior Lecturer, Western General Hospital, Edinburgh, UK

Stephen Lock
Former Editor, *British Medical Journal*, London, UK

Sheila AM McLean
School of Law, University of Glasgow, UK

Paul McNeill
Associate Professor, School of Community Medicine, University of New South Wales, Sydney, Australia

Eric M Meslin
Executive Director, National Bioethics Advisory Commission, Bethesda, USA

Jonathan Montgomery
Reader in Health Care Law, The Department of Law, University of Southampton, UK

Prushini Moodley
Faculty of Medicine, University of Natal, Durban, South Africa

David JJ Muckart
Faculty of Medicine, University of Natal, Durban, South Africa

Richard Nicholson
Editor, *Bulletin of Medical Ethics*, London, UK

Suzanne O'Rourke
Department of Clinical Neurosciences, University of Edinburgh, Western General Hospital, Edinburgh, UK

Naomi Pfeffer
Professor of Social and Historical Studies of Health, School of Community Health, Psychology and Social Work, University of North London, UK

Lisa Power
Terrence Higgins Trust, London, UK

YK Seedat
Medical School, University of Natal, Durban, South Africa

Jim Slattery
Department of Clinical Neurosciences, University of Edinburgh, Western General Hospital, Edinburgh, UK

Richard Smith
Editor, *British Medical Journal*, London, UK

Ann Sommerville
Head of Medical Ethics, British Medical Association, London, UK

Trish Staniforth
Department of Clinical Neurosciences, University of Edinburgh, Western General Hospital, Edinburgh, UK

Chris Ward
Consultant Plastic Surgeon, Surrey, UK and Honorary Senior Lecturer in Medical Ethics, Imperial College School of Medicine, London, UK

Charles Warlow
Department of Clinical Neurosciences, University of Edinburgh, Western General Hospital, Edinburgh, UK

Mary Warnock
Former Chair of the Committee of Inquiry into Human Fertilisation

Paul Weindling
Humanities Research Centre, Oxford Brookes University, Oxford, UK

Kulsum Winship
Breast Cancer Advisory Committee, Barnet Health Authority, UK

Simon Woods
Lecturer in Bioethics, Institute of Medicine, Law and Bioethics, University of Manchester, UK

Foreword

I'm thinking of starting a new political party. Its working title is the "Life is hard; we have no solutions" party. It will work in a completely different way from traditional parties. They promise everything. We will promise nothing. Our manifesto, which is still under development, is shown in the box on page xiii. It seems unlikely that we will come to power soon, but we will eventually when the electorate tires of the political cycle of a party promising everything, getting elected, failing to deliver, and being replaced by its opponents who in their turn promise everything.

One of the stimuli to the new party is this magnificent book. It grew out of our uncertainty and confusion at the *BMJ*, and it's a book that provides no easy answers but will hugely deepen your understanding of informed consent. The book is a tribute to sharing uncertainty and confusion.

The *BMJ* had to decide three years ago whether to publish two original studies where the participants had not given informed consent. Publication is of course a binary event. Either we published or we didn't publish. We had intense arguments over what to do, and several advisers told us that we would be disgraced if we published. Nevertheless, we thought that there was much to be gained and little to be lost by sharing our uncertainties. I hesitate to say that we were right, but this book had its roots in our uncertainty.

We published the studies together with a series of commentaries, and we invited Len Doyal, the five star ethicist, and Jeff Tobias, the clinician at the coalface, to write opposing articles on whether we were right to publish some studies that didn't include fully informed consent. They thus started as opponents but then came together to edit this rich book. The book is made especially compelling and interesting by their dialectic running right through it.

The issue of the *BMJ* that included this collection of material produced a flood of well argued correspondence, and we recognised that we had touched a nerve. The *BMJ* issue was followed by a conference, where the focus began to shift from informed consent in research to informed consent in clinical practice and teaching. It became very clear that standards in clinical practice and teaching are considerably below those in research. Yet the spotlight continues to be shone on research because it must be approved by ethics committees and the results are held up to the world to be scrutinised. Clinical practice and teaching have nothing like the same exposure.

This book gathers together much of the material that arose from the *BMJ* and the conference and moves it on. Our small scale confusion is embedded in its historical context and then developed with a series of profound pieces on all aspects of informed consent.

An issue that becomes more central every day

Books take a long time to put together, and publishers always worry that the world may have lost interest in the subject of their book by the time that it is published. Here, I would argue, the opposite has happened. With every day that goes by the issue of informed consent becomes more central in health care. The driver is the changing relationship between clinicians and patients.

Clinicians were like politicians. They knew best. They would solve the patient's problems. So long as patients and society trusted them to do what was best then they would get on with their mysterious processes, including some judicious research without consent, and everything would be alright. In those days trust and ignorance went together. Now that's unacceptable. Patients are better educated. Deference is outdated. A series of scandals have exposed serious abuses within medicine and research. We now live in a world where what is closed is immediately suspect. Lack of transparency implies incompetence, corruption, or bias.

So clinicians increasingly relate to patients as partners, and there is growing evidence that this partnership brings better clinical outcomes, greater patient satisfaction, and reduced costs. It can also be beneficial to clinicians. They do not have to pretend to know what they do not know and be able to do what they cannot do.

A successful partnership depends on effective interchange of information. If the doctor keeps something from the patient then trust is likely to be broken, particularly if the doctor does something to the patient without consent. Trust comes now not from ignorance but from sharing uncertainty.

Here I must confess that this is more the view of an informed patient than a practising doctor. It's 20 years since I saw patients, and some of my friends who are seeing patients everyday tell me that I'm out of touch. I've spent too much time with ethicists and the chattering classes. I've forgotten the realities of practice, which include dealing with frightened and impaired patients who don't want to be overloaded with information and patients who for one reason or another have great difficulties handling complex information.

But even if it's true that some patients chose to know little, most do want to know – and there is no going back. Informed consent is coming ever more to the fore, and often it's a battleground. I'm writing this in July 2000, and one news page in this week's *BMJ* contains two stories that relate directly to consent. A new federal agency in the United States has stopped all government sponsored clinical trials at the University of Oklahoma Health Sciences Center at Tulsa. Researchers conducting a trial of a vaccine for malignant melanoma had failed to tell the patients of the vaccine's safety problems. They had also allegedly misled candidates for the trial by telling them that the vaccine might reduce the size of their tumours when the aim of the study was to test the toxicity of the vaccine.

The story underneath tells how researchers in Britain are having great difficulty recruiting patients to a big trial that aims to assess the effectiveness of chemotherapy in non-small cell lung cancer. Of 253 eligible candidates only 63 (25%) have agreed to enter the trial. Patients seem less willing than in previous studies to accept a high degree of toxicity. The possibility arises in my mind that these patients may be being told more about the possible side effects than participants in previous trials.

Clinicians and researchers

Some of those who read this book, particularly those who are researchers, will feel sympathy for the researchers in the lung trial. They are addressing a difficult and important clinical problem. Many patients with non-small cell lung cancer are treated every day all over the world, yet, as the lead researcher in the trial says, considerable uncertainty remains over the effectiveness of adding chemotherapy over standard treatment. That's why they are doing a trial.

But what do clinicians all over the world say to these patients? It's unlikely, I suggest, that they share all the uncertainty with their patients. The clinicians may pretend that they know more than they do, or – most likely – they pretend to themselves. They can then with a good conscience recommend a particular line of treatment. If, however, they choose to acknowledge the uncertainty (and perhaps join my new political party) then they are into something difficult. They will have to share their uncertainty with the patients. They might also feel an ethical obligation to start a trial to answer their uncertainty. Then they have to design a protocol, seek approval from an ethics committee, and seek from patients not only consent for treatment but also for randomisation.

Researchers, many of whom are clinicians, resent what they see as these "double standards". Some want to be able to adopt the "lower" standards that apply to the clinicians, but I think they misread the zeitgeist. What is more likely is that clinicians will have to learn to share their uncertainty.

From Pappworth to COPE

This territory in health care where all is uncertain and where clinicians and researchers are both found is the source of many difficulties. Clinicians want to help patients. Researchers want to reduce the uncertainty. Patients would like things to be certain but mostly, evidence suggests, want to know about the uncertainty. It's easy to take a wrong step in such territory, which covers much of health care.

I thought about this territory when I read the beginning of Maurice Pappworth's preface (reproduced here) to his important book *Human Guinea Pigs* in which he exposed the wide extent of experimentation without consent in Britain (p. 39). The book was published in 1967, but his words are as applicable now as then.

"The main purpose of this book is to show that the ethical problems arising from human experimentation have become one of the cardinal issues of our time…I believe that only by frank discussion among informed people, lay as well as medical, can a solution be reached."

To bring the words completely up to date I would broaden Pappworth's phrase about "ethical problems arising from human experimentation" to "ethical problems arising from managing uncertainty in clinical practice and research". It also sounds old fashioned to me to think that "a solution can be reached". In the postmodern world, all truths are provisional and all solutions are not only incomplete but also suspect.

Thirty years after Pappworth wrote his book, the Committee on Publication Ethics was formed, and anybody reading COPE's annual reports might be reminded of Pappworth's book. COPE advises editors of medical journals on ethical problems thrown up by papers they are considering or have published, and the annual reports describe these cases. The cases are rarely as shocking as those included in *Human Guinea Pigs*, but they have similarities.

I have dealt with several cases where clinicians have developed theories on new treatments, including surgical treatments, and have tried them out on patients without getting any approval from an ethics committee. They have also conducted their experiments in ways that I believe do not allow for any confident conclusion, which in itself raises ethical problems. Research that is scientifically unsound may be regarded as automatically unsound ethically. When I challenge these authors they usually tell me that patients have consented to the treatment. Clearly they have in the sense that they have taken the tablets or undergone the operation, but did they understand that they were part of an unscientific experiment? I doubt they did because surely then they would not have consented. But then the doctors did not regard what they were doing as experiments, even though they have written up their studies for the *BMJ*. They think of them as accounts of clinical practice. I think of them as explorations of uncertainty, and I think that they should share their uncertainty with the patients. They think I'm an ethically obsessed editor. We don't agree.

Readers of this book are not expected to agree with everything it contains. Indeed, they couldn't because the book is full of disagreement. I hope, however, that readers will agree that informed consent is a central issue for health care, that the problems are real and pressing, that no solution will be found, and that this is a marvellous book.

Richard Smith
Editor, *BMJ*

Competing interest statement: I am the chief executive of the BMJ Publishing Group, which is publishing this book, and I am the editor of the *BMJ*, from which some of the material comes. I am, however, paid a fixed salary and will not benefit financially from any success this book might have.

Manifesto of the "Life is hard; we have no solutions" party

Death is inevitable. Prepare for it.

We live in a world of competing sorrows.

You will rarely understand and will be constantly misunderstood.

You identify the problems. You do something about them, recognising that all solutions tackle only part of the problem and give rise to other problems.

Life is full of inevitable contradictions.

When things go wrong, as they will, little is gained by blaming somebody.

Introduction

Len Doyal and Jeffrey S Tobias

Belief in the right of individuals to good healthcare, a fundamental precept of the National Health Service in the United Kingdom, goes hand in hand with a moral commitment to support medical research. Without it, how can we claim to have minimised the ill-effects of disease? Since all of us are potential or actual patients at some point during our lives, a public commitment to well designed clinical studies offering reliable information about new treatment methods, must surely be in the common interest. Yet it is also true that in their zeal to make progress, some medical researchers have behaved unethically, sometimes exposing patients to unacceptable risks of further ill health: the polar opposite of what good medicine seeks to promote. As a result of concern about such unethical practice, medical research has become highly regulated over the past three decades.

One component of this regulation is the general duty of researchers to obtain the consent of patients or healthy volunteers before they participate in medical experiments. This emphasis on choice is based on the moral and legal importance of individuals exercising control over what happens to their bodies, especially when they may be subject to the risk of physical or mental harm. Choice to participate in medical research, it is argued, cannot be rationally exercised without information about what is proposed and why, together with the main side-effects and hazards that might occur as a result. Since the capacity to exercise such choice – to act with autonomy – is commonly regarded as the most important attribute which sets humans apart from other animals, not to respect this capacity could be seen as an affront to human dignity.

This book is about the principle of informed consent in medical research. It was most notably articulated by the Nuremberg Code in the aftermath of Nazi medical atrocities and has since been adopted both in the Helsinki Declaration of the World Medical Association and by a wide range of other promi-

nent national and international organisations involved in the professional regulation of medical research. The consensus of professional opinion about the general importance of informed consent in research has been fuelled by a number of widely criticised medical experiments over the past 50 years where irrespective of any other harm that may have befallen participants, informed consent was not obtained. As a result, in North America and the United Kingdom, for example, great emphasis is now placed by research ethics committees on ensuring that researchers will routinely obtain informed consent. Yet despite this consensus about the importance, in principle, of respecting the right of participants in medical research to informed consent, there is much less agreement about how to interpret this rule in practice.

On the one hand, some argue that if the principle is interpreted rigidly then it becomes inconsistent with other moral duties. For example, if patients have a strict right to information about potentially distressing aspects of participating in research, does this not then conflict with the clinical duty of researchers not to distress them with information which may be unwanted and might cause considerable harm? Equally, if it is accepted that we all have a right to optimal healthcare, and thus to the benefits of the participation of past volunteers in medical research, do we not have a corresponding duty to participate in such research for the public good and for future generations – whatever our preferences might be to the contrary? Others argue in return that the right to exercise autonomous choice over participation in research trumps any of our other rights and duties, even when these are also accepted as morally important. For example, patients may be more upset by having potentially distressing information withheld about their participation in research than they would be by the information itself. Equally, while it may be accepted

– or at least argued – that we do all have a duty to participate in medical research in the public interest, it does not follow that we should be manipulated through lack of information to do so.

Because of such differences of opinion, the *BMJ* asked us in 1997 to write position papers which would explore both sides of the argument. At that point, our focus was to be the question of whether or not the *BMJ* should publish the results of research which had been done without the informed consent of participants. These papers, along with other accompanying articles and editorial comment, generated the largest "mail bag" of letters in the history of the *BMJ*. As a result of this enormous interest, a successful national conference was held in 1998 to debate the issues. In the heady aftermath of this gathering, we decided to create a book which would take the discussion and debate further still, as well as providing a practical guide to researchers about their current obligations concerning informed consent. The book is divided into five parts.

Part 1 explores the historical evolution of the doctrine of informed consent in medical research. The development of international and national regulation concerning consent is outlined, along with its relationship to a variety of examples of unethical research. The impact of the infamous Nazi experiments is described, including an interesting and surprising description of some of the contemporary controversy surrounding the Nuremberg trial.

This general background is followed by the exciting re-publication for the first time of two of the most important works on the ethics of medical research and the principle of informed consent. These often referred to, but seldom seen contributions, are Henry Beecher's famous article in the 1966 *New England Journal of Medicine* which is reprinted in full and Maurice Pappworth's equally devastating contribution of the following year, *Human Guinea Pigs*, from which we have chosen representative selections. Both works exhaustively documented examples of unethical research in Britain and the United States during the 1950s and 1960s and influenced current national and international patterns of regulating research. Interestingly, the dramatic impact of Beecher's work on the development of North American regulation was only matched by the relatively deaf ears on which Pappworth's efforts fell in Britain. Both contributions are introduced by fascinating historical analyses of the background to these different national responses. Finally, to bring readers up to date, we have included a detailed exposition of more recent and questionable research practice pertaining to informed consent. This chapter outlines research which has been consistently criticised in the United States, Australia, New Zealand, the United Kingdom and elsewhere.

Part 2 includes the publications within the *BMJ* that generated such an enormous correspondence. First, there are two studies that took place without informed consent and which the *BMJ* decided to publish anyway. These concern an assessment of a family care worker for patients in the aftermath of a stroke and a study in South Africa concerning rates of HIV admission to surgical intensive care. The reasons why the researchers believed informed consent to be inappropriate are outlined by them, with some preliminary critical reactions of others.

Then our two papers are reproduced, debating whether or not the *BMJ* should ever publish such research. While fully respecting each other as fellow professionals, we strongly disagree in our arguments and conclusions about this matter. Our contributions are followed by the complete publication of the extraordinary (and for us gratifying) breadth of letters published by the *BMJ*, representing a huge diversity of perspectives on the moral, legal and professional importance of informed consent in medical research. Finally, a range of other types of responses to the debate also published by the *BMJ* – editorials, short articles and other forms of comment – are also included. *In toto*, this is a unique collection of material, highly useful for undergraduate and postgraduate teaching.

The many contributions to Part 2 raise important issues about the appropriate professional boundaries of the principle of informed consent within medical research. However, because of their brevity, most contributions unavoidably lack the detail which justice to these issues demands. Consequently, for **Part 3** of the book, we commissioned well-known experts to explore how different countries approach the problem of informed consent in regulating medical research and how this regulation impacts upon the practice of medical research in a variety of clinical disciplines.

Three interesting problems emerge from these contributions:

1 While the general approach to regulating research through North America and Europe continues to support the general appropriateness of informed consent, this does not amount to a blan-

ket endorsement or mandate. Most regulations recognise the acceptability of exceptions to the rule, with respect to other circumstances, where it is believed that there is no risk to patients who participate without their knowledge or where patients are unable to consent and the risk–benefit ratio of doing so is very much in their favour.

2 Several contributors raise practical problems about obtaining consent, even where it is accepted that it should generally be attempted. For example, these often concern difficulties in communicating complex information to patients who may be under enormous stress because of their illness or who have other personal problems about understanding such information.

3 Some contributors note that to overly emphasise the individual right to consent (or not) to participate in research can lead to an underemphasis on the moral responsibility of healthy volunteers and patients to do so.

In **Part 4** other experts analyse these three – and other – problems in more detail. For example, the chapters argue in sequence that:

• Respect for the right of patients to give their informed consent to medical research should be understood in the context of broader, internationally recognised human rights. Any compromises which are reached with respect to the specific issue of informed consent should always be understood against the background of the potential abuses of human rights to which they could lead.

• A rigid emphasis on informed consent can itself lead to violations of human rights. If patients have a right to be given certain information before they participate in medical research then does it not follow that they also have a right to refuse unwanted and potentially distressing information? Why should they not simply be able to trust their doctor/researcher to act in their best interests.

• Conventional analyses of informed consent in medical research risk dangerously overemphasising the hazards of participation. In fact, much ordinary clinical care is administered without the same attention to evidence and control over clinical administration that is usually found in the conduct of medical research. Without understanding this, patients cannot give proper informed consent to conventional treatment, much less understand why it might be always in their best interests to choose to participate in research.

• Placing too much moral emphasis on informed consent detracts from the responsibility of citizens to contribute to the public good through not becoming "free riders" in their use of medical advances. This will result inevitably from refusing to participate in medical research. While not concluding that participation in medical research should be compulsory, these authors do point in the direction of how this might be argued.

Finally, it makes little sense to emphasise the moral and legal importance of informed consent without paying equal attention to the practical problems associated with obtaining it. Thus the final chapters reason that:

• There should be more consumer participation in the planning and execution of medical research. Here it is maintained that just as patients can have personal difficulties in understanding information, the same applies to clinical researchers with respect to their communication skills and their understanding of the moral importance of an acceptable level of disclosure of information. For this reason, informed consent in medical research should not just be understood as an ethical issue – it also raises problems about education and professional training.

• There is extensive evidence that some healthcare researchers have poor communication skills as regards obtaining informed consent and that these can – and should – be improved.

• There is a variety of ways in which the moral importance of informed consent and the practical importance of related communication skills can and should be taught within undergraduate and postgraduate education.

In **Part 5**, we reflect on the arguments which have been developed in the book, relating these back to the themes we explored in our original *BMJ* chapters. While we have not altered many of our fundamental tenets, we have certainly sharpened and clarified them by considering the many new arguments of our contributors. Whatever remains unresolved in the debate between us, future discussions about informed consent will doubtless be far better informed by the labour of the their contributions.

Throughout the development of this book, our goal has been to help researchers understand the moral, legal and professional demands concerning the provision of informed consent by participants in medical research. We have also attempted a fair and incisive analysis to help explain why the principle of informed consent is now taken so seriously, along with the obligation to obtain such consent. We have been consistently gratified by the extremely high quality of the chapters and by the enthusiasm and commitment of the contributors. We thank Janet Bennett, Lesley Doyal, Jayshree Kara, Christine Sinclair, and especially appreciate the advice and support that we received from Mary Banks, Christina Karaviotis and Alex Stibbe at BMJ Books.

Part 1

Informed consent and medical research: a historical perspective

1 • The Nuremberg Code* and the Helsinki Declaration†

The Nuremberg Code (1947)

The judgment by the war crimes tribunal at Nuremberg laid down 10 standards to which physicians must conform when carrying out experiments on human subjects.[1]

PERMISSIBLE MEDICAL EXPERIMENTS

The great weight of the evidence before us is to the effect that certain types of medical experiments on human beings, when kept within reasonably well-defined bounds, conform to the ethics of the medical profession generally. The protagonists of the practice of human experimentation justify their views on the basis that such experiments yield results for the good of society that are unprocurable by other methods or means of study. All agree, however, that certain basic principles must be observed in order to satisfy moral, ethical and legal concepts:

1. The voluntary consent of the human subject is absolutely essential. This means that the person involved should have legal capacity to give consent; should be so situated as to be able to exercise free power of choice, without the intervention of any element of force, fraud, deceit, duress, overreaching, or other ulterior form of constraint or coercion; and should have sufficient knowledge and comprehension of the elements of the subject matter involved as to enable him to make an understanding and enlightened decision. This latter element requires that before the acceptance of an affirmative decision by the experimental subject there should be made known to him the nature, duration, and purpose of the experiment; the method and means by which it is to be conducted; all inconveniences and hazards reasonably to be expected; and the effects upon his health or person that may possibly come from his participation in the experiment. The duty and responsibility for ascertaining the quality of the consent rests upon each individual who initiates, directs, or engages in the experiment. It is a personal duty and responsibility that may not be delegated to another with impunity.

2. The experiment should be such as to yield fruitful results for the good of society, unprocurable by other methods or means of study, and not random and unnecessary in nature.

3. The experiment should be so designed and based on the results of animal experimentation and a knowledge of the natural history of the disease or other problem under study that the anticipated results justify the performance of the experiment.

4. The experiment should be so conducted as to avoid all unnecessary physical and mental suffering and injury.

5. No experiment should be conducted where there is an *a priori* reason to believe that death or disabling injury will occur; except, perhaps, in those experiments where the experimental physicians also serve as subjects.

6. The degree of risk to be taken should never exceed that determined by the humanitarian importance of the problem to be solved by the experiment.

7. Proper preparations should be made and adequate facilities provided to protect the experimental subject against even remote possibilities of injury, disability or death.

8. The experiment should be conducted only by scientifically qualified persons. The highest degree of

*BMJ 1996; **313**: 1448.
†Bull Med Eth 1999; August: 16–17.

skill and care should be required through all stages of the experiment of those who conduct or engage in the experiment.

9. During the course of the experiment the human subject should be at liberty to bring the experiment to an end if he has reached the physical or mental state where continuation of the experiment seems to him to be impossible.

10. During the course of the experiment the scientist in charge must be prepared to terminate the experiment at any stage, if he has probable cause to believe, in the exercise of the good faith, superior skill and careful judgment required of him, that a continuation of the experiment is likely to result in injury, disability, or death to the experimental subject.

Declaration of Helsinki (Doc. 17.c)(1996)

World Medical Association

Recommendations guiding physicians in biomedical research involving human subjects
Adopted by the 18th World Medical Assembly, Helsinki, Finland, June 1964 and amended ... Tokyo, Japan, October 1975, ... Venice, Italy, October 1983, ... Hong Kong, September 1989, *and ... Somerset, Republic of South Africa, October 1996.**

INTRODUCTION

It is the mission of the *physician** to safeguard the health of the people. His or her knowledge and conscience are dedicated to the fulfilment of this mission.

The Declaration of Geneva of the World Medical Association binds the physician with the words, "The health of my patient will be my first consideration," and the International Code of Medical Ethics declares that, "*A physician shall act only in the patient's interest when providing medical care which might have the effect of weakening the physical and mental condition of the patient.*"

The purpose of biomedical research involving human subjects must be to improve diagnostic, therapeutic and prophylactic procedures and the understanding of the aetiology and pathogenesis of disease.

In current medical practice most diagnostic, therapeutic or prophylactic procedures involve hazards. This applies *especially* to biomedical research.

*Amendments since 1975 are shown in italics.

Medical progress is based on research that ultimately must rest in part on experimentation involving human subjects.

In the field of biomedical research a fundamental distinction must be recognised between medical research in which the aim is essentially diagnostic or therapeutic for a patient, and medical research, the essential object of which is purely scientific and without *implying* direct diagnostic or therapeutic value to the person subjected to the research.

Special caution must be exercised in the conduct of research that may affect the environment, and the welfare of animals used for research must be respected.

Because it is essential that the results of laboratory experiments be applied to human beings to further scientific knowledge and to help suffering humanity, the World Medical Association has prepared the following recommendations as a guide to every physician in biomedical research involving human subjects. They should be kept under review in the future. It must be stressed that the standards as drafted are only a guide to physicians all over the world. Physicians are not relieved from criminal, civil and ethical responsibilities under the laws of their own countries.

I. BASIC PRINCIPLES

1. Biomedical research involving human subjects must conform to generally accepted scientific principles and should be based on adequately performed

laboratory and animal experimentation and on a thorough knowledge of the scientific literature.

2. The design and performance of each experimental procedure involving human subjects should be clearly formulated in an experimental protocol, which should be transmitted *for consideration, comment and guidance to a specially appointed committee independent of the investigator and the sponsor, provided that this independent committee is in conformity with the laws and regulations of the country in which the research experiment is performed.*

3. Biomedical research involving human subjects should be conducted only by scientifically qualified persons and under the supervision of a clinically competent medical person. The responsibility for the human subject must always rest with a medically qualified person and never rest on the subject of the research, even though the subject has given his or her consent.

4. Biomedical research involving human subjects cannot legitimately be carried out unless the importance of the objective is in proportion to the inherent risk to the subject.

5. Every biomedical research project involving human subjects should be preceded by careful assessment of predictable risks in comparison with foreseeable benefits to the subject or to others. Concern for the interests of the subject must always prevail over the interests of science and society.

6. The right of the research subject to safeguard his or her integrity must always be respected. Every precaution should be taken to respect the privacy of the subject and to minimise the impact of the study on the subject's physical and mental integrity and on the personality of the subject.

7. Physicians should abstain from engaging in research projects involving human subjects unless they are satisfied that the hazards involved are believed to be predictable. Physicians should cease any investigation if the hazards are found to outweigh the potential benefits.

8. In publication of the results of his or her research, the physician is obliged to preserve the accuracy of the results. Reports of experimentation not in accordance with the principles laid down in this Declaration should not be accepted for publication.

9. In any research on human beings, each potential subject must be adequately informed of the aims, methods, anticipated benefits and potential hazards of the study and the discomfort it may entail. He or she should be informed that he or she is at liberty to abstain from participation in the study and that he or she is free to withdraw his or her consent to participation at any time. The physician should then obtain the subject's freely-given informed consent, preferably in writing.

10. When obtaining informed consent for the research project, the physician should be particularly cautious if the subject is in a dependent relationship to him or her or may consent under duress. In that case the informed consent should be obtained by a physician who is not engaged in the investigation and who is completely independent of this official relationship.

11. In the case of legal incompetence, informed consent should be obtained from the legal guardian in accordance with national legislation. Where physical or mental incapacity makes it impossible to obtain informed consent, or when the subject is a minor, permission from the responsible relative replaces that of the subject in accordance with national legislation.

Whenever the minor child is in fact able to give a consent, the minor's consent must be obtained in addition to the consent of the minor's legal guardian.

12. The research protocol should always contain a statement of the ethical considerations involved and should indicate that the principles enunciated in the present Declaration are complied with.

II. MEDICAL RESEARCH COMBINED WITH PROFESSIONAL CARE (CLINICAL RESEARCH)

1. In the treatment of the sick person, the physician must be free to use a new diagnostic and therapeutic measure, if in his or her judgement it offers hope of saving life, re-establishing health or alleviating suffering.

2. The potential benefits, hazards and discomfort of a new method should be weighed against the advantages of the best current diagnostic and therapeutic methods.

3. In any medical study, every patient – including those of a control group, if any – should be assured of the best proven diagnostic and therapeutic method. *This does not exclude the use of inert placebo in studies where no proven diagnostic or therapeutic method exists.*

4. The refusal of the patient to participate in a study must never interfere with the physician – patient relationship.

5. If the physician considers it essential not to obtain

informed consent, the specific reasons for this proposal should be stated in the experimental protocol for transmission to the independent committee (I.2).

6. The physician can combine medical research with professional care, the objective being the acquisition of new medical knowledge, only to the extent that medical research is justified by its potential diagnostic or therapeutic value for the patient.

III. NON-THERAPEUTIC BIOMEDICAL RESEARCH INVOLVING HUMAN SUBJECTS (NON-CLINICAL BIOMEDICAL RESEARCH)

1. In the purely scientific application of medical research carried out on a human being, it is the duty of the physician to remain the protector of the life and health of that person on whom biomedical research is being carried out.

2. The subjects should be volunteers – either healthy persons or patients for whom the experimental design is not related to the patient's illness.

3. The investigator or the investigating team should discontinue the research if in his or her or their judgement it may, if continued, be harmful to the individual.

4. In research on man, the interest of science and society should never take precedence over considerations related to the wellbeing of the subject.

REFERENCE

Taken from *Bull. Med. Eth.* August 1999; pp. 16–17.

2 · A historical introduction to the requirement of obtaining informed consent from research participants

Baruch A Brody

Current debates about consent in research require a historical understanding of how the need developed to obtain voluntary informed consent from research subjects. This chapter presents a brief account of that development, focusing on several major episodes: the trial at Nuremberg, the development of standards for ethical research by the World Health Organization, the USA and the UK, the elaborations on these standards throughout the world in the 1980s in response to further revelations of problematic research, and the recent discussions of exceptions to those requirements.

Although the development of the requirement of obtaining informed consent from research subjects paralleled in many ways the requirement of obtaining informed consent from patients in the therapeutic setting, this chapter will be confined to the research setting.

THE NUREMBERG CODE

In the immediate aftermath of World War II, a series of military tribunals were convened to judge the guilt of those Germans accused of war crimes and atrocities. Among those indicted were 23 individuals (20 of whom were physicians) charged with atrocities committed in the form of medical experimentation. Fifteen were found guilty, and seven (including the three non-physicians) were hung on June 2, 1948.[1]

The final judgement in that trial[1] asserted (p. 102) that "all agree, however, that certain basic principles must be observed in order to satisfy moral, ethical and legal concepts." It then listed 10 basic principles, most concerned with risks and benefits. These constitute the Nuremberg Code, which is the foundation of all later discussions of research ethics. Two of the

principles relate to consent. Principle Nine discusses the liberty of the subject to withdraw from the research protocol. Principle One is the more fundamental principle, and it became the focus of much attention (pp. 102–3):

> The voluntary consent of the human subject is absolutely essential. This means that the person involved should have legal capacity to give consent; should be so situated as to be able to exercise free power of choice, without the intervention of any element of force, fraud, deceit, duress, over-reaching, or other ulterior form of constraint or coercion; and should have sufficient knowledge and comprehension of the elements of the subject matter involved as to enable him to make an understanding and enlightened decision. This latter element requires that before the acceptance of an affirmative decision by the experimental subject there should be made known to him the nature, duration, and purposes of the experiment; the method and means by which it is to be conducted; all inconveniences and hazards reasonably to be expected; and the effects on his health and person which may possibly come from his participation in the experiment. The duty and responsibility for ascertaining the quality of the consent rests upon each individual who initiates, directs, or engages in the experiment. It is a personal duty and responsibility which may not be delegated to another with impunity.

This is a very strong requirement. It requires:

- voluntary
- informed
- prospective

consent from

- subjects with legal capacity, with
- the quality of that consent being ascertained by the experimenter himself.

Moreover, there is a full discussion of what information must be provided to the potential subject before his consent is accepted.

Where did this requirement come from? There has been much historical discussion about this question.[2] A general consensus has emerged that, whilst there were precedents, the court was primarily influenced by two of its expert witnesses, Andrew Ivy and Leo Alexander. Ironically, the most explicit precedents for this requirement come from pre-Nazi Germany. In 1900, the responsible Prussian ministry required that research not be conducted on minors or others who are incompetent, but only on someone who has "declared unequivocally that he consents to the intervention" after "a proper explanation of the adverse consequences that may result from the intervention." A later 1931 Reich Health Council Circular modified this requirement to allow for proxy consent by legal representatives for innovative therapies, but otherwise maintained the same strict requirements on all forms of research.[2]

THE DEVELOPMENT OF INTERNATIONAL AND NATIONAL STANDARDS

Whatever the origin of the requirement for informed consent from research subjects, its adoption in the Nuremberg Code was followed by its adoption in many other codes of research ethics, both international and national.

Declaration of Helsinki

Perhaps the most influential adoption was in the Declaration of Helsinki, first confirmed by the World Medical Association in 1964 at its 18th Assembly in Helsinki, and modified on several occasions since then. What is often forgotten is that the World Medical Association had already addressed some of the issues in a 1954 *Resolution on Human Experimentation*. It is important, in studying the history of the informed consent requirement, to differentiate its treatment in the 1954 resolution, in the 1964 Declaration, and in the Declaration's first modification in 1975 in Tokyo at the 29th Assembly.

The 1954 Resolution[3] required the researcher to explain to the potential subject the nature of the research, the reasons for it, and the risks. In the case of experimentation involving healthy subjects, this explanation would be the basis of informed and free

consent by the subjects. In the case of experimentation involving sick subjects, consent could be given by the subjects or their next of kin. In drawing this distinction, the Assembly of the World Medical Association began to allow for proxy consent in some cases. This differentiated its approach from the requirement of informed consent in the Nuremberg Code.

This approach was continued in the 1964 Declaration, but that Declaration is rooted in a differentiation between therapeutic research and non-therapeutic research. The requirement for informed consent for therapeutic research is ambivalent[1 (pp. 331–3)]:

> If at all possible, consistent with patient psychology, the doctor should obtain the patient's freely given consent after the patient has been given a full explanation. In case of legal incapacity consent should also be procured from the legal guardian; in case of physical incapacity the permission of the legal guardian replaces that of the patient.

The ambivalence relates to the issues of consistency with patient psychology and of the role of the legally incapable but physically capable research subject. These issues are not found in the requirements for non-therapeutic research, although proxy consent is allowed in that case as well:

> 2. The nature, the purpose, and the risk of clinical research must be explained to the subject by the doctor.
> 3a. Clinical research on a human being cannot be undertaken without his free consent, after he has been fully informed; if he is legally incompetent the consent of the legal guardian should be procured.
> 3b. The subject of clinical research should be in such a mental, physical and legal state as to be able to exercise fully his power of choice.

However, it is not clear how the acceptance of proxy consent in 3a is compatible with the requirement of 3b.

Many of these issues were clarified in the 1975 Modification[1 (pp. 333–6)]. The requirement of informed consent becomes a basic principle, proxy consent is allowed for minors as well as for patients with physical or mental incapacities that preclude their consenting, and doctors who wish to avoid obtaining informed consent for therapeutic research must justify this to an independent committee. The content of the information to be supplied is amplified, as "anticipated benefits" must now be discussed. Finally, there is a new requirement for the consent process, when the research involves subjects who "are in a dependent relation" to the researcher or who may "consent under duress". In such cases, "the informed consent should be obtained by a doctor who is not engaged in the investigation and who is completely independent of this official relationship."

The 1975 Modification involves an additional component:

> I.2 The design and performance of each experimental procedure involving human subjects should be clearly formulated in an experimental protocol which should be transmitted to a specially appointed independent committee for consideration, comment and guidance.

This component of independent review has, of course, become widely accepted throughout the world, but its relation to the requirement of informed consent has not been adequately defined. It is well understood that one, but only one, of the tasks of the independent review of the protocol is to examine its provisions for obtaining informed consent. However, what also needs to be understood is that we now have a system in which there are two separate protections of the rights and interests of research subjects: subjects protect themselves through the informed consent process and they are further protected by the independent review. Normally, each of these protective processes are necessary for the licitness of research, and only the satisfaction of both is sufficient for the licitness of research. The importance of this point to contemporary discussions of exceptions to the requirement of informed consent will emerge below.

Development of US Standards

The Declaration of Helsinki was accompanied, and sometimes preceded, by similar standards adopted at the national level. The development of US standards began with a policy adopted in 1953 at the National Institute of Health's (NIH) Clinical Center, where intramural research is conducted. This early policy mandated the following[4]:

> The principal investigator personally provides the assigned volunteer, in lay language and at the level of his comprehension, with information about the proposed research project. He outlines its purpose, methods, demands, inconveniences and discomforts, to enable the volunteer to make a mature judgment as

to his willingness and ability to participate. When he is fully cognizant of all that is entailed, the volunteer gives his signed consent to take part in it.

There were also provisions in this early policy for independent review of protocols raising ethical issues, but this policy only covered research at the Clinical Center, and its approach was not widely followed.

This changed in the early 1960s as a result of efforts both at the Food and Drug Association (FDA) and the NIH. The FDA was mandated to deal with these issues by the 1962 statute, which greatly expanded its authority over the drug testing and approval process. As part of the drug and device testing process leading to FDA approval, investigators were required by the statute to "obtain the consent of such human beings or their representatives, except where they deem it not feasible or, in their professional judgment, contrary to the best interests of such human beings."[5] This statutory provision was clarified in regulations issued in 1967.[6] Among the provisions about the information to be provided were the requirements to tell the subject about "his possible use as a control" and "about the existence of alternative forms of therapy, if any". Extremely important as historical background to the current debates about the exceptions to the requirement of obtaining informed consent is the clarification of the "not feasible" exception:

> "Not feasible" is limited to cases wherein the investigator is not capable of obtaining consent because of inability to communicate with the patient or his representative; for example, the patient is in a coma or is otherwise incapable of giving consent, his representative cannot be reached, and it is imperative to administer the drug without delay.

In the period 1965–74, the NIH developed policies on the ethics of extramural research funded by the agency. The fundamental principle of its policies was articulated by the National Advisory Health Council in 1965[7] (p. 208):

> ... Public Health Service support of clinical research and investigation involving human beings should be provided only if the judgment of the investigator is subject to prior review by his institutional associates to assure an independent determination of the protection of the rights and welfare of the individual or individuals involved, of the appropriateness of the methods used to secure informed consent, and of the risks and potential medical benefits of the investigators

As the policies were developed from 1965–74 and turned into regulations, there was considerable debate about the parameters of the informed consent requirement, particularly as it applied to interviews, questionnaires, and the use of stored records and data. These debates are an important part of the historical background to the contemporary discussion of these types of research as an exception to the requirement of obtaining informed consent.

Development of UK Standards

The USA was not the only country to develop such standards for research on human subjects in this time period. As early as October of 1953, the British Medical Research Council (MRC) had issued a *Memorandum on clinical investigations*, which was supplemented by its 1963 report on *Responsibility in investigations on human subjects*. However, a somewhat different attitude pervaded some of that earlier British activity. There was far greater scepticism about the requirement of obtaining informed consent. To quote the 1953 document[4] (p. 847):

> To obtain the consent of the patient to a proposed investigation is not in itself enough. Owing to the special relationship of trust which exists between a patient and his doctor, most patients will consent to any proposal that is made. Further, the considerations involved are nearly always so technical as to prevent their being adequately understood by one who is not himself an expert. It must, therefore, be frankly recognized that, for practical purposes, an inescapable responsibility for determining what investigations are, or are not, undertaken on a particular patient will rest with the doctor concerned.

In 1993, commenting on this approach, the MRC[8] said "that the concept stated then – that consent could simply be assumed to a new procedure that the doctor believed would benefit the patient – seems outmoded ..." Moreover, there certainly is an unqualified commitment to the general requirement of obtaining informed consent not merely in these later guidelines from the MRC but also in the extremely influential reports from the Royal College of Physicians.[9] It may well be that much of the contemporary debate in the UK about exceptions to the requirement of informed consent has, as part of its background, this earlier scepticism about the meaningfulness of informed consent in research, especially in the therapeutic setting.

Conclusions

Much more can be said about the initial development in the period 1950–75 of international and national standards for obtaining informed consent from research subjects. However, enough has been said to document the following conclusions:

- The Declaration of Helsinki's requirement of obtaining informed consent was widely accepted, even if doubts were sometimes expressed about its meaningfulness. This requirement was in addition to the requirement of an independent review of the research protocol.
- The concept of proxy consent for those who could not give their own consent was accepted.
- There emerged the idea of exceptions to the requirement of obtaining anyone's consent, either in the context of medical emergencies or in the context of interviews and stored data.

These developments would be modified in the years that followed, in part in response to further revelations of disturbing breaches of research ethics.

REVELATIONS OF PROBLEMATIC RESEARCH

As I have shown in a recent book,[10] the acceptance of many of the requirements of research ethics has been promoted by the revelation of striking examples of problematic research. This is certainly true in the case of the requirement of obtaining informed consent. The Nuremberg Trial's shocking revelations and the resulting Nuremberg Code was one example, but it was not the only one. In the 1960s and early 1970s, further revelations of problematic research impacted the articulation and acceptance of the informed consent requirement.

In the United States, one extremely prominent example was Henry Beecher's 1966 article[11] documenting 22 problematic studies (he had collected 50, but only published a description of 22). These involved withholding known effective treatments, continuing study treatments after significant morbidities, and exposing subjects to significant risks for non-therapeutic purposes. This was a particularly troubling revelation, because Beecher suggested that these studies had been published in excellent journals (we now know, for example, that six appeared in the *New England Journal of Medicine*[12]). Beecher noted that "in only 2 of the 50 examples originally compiled for this study was consent mentioned." He himself believed that a "far more dependable safeguard than consent is the presence of a truly responsible investigator," but he nevertheless agreed that "it remains a goal toward which one must strive for sociologic, ethical, and clear-cut legal reasons."

In his article, Beecher refers to a personal communication from M.H. Pappworth who had collected 500 examples of what he took to be unethical research. Pappworth published his findings about unethical research by British investigators in 1967 in a book.[13] In Canada, the 1965 Halushka case attracted much attention.[14] In that case, a subject developed a cardiac arrest in response to a test of a new anesthetic agent, where a catheter had been advanced through his heart. The basis for his law suit was a lack of candid information in the consent process. The court articulated a strict standard, not allowing for exceptions, that in research it was the duty of a researcher to give a "full and frank disclosure of the facts, probabilities, and opinions which a reasonable man might be expected to consider before giving his consent."

These revelations were too late to impact the development of the above-discussed standards, but they undoubtedly contributed to their acceptance. There were further revelations that impacted directly upon the development of the next wave of standards for informed consent on research subjects. These were revelations discussed at hearings chaired by Senator Kennedy in 1973 about the Tuskegee Syphilis Study (where untreated patients with syphilis were followed in a study of the natural history of that disease long after effective treatments became available) and about the Willowbrook Hepatitis Study (in which institutionalised children were injected with a strain of the virus to study the disease and its possible treatment). These hearings led to the 1974 National Research Act, which created in the USA the National Commission for the Protection of Human Subjects[7 (pp. 213–14)]. Its report, and the ensuing 1981–83 US regulations, launched the second wave of international and national standards for obtaining informed consent from research subjects.

THE NEWER STANDARDS

The Commission produced an extensive set of reports. Perhaps the most influential was its *Belmont Report*, which articulated an ethical foundation for

the requirement of obtaining informed consent [10 (pp. 281–8)]. For many, this requirement was a way of giving potential subjects the possibility of protecting themselves against dangerous research. This would be in addition to the protection given by independent review and by the scruples of the investigator. This way of thinking promoted discussions, such as those by Beecher and by the British MRC, about the efficacy of these various forms of protection. The *Belmont Report* articulated an alternative. It postulated as a fundamental ethical principle "respect for persons" which it divided into two components: "first, that individuals should be treated as autonomous agents, and second, that persons with diminished autonomy are entitled to protection." It is the first, understood as giving people the "opportunity to choose what shall or shall not happen to them," which leads to the requirement of informed consent. The latter leads to proxy consent and to extra protections in the independent review process. On this way of understanding, informed consent is far more than a protection against exploitation in research. It is an acceptance that the research subject is an autonomous agent who has the right to decide, in a voluntary and informed manner, what shall or shall not happen to him.

This *Belmont Report*, and the extensive detailed reports suggesting how its principles should be implemented, heavily influenced (although not always successfully) the deliberations which led to the 1981–83 NIH regulations on human subjects research.[15] These are built around the dual requirements of independent review and informed consent. As far as informed consent is concerned, the following are the most notable provisions:

1. The elements of informed consent are carefully defined (identification and purpose of the experimental procedures, potential benefits, "reasonably foreseeable" risks, alternatives, protections of confidentiality, existence of compensation for injury, contact persons, and voluntariness of participation at all stages).
2. Two forms of documentation are accepted, a full form (where all the information is in the consent form) and a short form (where the consent form merely says that the information has been covered).
3. Emphasis is placed on the context and language of the informed consent process and form. The context must be one in which the prospective subject or the proxy has "sufficient opportunity to

consider whether or not to participate" and that "minimizes the possibility of coercion or undue influence," while the language of the form must be "understandable to the subject or the representative."

4. In addition to a general acceptance of proxy consent from the subject's "legally authorized representative," there are special authorisations for parental consent for paediatric research. Of particular importance is the emphasis on also obtaining the assent ("affirmative agreement to participate in research") of the paediatric subject when the independent review concludes, taking into account "the ages, maturity, and psychological state of the children involved," that they are capable of assenting. There are no analogous provisions for cognitively impaired adults because there are no special regulations covering them, even though such regulations were recommended by the National Commission.

5. Neither the requirement of independent review nor the requirement of informed consent apply to "research involving the collection or study of existing data, documents, records, pathological specimens, or diagnostic specimens, if these sources are publically available or if the information is recorded by the investigator in such a manner that subjects cannot be identified, directly or through identifiers linked to the subjects," or to "research involving the use of educational tests … survey procedures, interview procedures," unless the information can be linked to the subjects and, if disclosed, would subject them to liability or would damage their "financial standing, employability, or reputation". In addition, the independent review may waive the requirement of informed consent if the risks of the research are minimal, the waiver "will not adversely affect the rights and welfare of the subjects," the research could not be done otherwise, and the subjects are informed afterwards "whenever appropriate".

Much of this is an elaboration on what had appeared in earlier standards, but the discussions of assent and the elaboration of the various exceptions was breaking new ground.

These new US regulations were not the only standards to appear that incorporated these many detailed elements. In a recent book,[10] the Author compared the following important documents, all of which are in close agreement about these issues of informed consent:

- the 1993 (based on a 1982) CIOMS International Guidelines for Human Research[10 (pp. 223–6)]
- the 1996 International Conference on Harmonization Guideline for Good Clinical Practice[10] (pp. 219–24)
- the 1990 Council of Europe Recommendation[10] (pp. 241–50) Concerning Medical Research on Human Beings (supplemented by the 1996 Convention on Human Rights and Biomedicine[10] (pp. 251–2)
- 1992 British Guidelines from the Medical Research Council[8] and 1993 National Health Service Guidelines[16] on Local Research Ethics Committees (supplementing reports from the Royal College of Physicians[16 (sections V.6–V.9)], going back to the 1970s and updated in the 1990s)
- the 1988 national legislation in France[10 (pp. 336–8)]
- the 1998 Canadian Tri-Council Policy Statement[17] on Ethical Conduct for Research Involving Humans (replacing guidelines first developed in the 1970s), and
- the 1992 Australian National Health and Medical Research Council Statement on Human Experimentation.[10 (pp. 343–53)]

While there are subtle differences in details between all of these documents, there is overall complete agreement on the fundamental principle of informed consent. That is now a settled issue. In the current discussions of revising the Declaration of Helsinki, where many revisions have been suggested, the principle of informed consent has remained unchallenged.[18] Where there is room for disagreement is about exceptions.

THE DEBATE ABOUT EXCEPTIONS: SOME HISTORICAL REFLECTIONS

There are those who yearn for the absoluteness of the Nuremberg Code's insistence that no research can proceed without the informed consent of the subject. Historically, however, Nuremberg is an anomaly. The 1931 Reich Health Council Circular, the 1954 World Medical Association Resolution, the 1962 FDA statute and the initial guidelines from the Royal College of Physicians all recognised at least some exceptions, even if they did not agree on all the permissible exceptions. This pattern has continued in all of the more recent standards. Moreover, the type of absoluteness found in the Nuremberg Code has always seemed ethically suspicious. The moral life is a life of compromise among many important and legitimate values, none of them being absolute, and there is no reason why the requirement of obtaining informed consent for participation in research should be an exception to this. In some cases, when the public good (and perhaps the good of the subject) requires that research be conducted and when prospective voluntary informed consent cannot be obtained, the value of conducting the research may be sufficiently great to justify making an exception to the requirement that informed consent be obtained. From a moral perspective, the Nuremberg absoluteness is better seen as understandable rhetorical flourish rather than as valid moral insight.

Which exceptions have been recognised? As we have already seen, three prominent exceptions widely recognised are proxy consent for children and the cognitively impaired, research in emergency situations, and research involving no interventions on the subject (e.g. research on existing data or biological specimens).

As one reviews the more recent standards, one sees that there is room for disagreement about the details of these exceptions, even if one accepts their basic legitimacy. One example of disagreement about the details of each of these exceptions is provided here:

- *Proxy consent.* Is proxy consent sufficient if the incompetent subject (whether because of age or cognitive impairment) objects to the research intervention? The Council of Europe[10 (p. 241)] seems to think that it is not, since it says that, "If the legally incapacitated person is capable of understanding, his consent is also required and no research may be undertaken if he does not give his consent." On the other hand, the NIH regulations about children, while emphasising assent, insist that "if the IRB determines ... that the intervention or the procedure involved in the research holds out a prospect of direct benefit that is important to the health or well-being of the children and is available only in the context of research, the assent of the children is not a necessary condition for proceeding with the research.[15 (46.408)]
- *Emergency research.* Is this justified because of its potential benefit and the inability to get consent, or are further procedural safeguards required? The Council of Europe seems to adopt the former position, since it requires only the inability of the patient to give consent, the intention of direct health benefit, and the approval by independent

review of a protocol developed for such an emergency situation[10 (p. 242)]. On the other hand, the FDA, in its 1996 regulations allowing for this exception,[10 (pp. 298–9)] added additional procedural safeguards such as the establishment of a data monitoring committee and community notification/consultation. It is supported in this insistence by the Canadian Tri-Council Policy Statement.[17 (p. 2.12)]
- *Research on existing data or biological specimens.* Is any independent review or informed consent required for such research? The British Royal College of Physicians has said[19] that neither is required, so long as access is obtained from the custodian of the records or material, confidentiality is assured, and the recipient is a senior professional subject "to an effective disciplinary code enforced by his or her professional body over any breach of confidentiality." As noted above, the 1981 NIH regulations[15 (46.101)] adopt the same rule subject to the requirement that the investigator record the information without identifiers. CIOMS, in special 1991 guidelines on epidemiological research,[10 (pp. 225–32)] insists on independent review to insure that there are appropriate measures to protect confidentiality, and that individual consent is unnecessary or impractical.

CONCLUSIONS

What we have seen in this chapter is the emergence both of a near universal acceptance of the requirement of obtaining informed consent from research subjects and a near universal recognition that there are occasions in which exceptions to this requirement are justified. What we have entered into now is a period of time in which the major debate about informed consent in research is about how to structure the exceptions to that requirement. Before ending, however, the Author would like to make two additional personal observations:

- There is the need to do empirical research on how to strengthen the quality of the informed consent process, particularly in special populations (e.g. the less educated), where meeting the basic requirement is more problematic.
- There is the need to confront the ethical question of how to deal with subjects who, because of social understandings or personal anxieties, do not want to be consulted about participating in research,

even though they may want the benefits of being in research protocols.

The debate about informed consent should be about these questions, as well as about the structuring of the exceptions to the requirement, and not about the requirement itself.

REFERENCES

1. Annas G, Grodin M. eds. *The Nazi doctors and the Nuremberg Code*. New York: Oxford University Press, 1992, Part II.
2. Grodin M. Historical origins of the Nuremberg Code. In: Annas G, Grodin M. eds. *The Nazi doctors and the Nuremberg Code*. New York: Oxford University Press, 1992, Part II.
3. McNeill P. *The ethics and politics of human experimentation*. Cambridge: Cambridge University Press, 1992.
4. Katz J. *Experimentation with human beings*. New York: Russell Sage Foundation, 1972.
5. 21 *United States Code* 355(i).
6. 32 *Federal Register* 8753 (1967).
7. Faden R, Beauchamp T. *A history and theory of informed consent*. New York, Oxford University Press, 1986.
8. Medical Research Council. *Responsibility in investigations on human participants and material and on personal information*. London: Medical Research Council, 1992, Section 3.
9. Royal College of Physicians. *Research involving patients*. London: Royal College of Physicians, 1990, and *Guidelines on the practice of ethics committees in medical research involving human subjects*, 3rd. edn. London: Royal College of Physicians, 1996.
10. Brody B. *The ethics of biomedical research*. New York: Oxford University Press, 1998.
11. Beecher H. Ethics and clinical research. *N Engl J Med* 1966; **274**: 1354–60.
12. Rothman D. *Strangers at the bedside*. New York: Basic Books, 1991, Appendix A.
13. Pappworth MH. *Human guinea pigs*. Boston: Beacon Press, 1967.
14. Halushka v University of Saskatchewan 52 W.W.R. 608(1965).
15. 45 *Code of Federal Regulations* 46, reprinted in ref. 10 pp. 262–81.
16. Foster C. ed. *Manual for research ethics committees*, 3rd edn. London: King's College, nd section V.5.
17. Tri-Council Policy Statement. *Ethical conduct for research involving humans*. Ottawa: Medical Research Council of Canada, 1998.
18. Proposed revision of the Declaration of Helsinki. *Bull Med Ethics*; Aug: 18–22.
19. Royal College of Physicians. *Guidelines on the practice of ethics committees in medical research involving human subjects*. London: Royal College, 1996, Appendix B.

3 · Human guinea pigs and the ethics of experimentation: the *BMJ*'s correspondent at the Nuremberg medical trial*

Though the Nuremberg medical trial was a US military tribunal, British medical input was extensive. British forensic pathologists supplied extensive evidence for the trial. The *BMJ* had a correspondent at the trial, and he endorsed a utilitarian legitimation of clinical experiments, justifying the medical research carried out under Nazism as of long-term scientific benefit despite the human costs. The British supported an international medical commission to evaluate the ethics and scientific quality of German research. Medical opinions differed over whether German medical atrocities should be given publicity or treated in confidence. The *BMJ*'s correspondent warned against medical researchers being taken over by a totalitarian state, and these arguments were used to oppose the NHS and any state control over medical research.

Kenneth Mellanby, reader in medical entomology at the London School of Hygiene and Tropical Medicine, determined to "rescue the records" of German medical research during the Nazi era for evaluation by British scientists. In the period leading up to the Nuremberg medical trial in December 1946, however, visits to Germany were strictly controlled and the only way to gain entry was as a bona fide medical reporter. To this end Mellanby approached Hugh Clegg, editor of the *BMJ*, with the offer of articles on German human experiments, and Clegg appointed him as the *BMJ*'s first ever foreign correspondent. When the prosecution opened proceedings in Nuremberg on 9 December, Mellanby joined the ranks of medical reporters from Germany,

France, Belgium, and other nations.[1] (pp. 181–6) Despite Mellanby's later claims to have brought German experimental records back to Britain, none of these has ever been identified.

CONFIDENTIAL EVALUATION OF HUMAN EXPERIMENTS

The first trial of major German war criminals at Nuremberg was an international military tribunal of the four allies, Britain, France, Russia, and the USA. By contrast, the medical trial was constituted solely as a US military tribunal, organised and paid for by the USA. Behind the scenes, however, there was considerable liaison between British army and US medical war crimes investigators. British medical authority was represented by the forensic pathologists Professor Sydney Smith and Major Keith Mant. At a meeting with French and US counterparts at the Hoechst pharmaceutical offices in May 1946, these investigators assembled crucial evidence on German medical atrocities. The British handed over a group of German medical captives for trial, and in November 1946 Major Mant briefed the US prosecution's medical expert, the neurologist and Austrian emigré Professor Leo Alexander.[2, 3] The British came round to the view that medical scientists were best qualified to evaluate human experiments as an expert tribunal in closed session. Thus whereas the trial made German medical research publicly accountable to international justice, the British plumped for confidential evaluation by professional peers.[4]

BMJ 1996; **313**: 1467–70.

INTERNATIONAL SCIENTIFIC COMMISSION

From October 1946 Lord Moran, president of the Royal College of Physicians, chaired an international commission for the investigation of medical war crimes, based at the Pasteur Institute in Paris. The commission had dual ethical and scientific functions. Moran's approach was that medical experts should evaluate German medical research according to its scientific merit. He subsequently recruited a distinguished panel of British experts, including the bacteriologist Ronald Hare, the physiologists Henry Dale and Lovatt Evans, and the psychiatrist and eugenicist C P Blacker.[2, 5, 6]

MORAN CONDEMNS REPORTING

As journalists and film cameras at Nuremberg alerted the world to criminal abuses of medical science, Moran roundly condemned such publicity. He criticised Professor Alexander for "journalistic activities" and for publicising the medical trial in *Life*. In February 1947 Moran fulminated to a cabinet office civil servant how "both in America and in this country scientists of a sort are conducting private enquiries. The procedure is that they go to Germany for a short time, collect some material, and publish it with considerable advantage to themselves but with little or no profit to science."[7] One of Moran's targets was undoubtedly Kenneth Mellanby, who in January 1947 reviewed the trial in the *BMJ*.[8]

BRITISH STANCE ON THE PRINCIPLE OF CONSENT

In 1945 Mellanby had published the booklet *Human Guinea Pigs*, about British wartime scabies research at the Sorby Institute, Sheffield, on conscientious objectors who had volunteered.[9, 10] Mellanby defended research in human biology and suspected that innocent researchers were being treated unjustly at the Nuremberg medical trial, which he regarded as of "somewhat ambiguous legality."[1 (p. 184)] He defended the "serious research workers" among the accused, and criticised the *Lancet* for arguing that any value for scientific progress would be outweighed by condoning systematic murder.[11-13] For Mellanby the idea of human experiments entailing deliberate infection did not seem to be criminal if consent had been obtained.

In 1942 Mellanby had contacted his uncle, Edward Mellanby, secretary of the Medical Research Council, suggesting that his volunteers were prepared to allow themselves to be infected for typhus experiments. Edward Mellanby remarked that "the suggestion seems crazy." He referred the matter to Henry Dale, who replied that:

> If it were merely a question of vaccinating them and bleeding them to test the effect of the vaccine, I doubt whether they should be given the privilege of a rather fictitious herosim .... If it were a question, on the other hand, of subjecting them deliberately to a subsequent test of infection. I doubt whether it ought to be entertained, on account of the 'ballyhoo' in both directions, which would be liable to follow an inquest and unavoidable publicity.

The group had already undergone deprivation of water and food on behalf of the Committee on Care of Shipwrecked Mariners. Moreover, Dale had supported the widespread distribution of new American typhus vaccines and a vaccine derived from the Pasteur Institute in Tunis in 1941 to British medical officers, and asked that the effects should be monitored on an experimental basis. Thus for these MRC scientists human experiments without consent were permissible, provided that the risk of death was remote.[14, 15]

The MRC's stance on clinical research can further be illustrated by an incident in August 1945. Hans Krebs, a colleague of Kenneth Mellanby at the Sorby Institute, informed the MRC after a volunteer, receiving a depleted intake of vitamin C, had died of a heart attack. "Some of the volunteers come to the Institute with the express wish to take part in experiments which involve risks to life and limb. They do not wish to evade military service to get a 'soft' job. It is their intention to do something which is, in a way, comparable with military service, in that it is work for the good of the community, associated with some dangers." Krebs suggested that they were willing to sign a statement similar to one produced by Minnesota University in 1942.

The MRC's policy had not altered since 1933, when influenza trials were undertaken. The Treasury solicitor advised that liability for damages would be avoided if the patient gave full consent, that this should be given only after proper appreciation of the risk, and that any clinical trial should be performed with all due care and skill. The principle of consent was not enough to prevent criminal charges, which could be incurred for any operation not required on medical grounds that inflicted bodily injury. However, the assurance of the Director of Public Prosecutions was obtained that the risks of a criminal charge against the MRC were negligible.[16]

BRITISH RESEARCH ON SURVIVORS OF BELSEN

Shortly after the liberation of the concentration camp at Belsen, the MRC authorised nutritional research on survivors. The haematologist Janet Vaughan led the team, which experimented with an American preparation of protein hydrolysate for intravenous injection (Amigen). The research terrified the former prisoners, who believed that they were to receive a lethal injection:

> The majority of the patients were Russians, Poles, Yugoslavs, and Czechs – people with whom we had no common language, and to whom we could not explain what we were trying to do. Many of them were people who had come to regard the medical profession as men and women who came to torture rather than to heal. When we went up to our patients with a stomach tube they would curl themselves up and say, "Nicht crematorium." We gradually realised that it had been the custom, in the case of moribund patients, to inject them with benzene in order to paralyse them before they were taken to the crematorium. That attitude made treatment rather more difficult than it might of otherwise have been.[17]

Vaughan concluded that milk flavoured with tea or coffee would have been more appropriate than the products being tested. "What these people require is simple nursing and frequent small feeds. They want to be washed and made comfortable."[17, 18] In effect the camp inmates became experimental subjects for nutritionists who visited the camp to evaluate feeding methods and blood profiles.

IN PRAISE OF NAZI RESEARCH

Kenneth Mellanby was scathing about conscientious objectors but respected their selfless cooperation as clinical guinea pigs. His attitude to the victims of Nazi medical crimes was less indulgent: "The victims were dead; if their sufferings could in any way add to medical knowledge and help others, surely this would be something that they themselves would have preferred."[1 (pp. 181–6)] Mellanby questioned the pros-

ecution's claim that "practically no results of any value were obtained in any of the work," commenting, "From what we already know of the typhus work it is clear that a useful evaluation of the various vaccines was obtained; some of these results have already been published."

Mellanby praised the notorious paper on typhus vaccines, which an SS medical officer, Erwin Ding, published in 1943 in the Zeitschrift für Hygiene. This was an "important and unique piece of medical research" that "formed the basis not only of German, but also of British and Allied anti-typhus policy." Mellanby considered "for every victim of his experiments 20 000 others might have been saved."[1 (pp. 181–6)] This reflected the arguments of the defendants at Nuremberg. Mellanby's views had no historical basis, however, as the allies were firmly committed to using the American Cox vaccine whatever the results of any German research. As defendants eagerly cited Mellanby's apologetics, the prosecution tore Mellanby's arguments to shreds.[19]

Mellanby also justified the malaria experiments of the executed malariologist Claus Schilling at what he called the "reasonably humane" Dachau concentration camp. He considered that the reported numbers of deaths – several hundred among 1000 subjects – were exaggerated.[1 (p. 187)] Though agreeing that the Germans reprehensibly failed to obtain informed consent, Mellanby was convinced that the data were worth salvaging. He clung to the notion of the value of the experiments despite conceding from the testimony of victims that "little of the work had been properly planned, few of the investigators were competent, there was a lot of very inaccurate recording and even some deliberate falsification of results."[1 (pp. 181–6)] Overall, Mellanby endorsed a utilitarian legitimation of clinical experiments, justifying the medical research carried out under Nazism as of long-term scientific benefit despite the human costs.[20]

SEEDS OF CONFLICTING INTERESTS: THE BMA AND BEVAN'S NHS

Mellanby was concerned that too sweeping a condemnation at Nuremberg might endanger his scheme for an institute of human biology. At the same time he was resolutely against organised team research:

> I sometimes fear that many lavishly financed and effi-

ciently organised schemes will often be sadly sterile, for to my mind, in research inspiration and organisation by no means always go hand in hand. I hope that there will always be a place, and funds, for the individual who wishes to work in his own way, untrammeled as little as possible by the 'red tape' which seems to be a necessary accompaniment of any large-scale organisation.[1] (p. 8)

This reflected sentiments of the Society for Freedom in Science.

That society had been founded in 1940–41. After the war it gained influence in key journals like *Nature* as it doggedly denounced central state planning as totalitarian.[21] Faced by Labour government optimism about state direction of science as part of social planning, critics attacked this as ushering in a Nazi or Soviet style totalitarianism. Biologists were alienated by Soviet suppression of genetics, and Nazi science was perceived as synonymous with state regimentation. Protecting the scientist's autonomy meant shifting guilt for human experiments away from the scientifically trained physician seeking evidence-based medicine and on to the totalitarian state. As medical critics of the National Health Service denounced "Bevan or Belsen", it seemed that British medicine might be heading towards Nazi-style authoritarianism.[22]

An editorial in the *BMJ* diagnosed the problem as political: "the surrender, in fact, of the individual conscience to the mass mind of the totalitarian state." This verdict exonerated medical science by blaming advocates of state medicine for any medical atrocities.[23] As the BMA fought the introduction of the NHS, it interpreted Nazi medical crimes as the direct result of state intervention in healthcare. In November 1946 a BMA offical observed: "It is clear from the events of the past fifteen years that material achievement and scientific progress unless harnessed to a humanitarian motive and moral dynamic become the tools of totalitarian ideologies." In June 1947 the BMA gave its verdict on Nazi medical criminals: "Their amoral methods were the result of training and conditioning to regard science as an instrument in the hands of the state to be applied in any way desired by its rulers. It is to be assumed that initially they did not realise that ideas of those who held political power would lead to the denial of the fundamental values on which medicine is based." The BMA prescribed an increased sense of responsibility to individual patients by the physician; this remedy implied that ethical dangers lurked in the newborn NHS.[24]

LOW-KEY APPROACH TO NAZI MEDICAL CRIMES

As a ploy to soothe relations between the British medical establishment and the government, Lord Moran insisted on a low-key approach to German medical abuses. At times he displayed more interest in costs, remonstrating that he had received 50 guineas a day for five days for going to Nuremberg as part of a medical delegation to examine Rudolf Hess. He lamented that the international commission was underpaid, suggesting that a committee based in London would be more economic. Parsimonious civil servants eagerly accepted a solution of a nominal honorarium that combined economy with expediency.[25, 26]

Moran summed up in five pages the expert evaluations of German medical research in the Nazi era.[27] By contrast, the trial generated over 50 bulky volumes of evidence, condensed into two volumes published by the US government.[28] From the prosecution's opening speech to the concluding Nuremberg code requiring informed consent, the trial revised moral underpinnings for clinical research.[29] Moran marginalised French demands for ethical evaluation on the international commission. Moran's conciliatory stance on the NHS led to his appointment as chairman of the merit awards panel in 1949. At the same time he played down the Nuremberg medical trial for fear that it might undermine public confidence in British medicine.

INDIVIDUAL RESEARCH THREATENED BY DEMOCRACY

Whereas Moran remained somewhat sceptical of medical research as "medicine without patients", Mellanby advocated experimental medicine. He regarded the medical scientists prosecuted at Nuremberg as victims of a coercive totalitarian state. Though he conceded that much of their science was substandard, the moral issue was to keep the state from interfering in research. Resistance to public scrutiny was symptomatic of a broader resistance to the socialisation of medical services and to their modernisation on the basis of state-funded and organised scientific team research.[1 (p. 196), 30] For Mellanby the processes of democratising and modernising medicine were a threat to the individual freedoms of clinical researchers. Whereas debate on the trial passed into obscurity, the position advocated by Mellanby became an entrenched orthodoxy: medical researchers were keen to take public or charitable funds on condition that there should be as little scrutiny as possible of their privileged clinical position or research practices.

REFERENCES

1. Mellanby K. *Human Guinea Pigs*. London: Merlin Press, 1973, pp. 8, 181–187, 196.
2. International Scientific Commission for the Investigation of Medical War Crimes. *Protocol of FIAT meeting*. Kew: Public Records Office, WO 309–471.
3. Mant AK. Medical services in the concentration camp of Ravensbruck. *Med Leg J* 1949; **17**: 99–118.
4. Weindling, PJ. The Origins of Informed Consent. The International Scientific Commission for the Investigation of Medical War Crimes, and the Nuremberg Code. *Bull History Med* 2001 (in preparation).
5. Blacker CP. Eugenic experiments conducted by the Nazis on human subjects. *Eugen Rev* 1952; **44**: 9–19.
6. Weindling PJ. Ärzte als Richter: Internationale Reaktionen auf die medizinischen Verbrechen während den Nurnberger Ärzteprozess im Jahre 1946–47. In: Wiesemann C, Frewer A, eds. *Medizin und Ethik im Zeichen von Auschwitz*. Erlangen: Palm and Enke, 1966, pp. 31–44.
7. Public Record Office. Moran to Rowan, 13 February 1947; FO 371/66581.
8. Mellanby K. Medical experiments on human beings in concentration camps in Nazi Germany. *BMJ* 1947: **i**: 148–50.
9. Mellanby K. *Scabies*. London: Oxford University Press, 1943.
10. Mellanby K. Human guinea pigs. London: Victor Gollancz, 1945.
11. A moral problem. *Lancet* 1946; **ii**: 798.
12. Mellanby K. A moral problem. *Lancet* 1946; **ii**: 850.
13. A moral problem. *Lancet* 1946; **ii**: 961. Public Record Office.
14. MRC records FD 1/6627 Typhus CO Group, Sheffield, 1942: Kenneth Mellanby to E Mellanby, 15 June; H Dale to E Mellanby, 5 June; E Mellanby to H Dale, 3 June.
15. Weindling PJ. Victory with vaccines. The problem of typhus vaccines during the second world war. In: Plotkin SA, Fantini B, eds. *Vaccinia, vaccination, vaccinology, Jenner, Pasteur and their successors*. Paris: Elsevier, 1996, pp. 341–7.
16. Public Records Office. FD1/428: Experiments on human volunteers. Legal position. Treasury solicitor to secretary of the MRC, 21 June 1933; H Krebs to Landsborough Thompson, 13 August 1945; FR Fraser to MRC, 2 June 1933.
17. Contemporary Medical Archives Centre, Wellcome Institute of the History of Medicine. RAMC 792/3/4: Janet Vaughan report concerning the treatment of starvation, report to the War Office and MRC, 24 May 1945; Janet Vaughan papers, "Experiences of Belsen Camp," paper to the Inter-Allied Conference on Military Medicine, 4 June 1945; CE Dent, Rosalind Pitt Rivers, Janet Vaughan, "Report on the comparative value of hydrolysates, milk and serum in the treatment of starvation, based on observations made at Belsen Camp." Medical Research Council, Protein Requirements Committee.
18. Vaughan J. Experience at Belsen. *Lancet* 1945; **i**: 724.
19. The Medical Unit. *Trials of war criminals before the Nuremberg military tribunals*. Vol II. Washington, DC: US Government Printing Office, 1950, p. 91.
20. Caplan AL, ed. *When medicine went mad*. Totowa: Humana Press, 1992.
21. McGucken W. *Scientists, society, and state. The social relations of science movement in Great Britain 1931–1947*. Columbus: Ohio State University Press, 1984, p. 269–79, 295–300, 348–56.
22. Webster C. *Problems fo health care*. Vol 1. London: HMSO, 1988, p. 99–101, 110, 116.
23. Doctors on trial. *BMJ* 1947; **i**: 143.
24. British Medical Association. *War crimes and medicine. Statement by the Council of the Association for submission to the World Medical Association*. London: BMA, 1947.
25. Lovell R. *Churchill's doctor. A biography of Lord Moran*. London: Royal Society of Medicine, 1992, pp. 289–90.
26. Public Record Office. 317/66582: Moran to Leslie, 8 July 1947, and response of the Finance Comittee of the War Office.
27. Foreign Office. *Scientific results of German medical war crimes*. London: HMSO, 1949.
28. The Medical Unit. *Trials of war criminals before the Nuremberg military tribunals*. Vols. I, II. Washington, DC: US Government Printing Office, 1950.
29. Annas GJ, Grodin MA, eds. *The Nazi doctors and the Nuremberg code. Human rights in human experimentation*. Oxford: Oxford University Press, 1992.
30. Webster C. The metamorphosis of Dawson of Penn. In: Porter D, Porter RS, eds. *Doctors, politics and society: historical essays*. Amsterdam: Rodopi, 1993, pp. 212–28.

4 · Henry K Beecher and Maurice Pappworth: informed consent in human experimentation and the physicians' response

Paul J Edelson

BACKGROUND

At the end of the World War II, the US government, as one of the occupying powers in Germany, acting under Control Council Law no. 10 for the punishment of major war criminals under the former Nazi regime, brought to trial 23 Germans, including 20 high-ranking physicians, for their roles in carrying out medical experiments on concentration camp inmates and other prisoners of the Nazis. Marrus has given a useful description of the circumstances of the "Doctors' Trial", as it was called, as well as some very cogent criticisms of the entire approach to the ethical issues raised therein.[1] Although some of the "experiments" were little more than torture, some were genuine efforts to address important war-related medical problems, such as high altitude flying or survival in the cold or after prolonged immersion. However, many of the protocols led to the permanent injury or death of the subjects and, at least in some cases, were expected to do so. The defendants tried to justify their actions on the basis of wartime necessity, or the benefits to science that their work yielded, or used the defence of compulsion and fear for their own lives. None claimed that these cruelties had been undertaken with the consent of the subjects, something which would have been absolutely inconceivable given the nature of some of the protocols.

The "voluntary consent of the human subject" thus became the *sine qua non* in the codification of ethical precepts regarding "Permissible Medical Experiments", later known as the "Nuremberg Code", which was promulgated by the court in connection with its verdict,[2] and which was later adopted as the cornerstone of other post-war ethical codes on the

conduct of medical experimentation with human subjects, including those of the American Medical Association,[3] the World Medical Association,[4] and the British Medical Research Council.[5]

Although the trial was prosecuted by American lawyers, with the assistance of American and British medical experts, before American judges, under the overall authority of the American Occupation Forces, neither the trial itself nor the Nuremberg Code on medical experimentation stimulated, at the time, much discussion among medical scientists, government agencies that sponsored medical research, or the medical profession at large, in either the USA or Britain. Its principle rule, that all human experimentation required the consent of the subject, was echoed in a number of formal codes promulgated by medical associations over the next 20 years. The implications of the Nuremberg experience, however, that well-trained medical scientists could find the cruelest sorts of studies perfectly compatible with their own sense of the ethical demands of the medical profession, seemed to be consigned to oblivion among American researchers. Whilst a number of reasons have been offered by historians, ethicists, and the physicians themselves, to explain why the Nuremberg precepts were received so poorly in this country, I believe this continues to be an important historical question, and one that I want to begin to address in this chapter.

This lack of interest in the Nuremberg Code was not because American medical research at that time was a sleepy backwater with few active workers. On the contrary, as David Rothman explains so well in his book *Strangers at the bedside*,[6] medical research played an important role in the war effort, and was one of the major institutional beneficiaries of the new peace. Although it was clear that the huge wartime research enterprise – with projects ranging from the creation of the atomic bomb to the search for new antimalarials – had to be dismantled, it was felt that some parts of it, and particularly the medical program, had the potential to make similarly important contributions in peacetime. Intense lobbying and elaborate negotiations over the next several years eventually led to the medical research program being transferred to what was then a relatively modest laboratory component of the Public Health Service, the National Institute of Health. Over the next two decades, the NIH budget, supporting the vast majority of all the clinical medical research in this country, grew rapidly, going, as Rothman points out, from $700 000 in 1945 to $36 million dollars in 1955, to $436 million by 1965. Most of this money supported "extramural" research, work done outside of the NIH, and most of the extramural money went to medical centres and their associated universities. By 1965, medical schools were receiving over $450 million dollars from the federal government, accounting for about 86% of all their "sponsored" activities. Including payments for overheads, federal funds contributed about 53% of their total operating budgets.[6] The average pre-war budget for the entire university had been about $500 000; prices during the war had doubled, making this figure $1 000 000 in 1945 dollars.

By the mid-1960s American medicine, aided by an annual government research budget that had grown at a rate of 30% per year compounded over the previous decade (during the same time period, 1945–1965, inflation as based on the CPI was 175%)[7] had taken the world lead in the development of new medical diagnostic and therapeutic techniques. In addition, pharmaceutical companies had substantially expanded their own drug research programs and were beginning to develop entirely new categories of drugs – antibiotics beginning right after the war, psychoactive medications or "tranquilizers" in the 1950s, immunosuppressants and antitumour drugs somewhat later.

American medicine had clearly arrived. A nation that in the previous century had been taunted by the English journalist Sidney Smith for having made little contribution to the world's arts or sciences now led the world with such achievements as the eradication of polio with the Salk and Sabin vaccines, renal transplantation, and new techniques for studying the details of organ function in the living body. So it was with some irritation to the academic medical estab-

lishment that, among all the praise that medicine and medical scientists were receiving in the press, from political leaders, and in Congress – and not forgetting a fair amount of self-congratulation as well – two brief reports appeared that severely criticised the methods which some investigators had used to achieve these extraordinary feats.

BEECHER'S REPORT

One of the reports was written by Dr Henry Knowles Beecher, an experienced clinical scientist at the Massachusetts General Hospital and the Dorr Professor of Research in Anesthesia at the Harvard Medical School. The other was by Dr Maurice Pappworth, an English physician and private medical tutor. Both reports provoked responses from many physicians and medical scientists of denial of any wrong-doing, combined with tremendous anger that such laundry should be washed in public; ambivalent and defensive responses, which few might have expected from the leaders of so securely successful an enterprise as modern American medicine.

In order to understand the bases for these responses, and their significance for the development of modern research ethics, I believe it is important not only to examine the arguments offered by Beecher and Pappworth, but also to define who they were within the medical community, and the ways that they understood the professional identity of the physician and its relation to the culture of the larger society. I particularly want to look at the debate over the development of codes of conduct for the regulation of human experimentation, and to understand how positions regarding this apparently neutral policy issue were in fact very much involved in the attitudes of and responses to Doctors Beecher and Pappworth.

The story as I will present it is one which contrasts the quintessential "insider" with the very definite "outsider". I will argue that the responses to their work were intimately associated not primarily with the objective quality of the work, in which they were actually remarkably similar, but with the identity each of these men held within the medical community. However, those identities in turn shaped the solutions each man proposed for the ethical control of experimentation on humans.

Henry Knowles Beecher was at the pinnacle of a brilliant career in academic medicine when he sent his paper, "Ethics and clinical research", to the *New England Journal* in 1966. Trained in chemistry at the University of Kansas, Beecher, like so many other talented men and women, had migrated to Boston to seek his fortune. There, in 1928, he entered the Harvard Medical School. Although he seems to have shown a talent for research while still a medical student, Beecher did not originally plan a career in medical research – something still quite exceptional for a physician in those years – and instead went on to further clinical training as a "surgical house pupil", or resident, at the Massachusetts General Hospital. There, with the exception of one year of leave for a travelling fellowship, and military service in Europe during the war, he would spend the remainder of his extraordinary medical career.[8, 9]

In 1934, anaesthesiology did not exist as a recognised specialty in American medical practice; arrangements for anaesthesia were often quite casual, with the task often assigned to a medical student or a nurse, under the general supervision of a junior member of the Surgical Staff temporarily placed in charge en route to a career in surgery.[10, 11] Beecher, however, was selected by his chief, Dr Edward D Churchill, a Professor of Surgery at Harvard and chief of the West Surgical Service at the Mass General,[12] as the full-time head, to reorganise and develop a professional anaesthesia service at the hospital based on a solid program of basic physiologic and chemical studies. He appears to have taken to his new assignment with all of his rather formidable energy and focus. Over the next three decades he made major contributions to the management of severe battlefield trauma, to the safety of anaesthesia, and to the psychophysiology of pain relief. By 1960 he had published over 200 research papers and several books, and had established himself as head of the leading anaesthesiology training programme in the country, eventually training over 50 chairmen of other anaesthesiology programmes in the USA and abroad. He had also developed a deep interest in a subject, at that time just beginning to be discussed in medical circles in this country – the ethics of medical experimentation using human subjects. Beecher's own research was weighted heavily toward human experimentation; many of his studies on pain control, for example, could not have been accomplished in any other way. But, in the mid-1950s Beecher began a serious effort to rethink his understanding of the ethics of medical research, and between 1959 and 1966, when his landmark paper

"Ethics and clinical research" appeared in the *New England Journal of Medicine*,[13] Beecher became an active contributor to the medical literature on the ethics of human experimentation. His work appeared in such leading medical journals as the *Journal of the American Medical Association* and the *New England Journal of Medicine*, and he spoke frequently at medical conferences devoted to the subject of research ethics.

In his article in the *New England Journal* for June 16, 1966, Beecher reported on 22 medical studies, all but one published in widely read and highly respected medical journals, which he believed represented serious ethical breaches on the part of the physician investigators. In one, children who were institutionalised, either because of mental retardation or as a result of criminal behaviour, were exposed to an antibiotic that had been associated with significant liver abnormalities. In this study, the drug was nominally being used as an acne treatment, although safer choices were available for that purpose. The drug was continued past the point where subjects showed chemical evidence of liver dysfunction, and even after some had begun to show clinical signs of liver abnormalities. Eight of the most severely affected were hospitalised and underwent liver biopsies, in some cases twice, which showed evidence of liver damage. In four patients, once their clinical and chemical status had returned to normal, the researchers reintroduced the drug, causing a prompt reappearance of the toxic side effects in three. One subject underwent two such cycles of rechallenge, responding each time with symptoms of liver dysfunction. Evidence of liver function abnormalities persisted in some patients for as long as five weeks after the drug was discontinued.

In another study, of the potential dangers of cyclopropane anesthesia, 31 subjects undergoing what were described as 'minor" surgical procedures were placed under deep anaesthesia, and then allowed to breathe high concentrations of carbon dioxide until abnormalities in heart rhythm appeared. Serious, and potentially life-threatening cardiac arrhythmias, particularly abnormal ventricular beats, were induced, and in one patient persisted for an hour and a half before returning to normal. Such arrhythmias can cause sudden death in otherwise healthy young adults.

Other studies involved aggravating liver failure until patients began to manifest severe neurological symptoms, including hepatic coma; deliberately infecting institutionalised children, who were mentally retarded, with hepatitis virus; and injecting cancer cells from a young woman, dying of a malignant melanoma, into her healthy mother, thus transferring the cancer and leading to the mother's death about 15 months later. In this last case, the mother volunteered for the injection in the belief that it might lead to a serum that might be used to treat her daughter. The daughter, however, was described as being in the terminal stage of her illness at the time of this experiment.

What Beecher presented was a pattern of experimentation, almost uniformly without patient consent, carried out by physician scientists from, as Beecher described them, "leading medical schools, university hospitals, private hospitals, governmental military departments (the Army, the Navy and the Air Force), governmental institutes (the National Institutes of Health), Veterans Administration hospitals and industry."[13]

In fact, as David Rothman subsequently learned from Beecher's private paper, these studies came from the laboratories of some of the most respected investigators in the country, working at some of the most prestigious medical institutions, and were published in many cases in the leading medical journals. The research subjects in his examples included patients of both sexes, and of a wide variety of ages and medical conditions. The studies included a broad range of research activities, from the intentional production of serious drug toxicities, to the development and testing of new invasive diagnostic techniques, such as the direct puncture of the left ventricle of the heart, and cardiac catheterisation studies of the pulmonary and circulatory physiology of healthy newborns. As Beecher himself put it, "the basis for the charges [concerning these troubling research practices] is broad."[13] Beecher also recognized that the growth of medical research budgets, the development of a new type of academic medical career in full-time clinical investigation, and the increasing dominance of research and researchers in medical schools and teaching hospitals, all "can lead to unfortunate separation between the interests of science and the interests of the patient".[13] And yet, he did not see the issue as one of a systematic and expectable defect in modern scientific medicine, but rather as the result of "thoughtlessness and carelessness, not a willful disregard of the patient's rights ..."[13] and more likely to reflect an investigator's inexperience than his lack of standards. Indeed, despite presenting a strong case for certain institutional problems in medical research, he insisted that "...

American medicine is sound, and most progress in it is soundly attained."[13]

The response of his researcher colleagues, first exhibited about a year earlier at a private meeting of clinical researchers in Michigan,[14] was ferocious. Beecher, however, seems not to have been one to run from a fight. Indeed, after the original private meeting, and again with publication of his paper in the *New England Journal*, there was considerable attention given to his charges in the national press[15–17] – attention that he welcomed, had worked hard to get.[6] However, while he was glad to have the general public aware of these issues, he directed his comments primarily to his peers, and published his views almost entirely in the professional medical journals. In return, whilst many active clinical researchers objected strenuously to what he was saying, personal responses must have been made in private only, since, in the public debate he provoked, there is little evidence of personal attacks. Whilst Beecher may have been a "deviant" professional, as Judith Swazey has described all whistle-blowers,[18] he was able to maintain his standing as a responsible, indeed a distinguished, member of the medical profession and with that, the public respect and attention of his colleagues.

PAPPWORTH'S REPORTS

Maurice Pappworth's origins were in many ways similar to Beecher's. Unlike Beecher, Maurice Henry Pappworth (1910–1994) had little written about him either during his life, or after his death. The most useful biography appears in an obituary of him by a student and friend, himself a distinguished physician and medical journalist.[19] He, too, was brought up on the "periphery" – in his case, home wasn't Kansas but the English port city of Liverpool. Pappworth did very well in medical school, and succeeded in gaining his membership by examination in the Royal College of Physicians at the age of 26, in 1936. Despite a "distinguished career as a junior physician", Lock has written that Pappworth had been told that, as a Jew, he would never be appointed to a hospital consultancy, in effect ending his hopes of becoming a medical specialist. Instead, he became what Lock calls a "free-lance" medical teacher, specialising in preparing medical graduates for the examination for membership in the Royal College of Physicians – normally the first step in England away from General Practice and toward the more rarefied life of a consultant. He was, ironically, so talented in preparing men, and women, for this step, it is said that, in some years, over half of the successful candidates were students of his.

Not known as a man to mince words,[20] Pappworth first presented his observations on the "new ethics of medical research" in 1962, in a respected magazine for the general public,[21] followed soon after by several television appearances in which he discussed his concerns about the current ethical state of medical research work. He made several efforts to have his work published in the *Lancet*, the weekly medical journal most comparable, in England, in visibility and credibility with our *New England Journal of Medicine*. Pappworth recalled that having written to the *Lancet* on several occasions to complain about unethical studies published in their pages, he had always been told by the Editor that 'there is a wrong time and a right time to address issues like this publicly', and that one needed to be patient as each of these times was the wrong time to do so. Finally, when he had the manuscript of his book completed, he wrote again to the Editor, who told him in essence that it still was not the right time. Ultimately he was obliged to publish his work in a small non-specialist book, entitled *Human Guinea Pigs*, which appeared in 1967.[22] In it, he presents summaries of over 200 different clinical investigations carried out in Britain or the USA and published in respected medical and scientific journals, which, like Beecher's examples, represented cases of involuntary non-beneficial research on human beings. Pappworth gives details of studies involving infants, children, pregnant women, the elderly, persons in institutions, the retarded, and the desperately ill, all of which were carried out on people without their consent, and often without their knowledge.[22]

The responses to Pappworth were hardly the civil and temperate comments we might expect in public debates of the English professional classes. Although the book was initially ignored by most medical journals, it did receive a prompt and quite a thoughtful review in the *British Medical Journal*, apparently the only formal professional review his book received. In it, despite some reservations about Pappworth's specific recommendations, the reviewer reinforces Pappworth's concerns about the ethics of the studies he describes, and generally agrees with him about the extent to which career pressures and ambitions may drive clinical researchers to undertake unethical studies. Overall, the reviewer concludes that, "it would be a good thing for every clinician scientist to read this book."[23] An editorial in the *BMJ* a short time later was also generally favourable to the book, stating that, "There has been for some time public disquiet and uneasiness about investigations carried out in hospitals which have not always been in the interests of the subject of the investigation.[24]

The *Lancet*, however, a journal which, unlike the *BMJ*, was increasingly oriented to clinical research rather than to medical practice, was somewhat ambivalent about Pappworth's work – on the one hand, hostile to the book and to its author, whilst on the other recognizing the necessity of medicine to address the issues the book raised. Editorially, the *Lancet* called the book a "bitter analysis" by a "dissatisfied man", although they, in fact, accepted Pappworth's main contention, which was, as they put it: "that many researches would have been better left undone, that some were disastrous errors, and that the question of true consent by the patient was often glossed over or ignored."[25]

They were none the less of the opinion that:

> Shorn of such excesses [e.g. Pappworth's judgement of the morality of some of the research projects as comparable to that of those carried out by the Nazis] and some of its haughtiness, his book would have a greater impact on those he is presumably trying to influence.[25]

A year later, another editorial in the *Lancet*, concerning a recent programme at the Royal Society of Medicine that Pappworth had chaired, presented a similar attitude of resentment coupled with grudging respect, referring to Pappworth as having offered, "vitriolic amplification of some of the charges he has been more or less effectively firing at the medical profession over the years, especially in his cannonade of a book, published last year."[26]

The medical societies, and the official bodies responsible for regulating the medical profession in England, were also dismissive of Pappworth's charges. The Royal College of Physicians itself, and particularly its chairman, was unenthusiastic about addressing the issue of unethical human experimentation. The committee charged with reporting on these issues took until 1973, six years to present its recommendations, and, according to Pappworth, it was not until 1990, 23 years after they started, that the RCP finally published an "excellent" report on the problem.[26]

In England, it is the General Medical Council that has the responsibility of registering physicians to practise, and of disciplining them when necessary. In response to an inquiry by a patient advocacy group about its plans to act against any of the physicians Pappworth named in his book,[22] the Council wrote, "The Council [is] not empowered to deal with matters of professional conduct which, though they may be open to criticism, do not raise the question of infamous misconduct."[27] Unlike Beecher, Pappworth published full documentation, including the author's names, and their institutions, for each of the articles he cites.

The letter went on to suggest that, should the correspondents wish to bring a complaint of 'infamous conduct in a professional respect," they would be welcome to do so, but they would need to cite specific statutory violations, and "provide evidence of the matters complained of." Although in 1967 a working party of the GMC did make recommendations to the council regarding standards of ethical human experimentation, like the College of Physicians' work, the process was a slow one, taking some six years even before the recommendation were made public.

The last of the three major professional institutions responsible for medical research in Britain is the Medical Research Council. This body serves some of the same functions there which the NIH does in the USA – in particular, it is responsible for awarding the grants that support the research of most non-governmental medical investigators. The MRC had issued a memorandum concerning human experimentation in 1953, and again, in a stronger form in 1964, but there was no mechanism developed for identifying or punishing unethical behaviour, and little indication that the "voluntary self-regulation" of the medical profession had been terribly successful.

Perhaps some of the most interesting comments on Pappworth's accusations are those given as answers to parliamentary questions – questions asked during the period when members of the House may put questions to the government, or to particular responsible ministers, to stimulate government action or call attention to what they see as the government's shortcomings. Pappworth gives a substantial selection of these responses[27] concerning the status of medical research in hospitals; I will mention just a few to give some flavour of the attitudes of the "responsible authorities" to the outrageous ways in which some medical experiments were being conducted.

In 1955, responding to a question about a medical experiment in a Bristol hospital, the Minister of Health said, "Only the clinician in charge could say what is right and proper. It would be entirely improper for me to try to lay down what ethical principles should govern the conduct of professionals in the work they do in hospitals." Three years later, another member of the Government, responding to a question about experiments on the mentally retarded, answered in this way: "Investigations of this kind involve ethical matters which are not susceptible to control by legislation." And finally, responding to the same question about the cases that Pappworth present in *Human Guinea Pigs*, a single government spokesman offered the following several observations at different times: "Allegations that doctors in the UK have carried out unauthorized experiments of NHS patients are not based on fact", and "The allegations cannot be ground on which the apparatus of public scrutiny should be brought into play. They have been promptly denied by hospital authorities", and "The medical profession have for generations been guided by strict codes."

Other excuses from politicians and physicians included statements that the hospitals at which the experiments were carried out had denied the charges, that is was impossible to actually define a medical "experiment", that these things may go on in the US, but certainly not in Britain, and that while unethical studies may have been carried out in the past, they couldn't possibly occur at present. Some reassuringly pointed to the existence of research committees established in many institutions to pass on the acceptability of human experimentation, although, as Pappworth noted, these committees were of very limited value in asserting ethical values concerning human experiments, often being composed of the very hospital staff doing clinical research themselves, and so hardly likely to block a colleague's research application. In addition, they were often run very informally, and with little or no accountability to the medical profession or the public at large. The responsibilities of these committees were considered of such modest importance that about 10% of them conducted their business by 'phone, or via mail.

CONCLUSIONS

To a considerable extent, Beecher and Pappworth presented similar findings – in some cases they discussed the same cases – in generally similar ways, and for very similar reasons. Each referred to the other's work approvingly. Whilst the excuses given in

Britain for not addressing Pappworth's concerns were, in some cases, very similar to the excuses Americans gave for a similar lack of action in this country, the response to the authors of the reports was quite different. Pappworth was personally attacked – he was called "shrill", his work was described as "slanted", he was said to lack the "restraint" necessary to write a "more effective "book – in a way that Beecher, always referred to in print courteously as "Professor Beecher", or, as *Time Magazine* put it "Harvard's Dr. Beecher", never was.[28] Also, unlike Beecher, whose article has been widely cited and reprinted as a crucial piece in the evolution of the debate over medical experimentation, Pappworth's book has been cited in the medical literature less than a dozen times since its appearance in 1967. If, as some have said, Beecher's writings helped to promote a system for the review of medical experimentation in the USA, it is not at all clear that Pappworth's writings have had nearly the same impact on public policy in Britain. Although in private Pappworth's work, and the courage it took for him to present it publicly, may have been appreciated, for example, in this quotation from a letter written to him by a very senior physician involved in the College's review of medical experimentation:

> I would very much like to take this opportunity personally to say how very much I appreciate the effort you have made in recent years to focus attention on this very important problem [of human experimentation]. You did a very good job, and I am sure that others think so too[27]

publicly he was repeatedly dismissed as being a trouble maker who lacked the polish of a gentleman. It may be that, as a result, he was not an acceptable person to refer to publicly at meetings or professional discussions, regardless of the substance of his remarks. Beecher, on the other hand, whilst he may have been pilloried in private, was generally treated respectfully in public, which, perhaps, allowed people to use him both substantively and symbolically as a sponsor of medical reforms in which they were interested.

I would take the differing responses of the medical profession to Beecher and to Pappworth to underline that medical ethics, like all other aspects of medicine, emerges out of a social context in which the personal and the professional are not rigidly separated. The acceptance of a thesis, no matter how strongly it is supported by objective data obtained in a logical and systematic way, is dependent upon more

than just the scientific probity of that data. It also reflects the personal judgements, preferences, and prejudices of medical men and women living in specific cultures, and at specific historical times. Such contingency is not often discussed as affecting the community's judgement of ethical norms, but it should be no surprise that, whatever activities human beings participate in, they are clearly coloured by human culture.

ACKNOWLEDGEMENTS

I thank Mr Geoffrey Sea for his invaluable research assistance, and Dr Francis P Chinard for his kindness in providing a copy of Pappworth's "Supplement" written for the Pelican edition of his book. Earlier versions of this manuscript were presented at the Conference on Public Health and Medicine, History and Ethics, Columbia University School of Public Health, The New York Academy of Medicine Interinstitutional Seminar in Medical History, and at the Annual Meeting of the American Society for Bioethics and the Medical Humanities, October 28, 1999, in Philadelphia PA. This work was supported in part by NIH grant HD-01302.

REFERENCES

1. Marrus MR. The Nuremberg doctors' trial in historical context. *Bull Hist Med* 73 (1999): 106–123.
2. US Army Adjutant General's Office. Trials of war criminals before the Nuremberg military tribunals under control council law No. 10 (October, 1946 – April, 1949). *The Medical Case* 1949; **2**: 181–4 (US Government Printing Office).
3. Requirements for experiments on human beings. *JAMA* 1946; **132**: 1090.
4. Principles for those in research and experimentation formulated by the Committee on Medical Ethics, and adopted by the Eighth General Assembly of the World Medical Association, 1954. *World Med J* 1955; **2**: 4–15.
5. Memorandum on clinical investigations. Medical Research Council Memorandum 53/649 (October 16, 1953), reprinted in I Ladimer, RW Newman. *Clinical investigation in medicine: legal, ethical, and moral aspects. An anthology and bibliography*. Boston: Law-Medicine Research Institute, Boston University, 1963.
6. Rothman DJ. *Strangers at the bedside*. NY: 1991, pp. 51–4.
7. McCusker JJ. How much is that in real money? A historical price index for use as a deflator of money values in the economy of the United States. American Antiquarian Society, 1992.

8. Henry Knowles Beecher (1904–1976). In: Kaufman M, Galishoff S, Savitt TL (eds). *A dictionary of American medical biography*, Vol. I. Greenwood Press, 1984, pp. 53–4.

9. Welch CE. Henry K Beecher MD. *New Engl J Med* 1976; **295**: 730.

10. Beecher HK. The specialty of anesthesia. *Ann Surgery* 1947; **126**: 486–99.

11. Gravenstein JS. Henry K Beecher: the introduction of anesthesia into the university. *Anesthesiology* 1998; **88**: 245–53.

12. Beecher HK. Edward D Churchill and anesthesia at Harvard. *Ann Surgery* 1963; **158**: 872–6.

13. Beecher HK. Ethics and clinical research. *New Engl J Med* 1966; **274**: 1354–60.

14. *Problems and complexities of clinical research*. A Symposium for Science Writers, held at Brook Lodge, Kalamazoo MI, and sponsored by the Upjohn Corporation, as reported in Osmundsen JA. Physician scores tests on humans, *New York Times*, March 24, 1965.

15. Brody JE. Some drug tests on people scored, *New York Times*, June 17, 1977, section 1, p. 17.

16. Carley WK. Medical ethics violated by some research with patients, Harvard Professor charges, *Wall Street J*, June 16, 1966.

17. The ethics of human experimentation, *Time Magazine*, July 8, 1966, p. 42. [This refers to Beecher as "Harvard's Dr. Henry K Beecher."]

18. Swazey JP, Scher SR. The whistle-blower as a deviant professional: Professional norms and responses to fraud in clinical research. In: *Whistleblowing in biomedical research*. Washington: US Government Printing Office, 1982, pp. 173–92.

19. Lock S. Obituary: Dr Maurice Pappworth. *The Independent* (London), November 12, 1994, p. 42. See also Lock S, this volume, pp. 47–8.

20. Editorial. More or less screening? *Lancet* 1968; **1**: 1020.

21. Pappworth MH. Human guinea pigs – a warning. *Twentieth Century* Autumn, 1962.

22. Pappworth MH. *Human Guinea Pigs. Experimentation in man*. London: Routledge and Kegan Paul, 1967, p. 3. (An American edition was published the next year by Beacon Press, and a paperback edition was published by Penguin Books in 1969.)

23. Witts LJ. Experiments on man. *BMJ* 1967; **2**: 689.

24. Editorial. Experimental medicine. *BMJ* 1967; **2**: 1108.

25. Editorial. Responsibilities of research. *Lancet* 1967; **1**: 1144.

26. Editorial. More or less screening. *Lancet* 1968; **1**: 1020.

27. MH Pappworth. Human guinea pigs – a history. *BMJ* 1990; **301**: 1456–60.

28. Medicine. *Time Magazine* 1966 July 8: 42–3.

5 · Extracts from Pappworth and Beecher

Introduction to Beecher's "Ethics and clinical research"

Len Doyal

The Nuremberg Code is often given prominence in the teaching of ethics and law applied to medical research. On the face of it, this seems plausible. After all, the Code was developed in response to Nazi doctors who had inflicted horrific cruelty on primarily Jewish prisoners, and who had defended their actions as examples of justifiable medical research. The Code was designed to keep physicians from ever engaging in such unethical research again. It placed particular emphasis on the importance of obtaining the informed consent of those asked to participate.

What is not always spelled out, however, is the lack of attention by medical researchers to the Nuremberg Code for two decades. It was rarely referred to or cited in the research literature. Researchers who knew about the Code often believed that it had little or nothing to do with them. They reasoned that they were not Nazis and should not be thought of, or expected to think of themselves, in these terms. Further, medical researchers were influenced by the conduct of potentially harmful experiments on American citizens as part of the war effort. These experiments – sometimes done on participants who were incompetent to give informed consent – were thought to be morally justified for the sake of public interest and patriotic duty. The consequence was a post-war institutional environment where some doctors felt able to continue to ignore the moral rights of patients whom they entered into research studies without their knowledge.[1]

One of the first major challenges to such moral complacency in the United States was the publication in 1966 by Henry Beecher of his classic paper, "Ethics and human experimentation". The structure of his paper was as simple as its content was devastating. Beecher outlined the academic and professional pressures on young researchers to prove themselves through the conduct of medical research: "Every young man knows that he will never be promoted to a tenure post, to a professorship in a major medical school, unless he has proved himself as an investigator." This was the age of "the ready availability of money" for medical research and as a result, its sheer volume was dramatically increasing. After indicating some evidence that "unethical experimentation" was occurring, Beecher highlighted one of his main moral concerns – "the problem of consent".

On the one hand, he argued that informed consent for participation in medical research "remains a goal toward which one must strive for sociologic, ethical and clear-cut legal reasons. There is no choice in the matter." Against the background of their trust for doctors, patients may be willing "to submit to inconvenience and some discomfort" for research purposes. However, there is no evidence to suggest that they will agree to place their lives or health in any serious risk "for the sake of 'science'". Therefore, by implication, if any such risk is posed by research, there is a strict duty to obtain consent from patients or other volunteers before involving them in it. Yet on the other hand, Beecher also underlined how difficult it can be to obtain consent that is properly informed. It follows that aside from the duty to try to give potential research participants an informed choice, it should not be forgotten that: "A far more dependable safeguard than consent is the presence of a truly responsible investigator."

Unfortunately, Beecher went on in his paper to give example after example of research that was potentially harmful or where potential harm clearly occurred, where there was no evidence that informed consent had been obtained, and thus where researchers had been grossly irresponsible. These examples had been published in a variety of journals. Beecher did not cite them but we now know that they included those of the highest prestige, including the *New England Journal of Medicine* itself! Much of the research to which Beecher drew attention was truly shocking and his paper had an enormous impact. While some medical researchers continued to bury their heads in the sand, many recognised the need for greater professional regulation of the moral and legal boundaries their work. This recognition was helped by the fact that Beecher himself was a pre-eminent academic physician whose own commitment to medical research could not be questioned.

Many readers of this book will already know something of Beecher's importance for the evolution of the ethics of medical research and for the moral emphasis that is now placed on the doctrine of informed consent. His work is commonly referred to and outlined. However, references to his historical importance should not be taken at face value, without actually reading his classic paper. It becomes too easy to forget the extraordinary willingness of clinical researchers at the time to abuse the basic rights of patients through giving them no informed choice about the unacceptable levels of risk to which they were being exposed. The emergence of the Helsinki Declaration and of varying national approaches to the regulation of research is rooted in the kinds of horrors that Beecher unearthed. We can still learn much from the details he published and we should certainly remember those who were forced to participate in, and suffer from, research about which they knew little or nothing at the time.

For this reason, we are reprinting Beecher's classic paper, along with a short reflection on his work by Dr John P Bunker who knew and worked with him.

REFERENCE

1. Rothman D J. Ethics and human experimentation: Henry Beecher Revisited. *New Engl J Med* 0000; **317**: 1195–9.

Ethics and clinical research*

Henry K Beecher

Human experimentation since World War II has created some difficult problems with the increasing employment of patients as experimental subjects, when it must be apparent that they would not have been available if they had been truly aware of the uses that would be made of them. Evidence is at hand that many of the patients in the examples to follow never had the risk satisfactorily explained to them, and it seems obvious that further hundreds have not known that they were the subjects of an experiment,

New Engl J Med 1966; **274**: 1354–60. Copyright © 1966 Massachusetts Medical Society.

although grave consequences have been suffered as a direct result of experiments described here. There is a belief prevalent in some sophisticated circles that attention to these matters would "block progress". But, according to Pope Pius XII,[1] "... science is not the highest value to which all other orders of values ... should be subordinated."

I am aware that these are troubling charges. They have grown out of troubling practices. They can be documented, as I propose to do, by examples from leading medical schools, university hospitals, private hospitals, governmental military departments (the Army, the Navy and the Air Force), governmental institutes (the National Institutes of Health), Veterans Administration hospitals and industry. The basis for the charges is broad.†

I should like to affirm that American medicine is sound, and most progress in it soundly attained. There is, however, a reason for concern in certain areas, and I believe the type of activities to be mentioned will do great harm to medicine unless soon corrected. It will certainly be charged that any mention of these matters does a disservice to medicine, but not one so great, I believe, as a continuation of the practices to be cited.

Experimentation in man takes place in several areas: in self-experimentation; in patient volunteers and normal subjects; in therapy; and in the different areas of *experimentation on a patient not for his benefit but for that, at least in theory, of patients in general*. The present study is limited to this last category.

REASONS FOR URGENCY OF STUDY

Ethical errors are increasing not only in numbers but in variety – for example, in the recently added problems arising in transplantation of organs.

There are a number of reasons why serious attention to the general problem is urgent.

Of transcendent importance is the enormous and continuing increase in available funds, as shown below.

Money Available for Research Each Year

Massachusetts general hospital		National Institutes of Health*
1945	$ 500,000†	$ 701,800
1955	2,222,816	36,063,200
1965	8,384,342	436,600,000

* *National Institutes of Health figures based upon decade averages, excluding funds for construction, kindly supplied by Dr. John Sherman, of National Institutes of Health.*
† *Approximation, supplied by Mr. David C. Crockett, of Massachusetts General Hospital.*

†At the Brook Lodge Conference on "Problems and Complexities of Clinical Research" I commented that "what seem to be breaches of ethical conduct in experimentation are by no means rare, but are almost, one fears, universal." I thought it was obvious that I was by "universal" referring to the fact that examples could easily be found in *all* categories where research in man takes place to any significant extent. Judging by press comments, that was not obvious: hence, this note.

Since World War II the annual expenditure for research (in large part in man) in the Massachusetts General Hospital has increased a remarkable 17-fold. At the National Institutes of Health, the increase has been a gigantic 624-fold. This "national" rate of increase is over 36 times that of the Massachusetts General Hospital. These data, rough as they are, illustrate vast opportunities and concomitantly expanded responsibilities.

Taking into account the sound and increasing emphasis of recent years that experimentation in man must precede general application of new procedures in therapy, plus the great sums of money available, there is reason to fear that these requirements and these resources may be greater than the supply of responsible investigators. All this heightens the problems under discussion.

Medical schools and university hospitals are increasingly dominated by investigators. Every young man knows that he will never be promoted to a tenure post, to a professorship in a major medical school, unless he has proved himself as an investigator. If the ready availability of money of conducting research is added to this fact, one can see how great the pressures are on ambitious young physicians.

Implementation of the recommendations of the President's Commission on Heart Disease, Cancer and Stroke means that further astronomical sums of money will become available for research in man.

In addition to the foregoing three practical points there are others that Sir Robert Platt[2] has pointed out: a general awakening of social conscience; greater power for good or harm in new remedies, new operations and new investigative procedures than was formerly the case; new methods of preventive treatment with their advantages and dangers that are now applied to communities as a whole as well as to individuals, with multiplication of the possibilities for injury; medical science has shown how valuable human experimentation can be in solving problems of disease and its treatment; one can therefore anticipate an increase in experimentation; and the newly developed concept of clinical research as a profession (for example, clinical pharmacology) – and this, of course, can lead to unfortunate separation between the interests of science and the interests of the patient.

FREQUENCY OF UNETHICAL OR QUESTIONABLY ETHICAL PROCEDURES

Nearly everyone agrees that ethical violations do

occur. The practical question is, how often? A pre-liminary examination of the matter was based on 17 examples, which were easily increased to 50. These 50 studies contained references to 186 further likely examples, on the average 3.7 leads per study; they at times overlapped from paper to paper, but this figure indicates how conveniently one can proceed in a search for such material. The data are suggestive of widespread problems, but there is need for another kind of information, which was obtained by examination of 100 consecutive human studies published in 1964, in an excellent journal; 12 of these seemed to be unethical. If only one quarter of them is truly unethical, this still indi-cates the existence of a serious situation. Papp-worth,[3] in England, has collected, he says, more than 500 papers based upon unethical experimentation. It is evident from such observations that unethical or questionably ethical procedures are not uncom-mon.

THE PROBLEM OF CONSENT

All so-called codes are based on the bland assump-tion that meaningful or informed consent is readily available for the asking. As pointed out elsewhere,[4] this is very often not the case. Consent in any fully informed sense may not be obtainable. Nevertheless, except, possibly, in the most trivial situations, it remains a goal toward which one must strive for soci-ologic, ethical and clear-cut legal reasons. There is no choice in the matter.

If suitably approached, patients will accede, on the basis of trust, to about any request their physician may make. At the same time, every experienced clin-ician investigator knows that patients will often sub-mit to inconvenience and some discomfort, if they do not last very long, but the usual patient will never agree to jeopardize seriously his health or his life for the sake of "science."

In only 2 of the 50* examples originally compiled for this study was consent mentioned. Actually, it should be emphasized in all cases for obvious moral and legal reasons, but it would be unrealistic to place much dependence on it. In any precise sense state-ments regarding consent are meaningless unless one knows how fully the patient was informed of all risks, and if these are not known, that fact should also be made clear. A far more dependable safeguard than

---

*Reduced here to 22 for reasons of space.

consent is the presence of a truly *responsible* investi-gator.

EXAMPLES OF UNETHICAL OR QUESTIONABLY ETHICAL STUDIES

These examples are not cited for the condemnation of individuals; they are recorded to call attention to a variety of ethical problems found in experimental medicine, for it is hoped that calling attention to them will help to correct abuses present. During ten years of study of these matters it has become appar-ent that thoughtlessness and carelessness, not a will-ful disregard of the patient's rights, account for most of the cases encountered. Nonetheless, it is evident that in many of the examples presented, the inves-tigators have risked the health or the life of their sub-jects. No attempt has been made to present the "worst" possible examples; rather, the aim has been to show the variety of problems encountered.

References to the examples presented are not given, for there is no intention of pointing to indi-viduals, but rather, a wish to call attention to wide-spread practices. All, however, are documented to the satisfaction of the editors of the *Journal*.

Known Effective Treatment Withheld

Example 1. It is known that rheumatic fever can usu-ally be prevented by adequate treatment of strepto-coccal respiratory infections by the parenteral administration of penicillin. Nevertheless, definitive treatment was withheld, and placebos were given to a group of 109 men in service, while benzathine penicillin G was given to others.

The therapy that each patient received was deter-mined automatically by his military serial number arranged so that more men received penicillin than received placebo. In the small group of patients stud-ied 2 cases of acute rheumatic fever and 1 of acute nephritis developed in the control patients, where-as these complications did not occur among those who received the benzathine penicillin G.

Example 2. The sulfonamides were for many years the only antibacterial drugs effective in shortening the duration of acute streptococcal pharyngitis and in reducing its suppurative complications. The investigators in this study undertook to determine if the occurrence of the serious nonsuppurative complications, rheumatic fever and acute glomerulonephritis, would be reduced by this treatment. This study was made despite the general experience that certain antibiotics, including penicillin, will prevent the development of rheumatic fever.

The subjects were a large group of hospital patients; a control group of approximately the same size, also with exudative Group A streptococcus, was included. The latter group received only non-specific therapy (no sulfadiazine). The total group denied the effective penicillin comprised over 500 men.

Rheumatic fever was diagnosed in 5.4 per cent of those treated with sulfadiazine. In the control group rheumatic fever developed in 4.2 per cent.

In reference to this study a medical officer stated in writing that the subjects were not informed, did not consent and were not aware that they had been involved in an experiment, and yet admittedly 25 acquired rheumatic fever. According to this same medical officer *more than 70* who had had known definitive treatment withheld were on the wards with rheumatic fever when he was there.

Example 3. This involved a study of the relapse rate in typhoid fever treated in two ways. In an earlier study by the present investigators chloramphenicol had been recognized as an effective treatment for typhoid fever, being attended by half the mortality that was experienced when this agent was not used. Others had made the same observations, indicating that to withhold this effective remedy can be a life-or-death decision. The present study was carried out to determine the relapse rate under the two methods of treatment; of 408 charity patients 251 were treated with chloramphenicol, of whom 20, or 7.97 per cent, died. Symptomatic treatment was given, but chloramphenicol was withheld in 157, of whom 36, or 22.9 per cent, died. According to the data presented, 23 patients died in the course of this study who would not have been expected to succumb if they had received specific therapy.

Study of Therapy

Example 4. TriA (triacetyloleandomycin) was originally introduced for the treatment of infection with gram-positive organisms. Spotty evidence of hepatic dysfunction emerged, especially in children, and so the present study was undertaken on 50 patients, including mental defectives or juvenile delinquents who were inmates of a children's center. No disease other than acne was present; the drug was given for treatment of this. The ages of the subjects ranged from thirteen to thirty-nine years. "By the time half the patients had received the drug for four weeks, the high incidence of significant hepatic dysfunction … led to the discontinuation of administration to the remainder of the group at three weeks." (However, only two weeks after the start of the administration of the drug, 54 per cent of the patients showed abnormal excretion of bromsulfalein.) Eight patients with marked hepatic dysfunction were transferred to the hospital "for more intensive study." Liver biopsy was carried out in these 8 patients and repeated in 4 of them. Liver damage was evident. Four of these hospitalized patients, after their liver-function tests returned to normal limits, received a "challenge" dose of the drug. Within two days hepatic dysfunction was evident in 3 of the 4 patients. In 1 patient a second challenge dose was given after the first challenge and again led to evidence of abnormal liver function. Flocculation tests remained abnormal in some patients as long as five weeks after discontinuance of the drug.

Physiologic Studies

Example 5. In this controlled, double-blind study of the hematologic toxicity of chloramphenicol, it was recognized that chloramphenicol is "well known as a cause of aplastic anemia" and that there is a "prolonged morbidity and high mortality of aplastic anemia" and that "… chloramphenicol-induced aplastic anemia can be related to dose …" The aim of the study was "further definition of the toxicology of the drug.…"

Forty-one randomly chosen patients were given either 2 or 6 gm. of chloramphenicol per day; 12 control patients were used. "Toxic bone-marrow depression, predominantly affecting erythropoiesis, developed in 2 of 20 patients given 2.0 gm. and in 18 of 21 given 6 gm. of chloramphenicol daily." The smaller dose is recommended for routine use.

Example 6. In a study of the effect of thymectomy on the survival of skin homografts 18 children, three and a half months to eighteen years of age, about to undergo surgery for congenital heart disease, were selected. Eleven were to have total thymectomy as part of the operation, and 7 were to serve as controls. As part of the experiment, full-thickness skin homografts from an unrelated adult donor were sutured to the chest wall in each case. (Total thymectomy is occasionally, although not usually part of the primary cardiovascular surgery involved, and whereas it may not greatly add to the hazards of the necessary operation, its eventual effects in children are not known.) This work was proposed as part of a long-range study of "the growth and development of these children over the years." No difference in the survival of the skin homograft was observed in the 2 groups.

Example 7. This study of cyclopropane anesthesia and cardiac arrhythmias consisted of 31 patients. The average duration of the study was three hours, ranging from two to four and a half hours. "Minor surgical procedures" were carried out in all but 1 subject. Moderate to deep anesthesia, with endotracheal intubation and controlled respiration, was used. Carbon dioxide was injected into the closed respiratory system until cardiac arrhythmias appeared. Toxic levels of carbon dioxide were achieved and maintained for considerable periods. During the cyclopropane anesthesia a variety of pathologic cardiac arrhythmias occurred. When the carbon dioxide tension was elevated above normal, ventricular extrasystoles were more numerous than when the carbon dioxide tension was normal, ventricular arrhythmias being continuous in 1 subject for ninety minutes. (This can lead to fatal fibrillation.)

Example 8. Since the minimum blood-flow requirements of the cerebral circulation are not accurately known, this study was carried out to determine "cerebral hemodynamic and metabolic changes ... before and during acute reductions in arterial pressure induced by drug administration and/or postural adjustments." Forty-four patients whose ages varied from the second to the tenth decade were involved. They included normotensive subjects, those with essential hypertension and finally a group with malignant hypertension. Fifteen had abnormal electrocardiograms. Few details about the reasons for hospitalization are given.

Signs of cerebral circulatory insufficiency, which were easily recognized, included confusion and in some cases a nonresponsive state. By alteration in the tilt of the patient "the clinical state of the subject could be changed in a matter of seconds from one of alertness to confusion, and for the remainder of the flow, the subject was maintained in the latter state." The femoral arteries were cannulated in all subjects, and the internal jugular veins in 14.

The mean arterial pressure fell in 37 subjects from 109 to 48 mm. of mercury, with signs of cerebral ischemia. "With the onset of collapse, cardiac output and right ventricular pressures decreased sharply."

Since signs of cerebral insufficiency developed without evidence of coronary insufficiency the authors concluded that "the brain may be more sensitive to acute hypotension than is the heart."

Example 9. This is a study of the adverse circulatory responses elicited by intra-abdominal maneuvers:

> When the peritoneal cavity was entered, a deliberate series of maneuvers was carried out [in 68 patients] to ascertain the effective stimuli and the areas responsible for development of the expected circulatory changes. Accordingly, the surgeon rubbed localized areas of the parietal and visceral peritoneum with a small ball sponge as discretely as possible. Traction on the mesenteries, pressure in the area of the celiac plexus, traction on the gallbladder and stomach, and occlusion of the portal and caval veins were the other stimuli applied.

Thirty-four of the patients were sixty years of age or older; 11 were seventy or older. In 44 patients the hypotension produced by the deliberate stimulation was "moderate to marked." The maximum fall produced by manipulation was from 200 systolic, 105 diastolic, to 42 systolic, 20 diastolic; the average fall in mean pressure in 26 patients was 53 mm. of mercury.

Of the 50 patients studied, 17 showed either atrioventricular dissociation with nodal rhythm or nodal rhythm alone. A decrease in the amplitude of the T wave and elevation or depression of the ST segment were noted in 25 cases in association with manipulation and hypotension or, at other times, in the course of anesthesia and operation. In only 1 case was the change pronounced enough to suggest myocardial ischemia. No case of myocardial infarction was noted in the group studied although routine electrocardiograms were not taken after operation to detect silent infarcts. Two cases in which electrocardiograms were taken after operation showed T-wave and ST-segment changes that had not been present before.

These authors refer to a similar study in which more alarming electrocardiographic changes were observed. Four patients in the series sustained silent myocardial infarctions; most of their patients were undergoing gallbladder surgery because of associated heart disease. It can be added further that in the 34 patients referred to above as being sixty years of age or older, some doubtless had heart disease that could have made risky the maneuvers carried out. In any event, this possibility might have been a deterrent.

Example 10. Starling's law – "that the heart output per beat is directly proportional to the diastolic filling" – was studied in 30 adult patients with atrial fibrillation and mitral stenosis sufficiently severe to require valvulotomy. "Continuous alterations of the length of a segment of left ventricular muscle were recorded simultaneously in 13 of these patients by means of a mercury-filled resistance gauge sutured to the surface of the left ventricle." Pressures in the left ventricle were determined by direct puncture simultaneously with the segment length in 13 patients and without the segment length in an additional 13 patients. Four similar unanesthetized patients were studied through catheterization of the left side of the heart transeptally. In all 30 patients arterial pressure was measured through the catheterized brachial artery.

Example 11. To study the sequence of ventricular contraction in human bundle-branch block, simultaneous catheterization of both ventricles was performed in 22 subjects; catheterization of the right side of the heart was carried out in the usual manner; the left side was catheterized transbronchially. Extrasystoles were produced by tapping on the epicardium in subjects with normal myocardium while they were undergoing thoracotomy. Simultaneous pressures were measured in both ventricles through needle puncture in this group.

The purpose of this study was to gain increased insight into the physiology involved.

Example 12. This investigation was carried out to examine the possible effect of vagal stimulation on cardiac arrest. The authors had in recent years transected the homolateral vagus nerve immediately below the origin of the recurrent laryngeal nerve as palliation against cough and pain in bronchogenic carcinoma. Having been impressed with the number of reports of cardiac arrest that seemed to follow vagal stimulation, they tested the effects of intrathoracic vagal stimulation during 30 of their surgical procedures, concluding, from these observations in patients under satisfactory anesthesia, that cardiac irregularities and cardiac arrest due to vagovagal reflex were less common than had previously been supposed.

Example 13. This study presented a technic for determining portal circulation time and hepatic blood flow. It involved the transcutaneous injection of the spleen and catheterization of the hepatic vein. This was carried out in 43 subjects, of whom 14 were normal; 16 had cirrhosis (varying degrees), 9 acute hepatitis, and 4 hemolytic anemia.

No mention is made of what information was divulged to the subjects, some of whom were seriously ill. This study consisted in the development of a technic, not of therapy, in the 14 normal subjects.

Studies to Improve the Understanding of Disease

Example 14. In this study of the syndrome of impending hepatic coma in patients with cirrhosis of the liver certain nitrogenous substances were administered to 9 patients with chronic alcoholism and advanced cirrhosis: ammonium chloride, di-ammonium citrate, urea or dietary protein. In all patients a reaction that included mental disturbances, a "flapping tremor" and electroencephalographic changes developed. Similar signs had occurred in only 1 of the patients before these substances were administered:

> The first sign noted was usually clouding of the consciousness. Three patients had a second or a third course of administration of a nitrogenous substance with the same results. It was concluded that marked resemblance between this reaction and impending hepatic coma, implied that the administration of these [nitrogenous] substances to patients with cirrhosis may be hazardous.

Example 15. The relation of the effects of ingested ammonia to liver disease was investigated in 11 normal subjects, 6 with acute virus hepatitis, 26 with cirrhosis, and 8 miscellaneous patients. Ten of these patients had neurologic changes associated with either hepatitis or cirrhosis.

The hepatic and renal veins were cannulated. Ammonium chloride was administered by mouth. After this, a tremor that lasted for three days developed in 1 patient. When ammonium chloride was ingested by 4 cirrhotic patients with tremor and mental confusion the symptoms were exaggerated during the test. The same thing was true of a fifth patient in another group.

Example 16. This study was directed toward determining the period of infectivity of infectious hepatitis. Artificial induction of hepatitis was carried out in an institution for mentally defective children in which a mild form of hepatitis was endemic. The parents gave consent for the intramuscular injection or oral administration of the virus, but nothing is said regarding what was told them concerning the appreciable hazards involved.

A resolution adopted by the World Medical Association states explicitly: "Under no circumstances is a doctor permitted to do anything which would weaken the physical or mental resistance of a human being except from strictly therapeutic or prophylactic indications imposed in the interest of the patient." There is no right to risk an injury to 1 person for the benefit of others.

Example 17. Live cancer cells were injected into 22 human subjects as part of a study of immunity to cancer. According to a recent review, the subjects (hospitalized patients) were "merely told they would be receiving 'some cells'" – "... the word cancer was entirely omitted ...."

Example 18. Melanoma was transplanted from a daughter to her volunteering and informed mother, "in the hope of gaining a little better understanding of cancer immunity and in the hope that the production of tumor antibodies might be helpful in the treatment of the cancer patient." Since the daughter died on the day after the transplantation of the tumor into her mother, the hope expressed seems to have been more theoretical than practical, and the daughter's condition was described as "terminal" at the time the mother volunteered to be a recipient. The primary implant was widely excised on the twenty-fourth day after it had been placed in the mother. She died from metastatic melanoma on the four hundred and fifty-first day after transplantation. The evidence that this patient died of diffuse melanoma that metastasized from a small piece of transplanted tumor was considered conclusive.

Technical Study of Disease

Example 19. During bronchoscopy a special needle was inserted through a bronchus into the left atrium of the heart. This was done in an unspecified number of subjects, both with cardiac disease and with normal hearts.

The technic was a new approach whose hazards were at the beginning quite unknown. The subjects with normal hearts were used, not for their possible benefit but for that of patients in general.

Example 20. The percutaneous method of catheterization of the left side of the heart has, it is reported, led to 8 deaths (1.09 per cent death rate) and other serious accidents in 732 cases. There was, therefore, need for another method, the transbronchial approach, which was carried out in the present study in more than 500 cases, with no deaths.

Granted that a delicate problem arises regarding how much should be discussed with the patients involved in the use of a new method, nevertheless where the method is employed in a given patient of *his* benefit, the ethical problems are far less than when this potentially extremely dangerous method is used "in 15 patients with normal hearts, undergoing bronchoscopy for other reasons." Nothing was said about what was told any of the subjects, and nothing was said about the granting of permission, which was certainly indicated in the 15 normal subjects used.

Example 21. This was a study of the effect of exercise on cardiac output and pulmonary-artery pressure in 8 "normal" persons (that is, patients whose diseases were not related to the cardiovascular system), in 8 with congestive heart failure severe enough to have recently required complete bed rest, in 6 with hypertension, in 2 with aortic insufficiency, in 7 with mitral stenosis and in 5 with pulmonary emphysema.

Intracardiac catheterization was carried out, and the catheter then inserted into the right or left main branch of the pulmonary artery. The brachial artery was usually catheterized; sometimes, the radial or femoral arteries were catheterized. The subjects exercised in a supine position by pushing their feet against weighted pedals. "The ability of these patients to carry on sustained work was severely limited by weakness and dyspnea." Several were in severe failure. This was not a therapeutic attempt but rather a physiologic study.

Bizarre Study

Example 22. There is a question whether ureteral reflux can occur in the normal bladder. With this in mind, vesicourethrography was carried out on 26 normal babies less than forty-eight hours old. The infants were exposed to X-rays while the bladder was filling and during voiding. Multiple spot films were made to record the presence or absence of ureteral reflux. None was found in this group, and fortunately no infection followed the catheterization. What the results of the extensive x-ray exposure may be, no one can yet say.

COMMENT ON DEATH RATES

In the foregoing examples a number of procedures, some with their own demonstrated death rates, were carried out. The following data were provided by 3 distinguished investigators in the field and represent widely held views.

Cardiac catheterization: right side of the heart, about 1 death per 1000 cases; left side, 5 deaths per 1000 cases. "Probably considerably higher in some places, depending on the portal of entry." (One investigator had 15 deaths in his first 150 cases.) It is possible that catheterization of a hepatic vein or the renal vein would have a lower death rate than that of catheterization of the right side of the heart, for if it is properly carried out, only the atrium is entered en route to the liver or the kidney, not the right ventricle, which can lead to serious cardiac irregularities. There is always the possibility, however, that the ventricle will be entered inadvertently. This occurs in at least half the cases, according to 1 expert – "but if properly done is too transient to be of importance."

Liver biopsy: the death rate here is estimated at 2 to 3 per 1000, depending in considerable part on the condition of the subject.

Anesthesia: the anesthesia death rate can be placed in general at about 1 death per 2000 cases. The hazard is doubtless higher when certain practices such as deliberate evocation of ventricular extrasystoles under cyclopropane are involved.

PUBLICATION

In the view of the British Medical Research Council[5] it is not enough to ensure that all investigation is carried out in an ethical manner: it must be made unmistakably clear in the publications that the proprieties have been observed. This implies editorial responsibility in addition to the investigator's. The question rises, then, about valuable data that have been improperly obtained.* It is my view that such material should not be published.[5] There is a practical aspect to the matter: failure to obtain publication would discourage unethical experimentation. How many would carry out such experimentation if they *knew* its results would never be published? Even though suppression of such data (by not publishing it) would constitute a loss to medicine, in a specific

---

*As far as principle goes, a parallel can be seen in the recent Mapp decision by the United States Supreme Court. It was stated there that evidence unconstitutionally obtained cannot be used in any judicial decision, no matter how important the evidence is to the ends of justice.

localized sense, this loss, it seems, would be less important than the far reaching moral loss to medicine if the data thus obtained were to be published. Admittedly, there is room for debate. Others believe that such data, because of their intrinsic value, obtained at a cost of great risk or damage to the subjects, should not be wasted but should be published with stern editorial comment. This would have to be done with exceptional skill, to avoid an odor of hypocrisy.

SUMMARY AND CONCLUSIONS

The ethical approach to experimentation in man has several components; two are more important than the others, the first being informed consent. The difficulty of obtaining this is discussed in detail. But it is absolutely essential to *strive* for it for moral, sociologic and legal reasons. The statement that consent has been obtained has little meaning unless the subject or his guardian is capable of understanding what is to be undertaken and unless all hazards are made clear. If these are not known this, too, should be stated. In such a situation the subject at least knows that he is to be a participant in an experiment. Secondly, there is the more reliable safeguard provided by the presence of an intelligent, informed, conscientious, compassionate, responsible investigator.

Ordinary patients will not knowingly risk their health or their life for the sake of "science." Every experienced clinician investigator knows this. When such risks are taken and a considerable number of patients are involved, it may be assumed that informed consent has not been obtained in all cases.

The gain anticipated from an experiment must be commensurate with the risk involved.

An experiment is ethical or not at its inception; it does not become ethical *post hoc* – ends do not justify means. There is no ethical distinction between ends and means.

In the publication of experimental results it must be made unmistakably clear that the proprieties have been observed. It is debatable whether data obtained unethically should be published even with stern editorial comment.

REFERENCES

1. Pope Pius XII. Address. Presented at First International Congress on Histopathology of Nervous System, Rome, Italy, September 14, 1952.

2. Platt (Sir Robert), 1st bart. *Doctor and Patient: Ethics, morals, government*. 87 pp. London: Nuffield provincial hospitals trust, 1963. pp. 62 and 63.
3. Pappworth, M. H. Personal communication.

4. Beecher, H. K. Consent in clinical experimentation: myth and reality. *J.A.M.A.* **195**: 34, 1966.
5. Great Britain, Medical Research Council. *Memorandum*. 1953.

Commentary on "Ethics and clinical research"

John P Bunker

The publication of Henry Beecher's paper in 1966 created quite a stir at the Massachusetts General Hospital, where he was Chairman of the Department of Anesthesia, and a still larger one in the Boston medical establishment. I worked in Beecher's department from 1950 to 1960, and by the time of the publication of "Ethics and clinical research" in the *New England Journal of Medicine*, I was away from the scene. Francis D Moore, Moseley Professor of Surgery Emeritus at Harvard, gave me his own first-hand memories. There were, he said, mixed reactions. Those of his colleagues involved in human research were offended, thinking that they were being criticised. Those of his surgical colleagues not involved in research shrugged it off, commenting, "There goes Harry shooting off again". Senior members of the Department of Medicine, such as Walter Bauer and Howard Means thought he was probably right. Younger investigators, including Moore, believed that he had a point, and there emerged a groundswell of opinion that he was, indeed, quite right. Dr Moore pointed out during our conversation that the Harvard Commission on Human Rights was established shortly after publication of his article, with Beecher as its chairman, thus largely vindicating his allegations, and that NIH regulations of ethical procedures for human research were published shortly afterwards.

One of the main criticisms Beecher made in "Ethics and clinical research" was that most of the experiments he described appeared to have been conducted without consent of the patients who were the subjects. One of his former colleagues recalls having suggested that consent may have been obtained but not so stated in the published report. "Just as bad," Beecher retorted. "It should be emphasized in all cases for obvious moral and legal reasons."

I had been a senior member of Beecher's staff and very much involved in clinical research during most of my tenure at the department. I have no memory of any discussion of the need for informed consent, nor do any of former colleagues with whom I have spoken. I myself had carried out two studies in surgical patients for which I did not obtain consent. Indeed, the need for consent had not occurred to me. It was not a topic that had reached the research agenda in academic circles.

A major focus of Beecher's own research had been on randomised trials of new and experimental analgesics, comparing them to placebos. The trials were conducted in good risk patients selected from the surgical schedule. Patients were informed that following surgery they would receive a new drug that was expected to give better relief than standard ones; and that, if did not receive relief, they would then be given another drug for which the analgesic properties were well established. Patients were not informed that they might receive a placebo, nor that selection of medication would be administered at random. While formal consent was not requested or obtained, patients could and on occasion did refuse to participate.

When research was to be carried out in human volunteers, Beecher insisted on informed consent. He appeared to believe, however, that in clinical research, thought not to involve significant risk, consent need not be obtained. It is of some interest, therefore, to note that early in his clinical trials of analgesics to control pain postoperatively, three very serious complications had occurred. A new long-acting analgesic was compared to placebo, and it was perhaps not recognised that there could be a large cumulative effect. Three patients, having received the new drug to relieve pain for the first 36 hours following surgery, proceded to sink into coma lasting several days. The cause of coma was not immediately recognised, but ultimately it was concluded that the experimental drug must have been responsible. (These events were probably never published.)

Beecher was clearly ambivalent as to the possibility of obtaining fully informed consent, as well as to the practical reality of its requirement. In an editorial in the *Journal of the American Medical Association*, published the same year as "Ethics and clinical research," he wrote that "The reality is that informed consent is often exceedingly difficult or impossible to obtain in any complete sense. The difficulties inherent in this complex situation are no excuse for giving up the effort: informed consent is a goal toward which we must strive." He considered the search for truly informed consent a moral imperative, but at the same time he found it an inconvenient obstacle in his own research.

An introduction to Pappworth's *Human Guinea Pigs*

Jeffrey S Tobias

No contribution to the continuing debate on informed consent could be regarded as complete, or even adequate, without reference to Pappworth's iconoclastic and influential book *Human Guinea Pigs* published by Routledge and Kegan Paul in 1967. Its subject, indeed its subtitle, was *Experimentation on man* and, like Beecher's damning critique published in the USA one year earlier (and reproduced later in this chapter), it caused a furore.

Pappworth's central points were that medical experimentation without adequate consent was far more commonly conducted than the public knew about; that such experimentation was morally offensive and, on occasion, dangerous to the subject; and that the profession itself was acting irresponsibly if it failed to recognise its responsibilities, both in the moral sense and also, in practical terms, as guardian of its own reputation. As he wrote in 1963:

- *Clinical research must go on, but there must be acknowledged and observed safeguards for the patients. At present such safeguards are virtually non-existent.*
- *The majority of those engaged in clinical research act with the highest moral integrity, but an expanding minority resort to unethical and probably illegal practices.*
- *Unless the medical profession itself stops the unethical practices of this minority, the public outcry will eventually be such as to cause opposition to all clinical research.*

Pappworth may now be remembered chiefly as a castigator of the medical profession but his views summarised above display a far more tolerant, indeed encouraging view of the importance of clinical research. Indeed Pappworth himself could be said to have occupied the "middle ground" and remained acutely aware of the dilemmas and tensions relating to clinical research on the one hand, coupled with the crucially important rights of individual patients, on the other.

This brief resumé of Pappworth's observations, and the book which became his epitaph, can only offer a relatively brief account of his views and the wide range of subjects he addressed. In contrast to reproducing Beecher's article in full (pp. 29–37), clearly there was no question in the present book of providing a complete picture of the practices that Pappworth criticised so strongly. Instead we have chosen to present parts of his introductory chapters and, as an illustration of his approach to the then totally uncharted territory of informed consent within a contemporary medical framework, extracts from the sections of his book entitled *What is being done*, and *Principles*. We have selected these relatively short sections partly in the interest of space, but also to give what we hope is an adequate flavour of Pappworth's style and careful annotation of references. How much has changed in the 30 years or so since publication of this remarkable book, which caused such an outcry particularly amongst the medical profession, when first published. We are grateful to Dr Stephen Lock, a previous editor of the *British Medical Journal*, who knew Pappworth, for commentary at the close of these extracts.

*Human Guinea Pigs** MH Pappworth

PREFACE

The main purpose of this book is to show that the ethical problems arising from human experimentation have become one of the cardinal issues of our time. That this is so, I hope no reader will doubt after completion of this book. I believe that only by frank discussion among informed people, lay as well as medical, can a solution be reached. The hope is that by presenting the facts in a dispassionate way this book will stimulate both the lay public and their doctors to seek a solution.

The vast majority of the medical profession are either genuinely ignorant of the immensity and the complexity of the problem or wish purposely to ignore the whole matter by sweeping it under the carpet. Even fewer lay people have any conception of the issues involved. But the medical profession must no longer be allowed to ignore the problems or to assert, as they so often do, that this is a matter to be solved by doctors themselves. The position has been well stated [p. 460] by a non-medical.[1]

> Modern medicine has provoked some serious moral questions, not through malignant perversity, but because of the enormous momentum medical science has gained in the past few decades ....
>
> There is the nagging question, What are the permissible limits and the proper conditions for experimentation on human beings?...
>
> These decisions cannot be postponed indefinitely. It is crucial at this historic juncture that the enormity of the problem of discovering clear moral insights to delineate some acceptable boundaries and limits to the use of human beings in research, should not produce either an impatience or moral cyncism.[1]

During private discussion of this subject I have frequently been attacked by doctors who contend that by such publication I am doing a great disservice to my profession, and, more especially, that I am undermining the faith and trust that lay people have in doctors. For a long time there have been rumours that I intended to publish this book and, as a result, I have been subjected to frequent telephone calls, almost entirely from strangers, in an attempt to persuade me to abandon the project.

Other doctors and lay people have attempted to persuade me that the wiser course would be to continue to attempt to publish my views in medical journals and so avoid completely any discussion outside professional circles. An important fact is that those journals which publish accounts of the worst types of experiments do not have correspondence columns. When I have spoken on this subject of human experimentation to medical societies, the usual reaction has been, "This does not concern us, as we do not do such things", and the problems posed are ignored. Mundane, material matters of pay, status and terms of service would, in contrast, produce a lively discussion.

I am fully aware of the fact that lay people may find the accounts of some of the experiments difficult to follow, indeed the complexity of many of them is such that it is difficult even for many doctors to understand everything. So I do not expect lay people to do so, but hope that the general gist of what the experiments involve will be obtained from these necessarily brief summaries. The diagrams of the circulation drawn by my wife should be consulted frequently.

Some readers may find that much appears to be repetitious. This has been done purposely in an attempt to convey a true picture of medical research, which indeed is frequently repetitious, almost identical experiments being performed time and time again by different research workers. This is partly due to the maniacal impulse which domi-

*Reproduced with permission from Pappworth MH. *Human Guinea Pigs*. London: Routledge and Kegan Paul, 1967, pp. ix–x, 3–5, 7–9, 12–13, 19–21, 25–7, 41, 51, 54–5, 66–7, 75–6, 90–1, 106–7, 159–60, 176–7, 190–1, 194, 211.

nates the medical world today to publish research papers, promotion and subsequent success often depending on it. But original ideas are rare, and the adage, "To be original you must not read – it has all been described before", is very true when applied to medical research. The apparently repetitious accounts in this volume serve to emphasize that most of the examples quoted are not isolated unusual instances but fairly common practice ....

INTRODUCTION

1. The subject

For several years a few doctors in this country and in America have been trying to bring to the attention of their fellows a disturbing aspect of what have become common practices in medical research. These practices concern experiments made chiefly on hospital patients and the aspect of them which is disturbing is the ethical one. In their zeal to extend the frontiers of medical knowledge, many clinicians appear temporarily to have lost sight of the fact that the subjects of their experiments are in all cases individuals with common rights and in most cases sick people hoping to be cured. As a result it has become a common occurrence for the investigator to take risks with patients of which those patients are not fully aware, or not aware at all, and to which they would not consent if they were aware; to subject them to mental and physical distress which is in no way necessitated by, and has no connexion with, the treatment of the disease from which they are suffering; and in some cases deliberately to retard the recovery from that disease so that investigation of a particular condition can be extended ....

The truth is that many investigations have been performed which have been harmful to many patients. How temporary that harm has been is usually not known. But sometimes it definitely has not been temporary, and sometimes it has been fatal ....

That some risk or some distress to the subject, which is quite unrelated to the treatment of his disease is a frequent concomitant of medical experiments is indicated, or suggested, by the fact that in Britain at least, such experiments are never carried out on private patients. They are reserved for what is known as the "hospital class".

The subject of this book is the relation between what is morally right and what is performed in medical experiments. My purpose in writing it is to enlighten the public about what is going on in such experiments; to stir the consciences of the doctors so engaged and to ask them to reflect on some of the ancillary results of what they are doing and the moral issues involved. I shall also try to indicate the principles on which medical experiments should be carried out, so that the ends of research may be effectively served without any of the harm done at present, and to suggest possible legislative changes and changes in accepted procedure in which these principles may be incorporated ....

Although a number of doctors have voiced their concern at the way in which medical experiments have been and are being carried out, I should stress the very important fact that few doctors, and this is particularly the case with general practitioners, are fully aware of what really happens especially in many teaching hospitals, to the patients whom they send to those hospitals. This I know from discussion with hundreds of doctors over the years. A large percentage of doctors who are themselves studying to be consultants, and who are not themselves engaged in the type of research which I have written about here, are also unaware of what is going on. Many conversations with postgraduates have convinced me of this. Nor is discussion about research experiments encouraged, in their fellow doctors, by those in charge of research. Rather the reverse. It is a recent and growing practice for some research workers to work behind closed doors, which not even their own junior medical staff are encouraged to enter.

2. Recent history

... Articles by individual research workers and by leaders of teams engaged on research reveal the frequency with which extremely unpleasant and often dangerous experiments are performed on unsuspecting patients. Most of those doctors who know that these things are common practice have felt powerless to stop them; while the public, for its part, has remained unaware of what is going on.

Some apologists for the kind of experiment I shall describe have quibbled about the meaning of the word "experiment". Their argument has been that every administration of medicine to a patient and every routine radiological or biochemical investigation is an experiment; that, therefore, experiment is inseparable from medicine; and that therefore any kind of experiment by any doctor is intrinsically jus-

tified. On this basis the empirical giving of an antibiotic to see if it will abate a high fever, or the performance of a barium X-ray to determine whether a
patient's dyspepsia is due to a pepetic [*sic*] ulcer are
experiments. So, in one sense, they are. But the
experiments with which I am concerned cannot, by
any stretch of the imagination, be deemed analogous. The first (such as administering an antibiotic
in the case of a high fever) are directed solely to the
treatment and cure of that one patient to whom they
are administered; the second are directed, solely in
some cases and chiefly in all cases, to the discovery
of what may help other patients ....

3. The risk to patients

... An often-repeated defence of the types of experiment described in subsequent chapters is that the
risk of death is very small and that any complications
which occur do so rarely and are generally "trivial",
and that the experiments sound much more gruesome than they really are. How gruesome an experiment may be, in fact, depends, among other things,
on the emotional make-up of its subject. What may
appear relatively innocuous to the hardened experimenter can produce extreme distress, including a
good deal of fear, in a patient who is being submitted to something he does not understand properly.
Usually he does not understand it at all. Such distress, endured by the subjects of experiments, is
rarely recorded in medical publications and often
appears to be of small concern to the experimenters
who have caused it.

For example, if a needle inserted into a patient
during the course of an experiment accidentally pen-
etrates, say, his spleen, kidney or liver and causes a
massive haemorrhage, the result will be severe physical and mental distress to that patient. In particular this will be the case if the patient realizes that
something has gone wrong. However, the experimenter is likely to record it as a trivial incident immediately corrected by blood transfusion.

... Indeed, what constitutes a minor and what a
major complication is often a matter of personal
opinion. The same applies to the consideration as to
what constitutes a reasonable risk. As a former president of the Royal Society of Medicine remarked,[2]

> All experiments involve some risk. It may be an infin-
> itesimally small one, but it is always there. If the exper-
> iment involves special techniques, then the risk is
> considerably enhanced.

In fact, to talk of completely innocuous experiments is a contradiction in terms. All experiments
by their very nature must have unknown potentiali-
ties, otherwise they would not be experiments. The
author of the last quotation has himself described
how he volunteered to receive an apparently
innocuous injection of pyrogen (a fever-producing
substance). The effect on him was "alarming", and
he considers a subsequent attack of jaundice as being
directly due to that experiment.

But when several different investigations, each
with its own separate risk, are done simultaneously,
then the possibilities of harm to the patient are
proportionately, or more than proportionately, increased.

The usual method of obtaining blood samples is
from a vein, but the reader will find many examples
in this book referring to the insertion of needles or
catheters into arteries. To the experimenter this is
often a very minor part of the whole procedure on
which he is embarked. But even this part of the
process is not free from the risk of unpleasant complications.

... A doctor may have developed a certain technical skill, for example, in passing cardiac catheters
or puncturing some viscus such as the liver or heart,
so that after many performances he can now do so
with hardly any risk of a patient dying and comparatively little risk of a major complication. While
acquiring this skill there have almost certainly been
major complications and even fatalities, but now that
the technique has been more or less mastered, the
chances of either are very much less. Does this justify him in continuing on many more patients for
experimental purposes? I consider that the answer
to this question is undoubtedly, "No".

... Many investigators who inject foreign substances into people forget the important fact that,
once having given the injection, they may be unable
to control its effects, as Professor McCance so rightly points out.

A non-medical has put the case [p. 460] even
stronger[1]:

> There is the obvious fact that some human being will
> always be the first one upon whom a medical tech-
> nique is tested or to whom a new medicine will be
> administered. But the question is, "When is it moral-
> ly justified to use the first human being for experi-
> mental purposes?"

I would like to emphasize that in this book, with
but very few exceptions, only experiments which have

been recorded in medical journals are discussed. Undoubtedly, and for obvious reasons, the worst experiments go unrecorded. That this is so is borne out by information given me by numerous postgraduate students of mine who have told me of what they themselves have witnessed.

... In the great majority of articles giving accounts of experiments on people, including most of those reported in this book, the authors do not mention whether consent was obtained. Therefore, in any particular example cited, unless definitely stated to the contrary, we must not assume that valid consent was, or was not, given. We do not know the truth.

It must be appreciated that it may be difficult to draw a sharp distinction between an investigation done in the patient's own interest, for the diagnosis or assessment of his own condition, and a purely experimental research investigation. This is especially true when the patient is suffering from the disease process being investigated. A great deal of the research into heart, liver and kidney disease is of this nature. The value to any individual patient of some of this type of investigation is often problematical, and this is especially so if the procedure is in any way novel. Some research doctors take advantage of this ambiguity, and this is likely to be particularly true in those hospitals where a multiplication of investigations is regarded as "routine".

4. The principle of medical morality

Many experiments are defended by those who carry them out on the grounds that, while admittedly of no help to the patient or other person who is the subject, the aim of such experiments is ultimately to help mankind. My contention is that it is immoral to perform experiments, especially dangerous ones, on unsuspecting patients not suffering from the disease being investigated, solely in the hope of making scientific discoveries. Science is not the ultimate good, and the pursuit of new scientific knowledge should not be allowed to take precedence over moral values where the two are in conflict. The statement which is not uncommonly heard among research workers, "It would be interesting to know", though natural and, doubtless, frequently true, is not in itself a justification for making experiments of whatever kind. The welfare of the subject must also and always be taken into account.

Any human being has the right to be treated with a certain decency, and this right, which is individual, supersedes every consideration of what may benefit science or contribute to the public welfare. No physician is justified in placing science or the public welfare first and his obligation to the individual, who is his patient or subject, second. No doctor, however great his capacity or original his ideas, has the right to choose martyrs for science or for the general good ....

PART I: WHAT IS BEING DONE

Experiments on Infants and Children

... A new method of X-ray visualization of the infant's heart was described in 1963.[3] The subjects were ten infants aged one to ten days, all of whom were "in poor to critical condition", because of severe congenital heart lesions, and nine of them were cyanosed (blue). Catheters were passed via the umbilical vein into the vena cava and so into the heart. In the older infants an incision had to be made over the navel to isolate the umbilical vein. In four cases the catheter was passed via the umbilical artery instead of the vein and thus into the aorta before it entered the heart. In all the infants a contrast medium was injected via the catheter and serial X-rays taken. Three deaths occurred within twenty-four hours of this procedure, but these, says the report, "were felt to be due to the underlying disease rather than the study itself." ...

Experiments on Pregnant Women

... In 1962 a doctor decided to test the effect of a certain drug on labour.[4] The drug used was Nialamide, which is a tranquilizer belonging to a group of compounds known chemically as monoamine oxidase inhibitors, and it was given to a large number of pregnant women. A matter of special importance is that the report quotes an authoritative statement[5] describing the results of administering a *related* drug to pregnant mice and rabbits. The results on these animals were either interference with the pregnancy or haemorrhage into the placenta. No ill effects were detected in the women; the course of their labour was normal and so were the infants when they were born. But in view of the known effects on animals of a related drug, the undertaking seems to me to have involved an unjustifiable risk. Furthermore, an important and serious matter is the danger of what is technically known as potentiation, namely, that even up to two weeks after the patient has received nialamide serious reactions may result if that patient should be given morphia or pethidine. These drugs are often administered to patients during labour, and the effect, in such a case, would be as though a very large (i.e. toxic) dose had been given. This whole experiment seems to me to have been very ill conceived ....

Experiments on Mental Defectives and the Mentally Sick

... In 1962 a new antibiotic designed to treat acne vulgaris (pimples) was investigated.[6] The subjects, all of whom had acne, were fifty in number and were either juvenile delinquents or mental defectives. After oral administration of the drug for two weeks no fewer than 50% of the children were found to have sustained liver damage. In spite of this, however, the doctors continued to administer the drug with the expected result, that "these liver abnormalities became more marked and in two children jaundice occurred". In eight of the children subsequent liver punctures showed severe liver damage, and in four cases liver puncture was done at least twice. The report adds,

> Four of the patients were challenged with a 1g. dose of the drug after liver function had returned to normal. Within 1 or 2 days hepatic dysfunction again developed in 3 of the 4.

An anonymous author wrote wittily in the *British Medical Journal*[7]:

> Juvenile delinquency in U.S.A. seems to carry with it hazards not previously suspected. The pimpled gangster of to-day may find himself the bilious guinea pig of tomorrow. It seems a little hard, perhaps, for a boy who has spent his formative years learning how to dodge flick knives to fall a victim to intercostal perforation by a liver puncture needle ....

Experiments on Prison Inmates

... In 1963 an interesting account appeared in the medical press of an experiment performed on volunteers from the Kansas State Penitentiary.[8] Originally eighty-four men aged between forty and sixty-five volunteered. Thirty-two of these were disqualified because they were found to have positive signs in their cardiovascular or nervous systems, or abnormal changes in the electrical tracings from their brains. Six changed their minds and declined "for personal reasons". For technical reasons three others had to be left out. The experiment was thus finally carried out on forty-three men, of whom thirty-six were Caucasians and seven were negroes.

The procedure was as follows. A needle was inserted into a brachial artery and a wire guide and catheter passed through the needle so as to enter the ascending aorta. A contrast medium was then injected through the catheter and serial X-rays taken to study the brain (and also, incidentally, the renal) circulation. There were no complications. Permission for this experiment was granted by the Chancellor of the University of Kansas, by the Board of Regents and the Director of Penal Institutions, and by the Attorney-General of the State of Kansas. The experiment was conducted by Dr. Faris and associates, who, in their report, "wish to express our appreciation to the inmates of Kansas State Penitentiary, without whose generous co-operation the study would not have been possible" ....

Experiments on the Dying and the Old

... A new method of measuring the blood flow of the collateral veins of the liver has been described.[9] According to the published report the safety of the technique, which had included the use of a radioactive compound, had been established by a preliminary testing which involved injecting this substance directly into the spleen of eight patients who had very large spleens, apparently without ill effects.

For the present experiment twelve patients were chosen. Of these seven had liver disease, three had severe diseases of the blood (thalasaemia [sic] and myelofibrosis), one had sarcoid and one Hodgkin's disease. Myelofibrosis and Hodgkin's disease are both fatal conditions and the investigation to which these two patients were submitted had no relation whatever to these diseases.

First, the patients were submitted to hepatic vein catheterization, a catheter being passed through an arm vein into and through the heart chambers and so into the liver vein. Second, a cannula was inserted into the femoral artery of the thigh. Third, a dye was infused[10] into an arm vein. Fourth, a large needle was inserted into the spleen, and through this a radio-active substance was "deeply injected into the spleen". Pressures within the spleen were measured before and after the injection. Blood samples were removed from the femoral and from the hepatic vein every five seconds during five minutes and a further single sample was taken from each at the end of ten minutes, i.e. at least 122 blood samples were taken from each patient ....

Experiments on Patients awaiting Operations

... Another experiment on twenty-two patients was to measure the amounts of circulating adrenaline under various specific conditions. Their ages ranged from fourteen to fifty-four, and they were either "normal" patients or had small lung lesions.[11] Three other patients were also used on whom the experiment was conducted at the time when they were operated on for tumours of the chest.

The procedure was as follows. A catheter was passed into the right side of the heart, a wide-bore needle was inserted into the main arm artery and a tightly fitting face mask was applied. A dye was then injected directly into the pulmonary artery. During the procedure "brachial artery blood was withdrawn at a constant rate". The three subjects who were studied at the time of their chest operations had needles inserted directly into their pulmonary artery and left atrial chamber of the heart and pressures recorded prior to and during a single rapid injection of adrenaline into the pulmonary artery. Otherwise the experiment consisted in measuring lung and heart function during four separate periods: (1) a control period immediately after the catheter had been inserted; this period lasted from ten to fifteen minutes; (2) a period of sixteen minutes during which the subject's respiration was markedly depressed by the inhalation of a special gas mixture; (3) a period lasting about an hour during which the patient received an intravenous infusion of noradrenaline; (4) a final period during which respiration was again depressed by the same technique while the noradrenaline infusion was still running. The authors explain that the patients were allowed to rest for fifteen to thirty minutes between each period. No doubt the three patients who were about to undergo surgery for tumours of the chest had given their permission for that operation. Had they also agreed to this lengthy, exhausing and unpleasant preliminary? Or did they imagine it was part of their necessary treatment? ...

Patients as Controls

... Complex heart and lung tests on thirty-three patients who, according to the report, had no "cardiac or pulmonary or other serious disease", and who may, therefore, be regarded as being purely controls, was [sic] reported in 1961.[12] First, a catheter was passed via an arm vein into the main chest vein, the superior vena cava, almost as far as the right atrial heart chamber. Face masks were then fitted together with nose clips so that samples of expired air could be obtained. A large needle was inserted into and kept in a main limb artery. A dye was then injected via the catheter. When the required estimations had been made, the patients, with catheter and face mask still in position, were made to exercise vigorously and the estimations were then repeated.

This completed the first stage of the experiment. For fourteen of the patients, however, a further stage followed immediately. This was the intravenous injection of a drug called lantoside C, which acts very powerfully on the heart. The cardiac output of these fourteen patients was then measured at "frequent intervals" for up to two hours after giving the injection". For thirteen other patients stage two of the experiment consisted in administering digitalis, which also has a powerful action on the heart, for seven days. At the end of that time the whole experiment, necessitating cardiac catheterization and lung function tests, was repeated....

Experiments on Patients with Heart Disease

... A complex investigation on twenty-three patients with valvular disease was carried out in 1961.[13] A catheter was passed via an arm vein into the right atrial heart chamber. A large needle was inserted into and kept in the brachial artery. A closely fitting face mask was applied. Cardiac and respiratory measurements were then made. With the instruments *in situ*, the patients were made to exercise vigorously and the measurements were repeated "in duplicate and triplicate". The patients were then turned on their faces and two needles were inserted, side by side, to a depth of six inches, by the side of the spine, until both entered the left atrial heart chamber. Catheters were then passed through both of these needles, so that one remained in the left atrium and the other went through the mitral valve, and so into the left ventricle. With these three catheters in the heart, a needle in the brachial artery and the breathing apparatus over the face, the patients were made to exercise yet again.

An additional part of the experiment was the infusion of the drug acetyl choline into the heart via one of the catheters, so that its effects on the circulation could be studied. That this drug can cause either heart stoppage or serious heart irregularity is well known ....

Experiments in which New Drugs are Tested

... A group of physicians wished to investigate the effects of the powerful heart drug, digoxin, on normal people. For this purpose twelve patients, two of whom were over sixty, were submitted to cardiac catheterization. In addition a needle was kept in a main artery of a limb and a face mask applied. The drug was injected through the cardiac catheter. As a result of this two of the patients developed serious abnormal heart rhythms, fibrillation or heart block. These presumably responded to treatment.[14]

A group of research workers experimented with a new drug called Persantin which was designed for the treatment of angina.[15] The particular aim of the experiment was to see what effect Persantin had on the coronary blood flow. Nine patients to whom "the nature of the experiment was explained" and from whom "written consent was obtained" were chosen as subjects. None of these had any cardiac disorder, their reasons for being in hospital being respectively: asthma, obscure blood spitting, hernia, neurasthenia, acute alcoholism, bronchiectasis, and bronchio-pneumonia, and two cases who were in surgical wards for observation.

A needle was inserted into a limb artery and a catheter into the heart. Measurements of cardiac output were then taken. The catheter was then made to enter the coronary sinus (the terminal part of the coronary vein) and the patients made to inhale nitrous oxide through a face mask. Further measurements were then taken and Persantin then injected intravenously. Measurements were repeated after the injection and yet again after the catheter had been replaced in the right atrium ....

PART II: PRINCIPLES

Ethical Principles

... What experimenter, hoping for whatever results

for research, would submit his own child, aged less than twelve months, and free from heart trouble, to cardiac catheterization? ... What experimenter would be happy that his own wife, pregnant and suffering no abnormality, should be subjected, in the interests of science, to translumbar aortography? ... And what experimenter, considering whatever advance might be made in research by his results, would agree to the subjection of one of his parents, who was fatally ill, to the development of a technique such as retrograde arterial catheterization ... in order that the experimenters may learn that particular technique? How comforted would he feel, after learning that a serious and painful complication had, in this case, resulted from the experiment, to learn from the experimenters' report that the number of such complications, while considerable, is regarded by them as "not prohibitively high" and that "New techniques encounter difficulties until they are perfected"?

If no experimenter would act in these ways towards someone close to him, surely it is wrong for him to do so towards someone he doesn't know – and is never going to know – "a case". For this reason I have called this principle ... the principle of equality.

Moreover, the number involved in any experiment is from an ethical point of view completely immaterial. If it is unethical for one, it is for the many. The reverse is also true, namely, if it is unethical to submit many to a proposed experiment, it is equally unethical to expose only one person.

The principle of valid consent

The importance of valid consent is emphasized in all codes of principles for human research. I am in full agreement with all the details concerning consent listed in the Nuremberg Code, which has been quoted fully previously.

... Two essential pieces of information are often deliberately withheld from "the consenting volunteer", namely, that the procedure is experimental and its consequences are unpredictable.

The medical research procedure by definition and by nature is a deviation from normal practice, even though all the specific elements involved may be well established, simply because medical practice ordinarily does not encompass employment of human beings primarily for advancement of knowledge. There is no implicit understanding that conventional methods will be used and that the patient will be released as soon as his condition warrants. Consequently, the researcher has a more specific responsibility for full disclosure of purpose, method and probable consequences.[16]

... The vast majority of published accounts of experiments on patients, including most of the reports quoted in this book, do not mention whether or not consent has been asked or obtained. This omission does not entitle us automatically to assume that consent was not sought or not obtained. We just do not know.

This ambiguity may cause injustice to experimenters who have obtained genuine valid consent. The fault lies with the writers themselves and the editors of medical articles, who should always not only state but give unequivocal evidence of having obtained genuine and legally valid consent ....

Proposed Legislation

... If medical editors themselves refused to publish papers which did not furnish evidence that the experiments they reported had been carried out in terms of the principles suggested, then the knowledge that the account of an unjustifiable experiment would not be published would, I believe, give considerable pause to those about to embark on such an experiment. I therefore suggest that this innovation might be made by all medical editors: no reports of experiments to be accepted for publication unless the editor is satisfied that what was done did not offend against any of the principles of medical experiments. This is not, of course, a novel idea. In the memorandum which I have already quoted a very similar recommendation is made[17]:

A further matter to which the Council would draw attention is that of propriety in publication. It cannot be assumed that it will be evident to every reader that the investigations being described were unobjectionable. Unless such is made unmistakably clear misconceptions can arise. In this connection a special

responsibility devolves upon the editors, and editorial boards, of scientific journals. In the Council's opinion, it is desirable that editors and editorial boards, before accepting any communication, should not only satisfy themselves that the appropriate requirements have been fulfilled, but may properly insist that the reader is left in no doubt that such indeed is the case.

REFERENCES

1. Stumpf SE. Some moral dimensions of medicine. *Ann Intern Med* 1966; **64**: 460–70.
2. McCance, *Proc Royal Soc Med* 1951; **44**: 189.
3. Ray RN, Chatterjea JB, Chaudhuri RN. *Bull Wld Hlth Org* 1964; **30**: 51.
4. Barron SL, *J Obstet Gynaecol* 1962; **69**: 443.
5. *Science* 1960; **131**: 1101.
6. Tickton, Zimmerman HJ. *New Engl J Med* 1962; **267**: 964.
7. *Anon. BMJ* 1962; **2**: 1536.
8. Faris, Poser, Wilmore OW, Agnew CH. *Neurology* 1963; **13**: 386.
9. Iber, Kerr DNS, Dolle, Sherlock S. *J Clin Invest* 1960; **39**: 1201.
10. Infusion of a dye is not the same procedure as the injection of a contrast medium for radiology. Dyes are infused into the circulation so that blood samples can be obtained later which will give some indication of the efficiency of a particular organ by assessing the extent to which the dye has been concentrated or absorbed.
11. Goldring, Turino, Cohen G, Jameson, Bass GB, Fishman AP. *J Clin Invest* 1962; **41**: 1211.
12. Rodman, Gorezyea, Pastor *Ann Intern Med* 1961; **55**: 620.
13. Samet, Bernstein and Litwak *Br Heart J* 1961; **23**: 616.
14. Selzer, Hultgren, Ebnother, Bradley HW, Stone AO. *Brit Heart J* 1959; **21**: 335.
15. Wendt, Sundermyer, den Bakker, Bing RJ. *Am J Cardiol* 1962; **9**: 449.
16. Irving Ladimer SJD. *J Public Law* 1955; **3**: 467.
17. *Medical Research Memorandum*, 1953/649.

Commentary on *Human Guinea Pigs*

Stephen Lock

To reread *Human Guinea Pigs* is to be reminded of how much a dedicated individual can still achieve. Almost 35 years later the excesses it records are unthinkable today, as is any human experimentation without approval by an ethics committee and truly informed consent by the patient. Yet Maurice Pappworth – who did "more for patients' interests than anyone of his time" – achieved what he did against the persistent opposition of his fellows, particularly the medical establishment concerned not to wash its dirty linen in public.

Fortunately, Pappworth was a quintessential outsider. Despite a distinguished academic record he had been denied a consultant job in his native Liverpool (and told privately that no Jew could ever be a gentleman). Despite distinguished war service, finishing as a lieutenant-colonel commanding a hospital in Bombay, he had then failed to secure a post in a London teaching hospital (largely he thought also on religious grounds). When he decided to survive by becoming a freelance postgraduate tutor of candidates for the MRCP (whose pass rate had fallen to 10%), the College grandees turned on him for interfering and ensured that he was not promoted to the Fellowship.

In Britain any discussion of the ethics of human experimentation started only after the close of World War II. Closed professional groups came to cosy conclusions, and the replies to the occasional question in Parliament were reassuringly bland: there was no problem and the details were a matter for the profession. At a meeting of an association of clinical professors in the early 1950s, for example, Sir John McMichael (the head of the professorial medical unit at the Postgraduate Medical School) insisted that the moral decision must be made by the experimenter, reinforced by a similar assertion by the MRC secretary, Sir Harold Himsworth: "Only a small branch of experienced investigators, who have devoted themselves to this branch of medicine, are likely to be competent to pass an opinion on the advisability of undertaking any particular investigation."

There were two main reasons why the public and the profession were not more concerned. Firstly, medical science was delivering not merely the new vaccines and antibiotics (promising the abolition of diphtheria and polio as well as cures for pneumonia and tuberculosis), but also new treatments for cancer and hypertension and the developments in anaesthetics, fluid balance, and surgical techniques, often coming from experience on the battlefield. Besides such rich dividends, the argument ran, any discomfort from research studies was minuscule: the Benthamite concept of the greatest good for the greatest number should prevail. The second reason was the revelation of the beastliness of the Nazi atrocities. How could humane fellow researchers be compared with concentration camp doctors? Anyway, wasn't potentially dangerous research seen off by the Nuremberg Code, developed after the war crimes trials to prevent such misconduct?

Thus the trials and the Code both backfired; in particular, the latter was seen as aimed at barbarians rather than physician-scientists. Moreover, there were other pressures not to constrain research. The number of researchers and their funding was increasing exponentially – the research budget of the National Institutes of Health rising from $17 million in 1948 to $803 million in 1967 – and tenure, promotion, and prizes were rapidly coming to depend on research productivity and publication (which some compared to an arms race).

Without the proselytising of two physicians, Henry Beecher, a Harvard anaesthesiologist, and Pappworth himself, events would have moved very differently – and certainly much more slowly. Their characters could hardly have been more different: Beecher, the dour Harvard insider, Pappworth the acerbic rootless dissident. Yet fortunately their concerns surfaced at much the same time, and soon both decided that the only way of winning the battle was to go public. Pappworth's worries came from what his students told him, particularly those from the Dominions working at the Postgraduate Medical School at Hammersmith Hospital. Not only were they anxious about the details of such research, but also in having to take part, whether actively or passively, in persuading a patient to volunteer, knowing that non-cooperation would jeopardise their careers.

Pappworth wrote letters to the editors of journals publishing research that he considered unethical, but these were often rejected for publication. "I know that there are times when good comes of speaking strongly and by giving maximum publicity to what appears to be public scandals," wrote the professedly liberal Quaker editor of *The Lancet*, Robbie Fox, to Pappworth, "but you haven't yet persuaded us that this is one of these occasions." Hence, he collected together 14 examples of ethically doubtful research, publishing them in 1962 in a special issue of the influential quarterly *The Twentieth Century*. The first part of his title, "*Human Guinea Pigs: a warning*", was used again for a subsequent book, but this included over 200, now fully referenced articles, including experiments on children, the mentally defective, and prison inmates. Often these involved cardiac or hepatic catheterization or metabolic manipulations, without any clear advantage to the patient or informed consent having been obtained. The sole reason seemed to be advancement of knowledge – and of the doctor's career through prestigious publications. As Pappworth commented later, "Medical research had become sacrosanct, based on the dubious dogma that its continuation must be the prime concern of teaching hospitals."

Mostly for legal reasons, Pappworth's book took five years to appear. During the interval he received telephone calls at different times from three men claiming to be senior physicians, all telling him that they knew the details of the proposed publication and urging him "for the good of the profession" to withdraw the manuscript. None would give his name or say how and why he had read the manuscript. Even when the earlier article had been published, there had been considerable media publicity, with banner headlines in the press and congratulatory or condemnatory letters from lay people or doctors. In a letter to *The Guardian* Sir John McMichael claimed that none of the 14 experiments described had been undertaken in his hospital (at Hammersmith); Pappworth was to riposte that, perhaps unknown to Sir John, no less than half of them had taken place there. In a television programme Pappworth asked Charles Fletcher, Consultant Physician at the Hammersmith, and a well-known TV medical personality what he thought about a study in which 43 diabetic patients (including children and those with complications) had their insulin deliberately withheld so that they became comatose, and then liver, and some renal, biopsies were done. His reply was, "The person was young and enthusiastic and should be forgiven", hitting the headlines of the national press the following day.

With the publication of the book this professional opposition intensified. Yet again *The Lancet* was irritated, rebuking Pappworth for his haughtiness in an unsigned editorial and continuing, "It is, after all, in the instant self-criticism by the profession that the patient secures his first and best protection." The new editor of the *New England Journal of Medicine*, Franz Ingelfinger, an ex-Harvard clinician-researcher (who one feels would have been unlikely to have published the earlier Beecher article), dismissed the problem, stating that what was really needed was a programme of "continuing and ever more intensive consensus building".

Eventually all this led, of course, to further debate both in the media and in government and, together with the belated cooperation of the medical Establishment, the setting up of institutional review boards and research ethics committees. The process was accelerated by society's questioning of the values and achievements of science, in part resulting from the thalidomide tragedy and from the success of the anti-science book by Rachel Carson *Silent spring*. Nevertheless, whatever the other influences, I doubt whether, without Pappworth's particular brand of vehemence, which he carried into the public domain, the profession would have been so ready to act, albeit at one minute to midnight. For cosy, inbred professions need people like him – as does society even more. He was a difficult man, to whom the concluding words of Beecher's obituary could also apply: "He was never convicted of a sense of humour." Yet, like Beecher, Pappworth was also a great man, fully deserving his inclusion in the forthcoming *New dictionary of national biography* – more, to be sure, than several of the time-servers to be recorded there. Even at the end of his life his principles did not desert him. As he remarked with characteristic bluntness: "My opinion remains that those who dirty the linen and not those who wash it should be criticised. Some do not wash dirty linen in public or in private, and the dirt is merely left to accumulate until it stinks."

6 · Learning from unethical research

Paul McNeill and Naomi Pfeffer

In May of 1997, President Clinton invited eight survivors of the Tuskegee study to the White House. They were lucky to be alive. Each of them had been diagnosed with syphilis and left untreated in a study that had a clear purpose: to observe and record the progress of syphilis as it ravaged their bodies.[1] In a public apology to these men President Clinton said,

"It is not only in remembering that shameful past that we can make amends and repair our nation, but it is in remembering that past that we can build a better present and a better future."[2]

The difficulty in remembering shameful cases from the past is that few researchers identify with extreme cases. They tend to dismiss them as aberrations. However, if lessons are to be learnt from outrages such as Tuskegee, they must be seen as logical extremes of a continuum, not as exceptions. This continuum ranges from a failure to comply with minor procedural requirements at one end, through to reckless disregard for the welfare of participants at the other.[3]

In this chapter we consider cases that lie towards the "reckless disregard" end of the continuum. At the extreme are the New Zealand Cervical Cancer case, and the Manchester Christie Hospital case, both of which led to many avoidable deaths. We also consider cases that did not lead to such serious consequences for the research participants. All of them, however, compromised participants' rights in some significant respect. None of these cases we review is of a trivial nature. The feature that is common to all of them is that research goals and convenience of investigators have been given priority over the welfare and rights of research participants. Yet this is against clear priorities expressed by the international community and many national codes for ethics of research.[4]

In most of the cases we examine, research participants have not been informed adequately of the research they were a part of. In some of those cases they had not even known they were included in a research program. Proper processes, it seems, for informing participants of their rights, and seeking their consent, are often lacking. In our view, this displays an attitude, on the part of researchers, that subjugates concerns for welfare of the human beings to the research goals and imperatives. Whilst none of the investigators in these studies had any intention to do harm, they (wittingly or otherwise) have treated people as a means to an end and given insufficient consideration to their rights and well being. The episodes we describe cast a shadow over the whole medical community. One of the results of unethical research, as the Tuskegee experiment revealed, is that people lose confidence in the purpose and safety of medical experiments and are reluctant to consent to participate in research. We describe the aftermath of some of these cases in order to draw attention to their effect on participants, patients, investigators, their sponsors, and to the whole community.

If we are to *"build a better present and a better future"*, we must study closely such cases, observe what went wrong, what failed, and why. Looking for causal factors also includes examining weaknesses in institutional structures and culture. We suggest that it may be counter productive to focus on individual fault. Human error, bias, and aberrant behaviour have always been with us and may never be eliminated. These are facts of life that need to be accepted if we are to create safer research environments. In most cases it will be more effective to focus on the whole system in which research takes place, and to devise approaches that minimise the harmful effect of errors and aberrant behaviour on those who volunteer to participate in research.

NEW ZEALAND NATIONAL WOMEN'S HOSPITAL

In New Zealand a scandal became public in 1986

concerning research at the National Women's Hospital, a large teaching hospital in Auckland.[5] We have gone into some detail in what follows as this is a "paradigm" case involving: poor research methodology; deception of patients and an abrogation of their rights; and a tendency for a researchers to be blinded by an unshakeable belief in their own hypothesis. It is also a typical example of what can happen when someone tries to expose unethical research. Those involved and their institutions may react against the person who "blows the whistle" and fail to address adequately the concerns raised and, in so doing, leave unprotected those most at risk.

The investigator, Associate Professor Herbert Green, believed that "carcinoma *in situ*" [CIS] left untreated, would *not* lead to invasive cancer of the cervix. To test his proposition (which was against international opinion at the time) conventional treatment was withheld from some of the women diagnosed with CIS, who were then observed for signs of progression of their disease. Those in the treatment group received normal treatment (essentially removal of suspect tissue). However, many more women in the "non-treatment" group advanced to invasive cancer. An official inquiry headed by Judge Silvia Cartwright found that at least 27 of the non-treatment group had died unnecessarily and many suffered the consequences of their disease for years without ever being informed of their initial diagnosis.[6]

In hindsight, it was clear that there were many breaches of accepted research principles and procedures. Women who had treatment withheld from them were not told of their condition or that they were part of a research program. Green maintained that it was not in the women's interests to tell them about what he was doing. "Patients", he said "were unnecessarily frightened if they heard the word cancer, and should be protected from doctors' uncertainties".[7] As they had not been informed that they were included in a research program, or even that they had been diagnosed with CIS, they had no opportunity to protect themselves by declining to participate or by carefully monitoring their own condition. This was a clear case of a researcher deciding his priorities were more important that those of his patients.

The research had been approved in 1966 by the National Women's Hospital Medical Committee (which functioned as an ethics committee) and continued until at least 1982. An academic journal article, written by concerned staff members, described the poor outcomes for women deprived of treatment. There was little reaction to ethical issues raised by that article. At least two of the authors, however, were treated as "whistleblowers" and "brought themselves trouble with the profession".[5 (p. 292)] It was not until two investigative journalists published an article in a popular magazine, the *Metro*, that effective action was taken. Within days of its publication, the then New Zealand Government announced a judicial inquiry, and, at its conclusion, adopted all its recommendations.[8]

The Inquiry found that members of the Hospital Medical Committee should have been aware of international opinion that CIS would progress to truly invasive cancer in a minority of women if left untreated (although Green had not informed them of relevant literature). There were major problems with the manner in which the research was conducted. Green, on finding evidence of invasive cancer of the cervix in some of the control group members, removed them from the control group on the ground that they must have been misdiagnosed in the first place. This selectively distorted the findings in favour of proving his hypothesis that CIS did not lead to invasive cancer and amounted to a complete breakdown of the empirical method.[8]

It is clear from the Inquiry Report that Green was blinded by his own belief that CIS did not lead to invasive cancer. Even the evidence could not persuade him otherwise. In his case, this led him to shoddy research, probably from ignorance rather than fraudulent intent. The temptation, however, to deny the evidence when it runs counter to strongly held beliefs, is common amongst researchers. In some circumstances this could be part of a laudable tenacity driving a researcher on to further investigation. Regrettably it has also led researchers to tamper with the evidence. The fact of such research bias is one of the reasons for independent review. When that is lacking, as in this case, subjects are exposed to harm.

Many others were implicated in the New Zealand case. A book written by Sandra Coney (one of the journalists who "broke" the story) detailed the extent to which doctors "closed ranks" in support of Green, many of them from fear of consequences to themselves professionally should they have been critical.[5] The findings of the Inquiry supported changes towards more independent review. It recommended adding a large proportion (half) of lay members to ethics committees, the appointment of patients' advocates, and the appointment of a Health Commissioner to receive complaints. It made recommendations about treatment in proposing the adoption of standardised treatment protocols, the improvement of the quality of information and consent procedures. It also made recommendations for the education of medical students by including ethics and communication skills into their training programs.[5]

COMMON FEATURES OF TUSKEGEE AND NZ CERVICAL CANCER

Both the Tuskegee study and the New Zealand Cervical Cancer Case involved doctors who, in the name of medicine, withheld accepted treatment from their patients. In both studies, many died who need not have died. Others needlessly suffered impairment and ongoing problems in their health. There was no opportunity for patients to consent or so little information given that their "consent" was meaningless. In both studies, research subjects were drawn from socially and economically disadvantaged, and relatively power less sections of the population.

The Tuskegee subjects were mostly poor and illiterate African Americans, living in the rural south. Told they had "bad blood", they were offered "incentives" such as free meals in exchange for their compliance.[1] A consequence is many African Americans are now reluctant to participate in medical research, which has led to concerns about the validity and generalisability of research to them. This, and a concern about the unequal distribution of the benefits of biomedical research, led to the National Institutes of Health (NIH) Revitalization Act of June 1993, which introduced a requirement for the inclusion of women and minorities in federally funded clinical studies, except where specific criteria for the exclusion of these groups can be satisfied.[9] In New Zealand, Maori women are overrepresented among women who die of cervical cancer and are overrepresented amongst public patients attending the National Women's Hospital. The Inquiry recommended a special program of screening, treatment and advice for Maori women, and, in the events following the Inquiry, new guidelines for appointing members to research ethics committees required authorities to consider the need for "cultural diversity" and a Maori perspective.[10 (p. 78)]

Both investigations involved practitioners who appeared to have abandoned (in Clinton's words) *"the most basic ethical precepts"* and to have lost sight of

"their pledge to heal and repair". The most basic ethical precept is that patients should not be exploited for research. Philosopher Mary Warnock considers that "non-exploitation" is the "most important principle that should govern research using human subjects".[3] Both Tuskegee and New Zealand Women's Hospital are clear cases of exploitation of unwitting people in service of research goals.

BLOWING THE WHISTLE ON UNETHICAL RESEARCH

One of the more disturbing features, of both Tuskegee and the New Zealand National Women's case, is that many others in the profession knew of deaths and harm resulting from the programs, and failed to take effective action to protect the unwitting research participants. To the contrary, the medical profession in New Zealand (with the exception of three National Women's Hospital staff members) acted to defend the aberrant doctors. As discussed above, the exception in the NZ case was the publication of outcomes for women by three concerned staff members. In this case, as in Tuskegee, officers of the relevant institutions and government took no effective action to safeguard patients even when they knew of problems. In both, publication of the scandals in the media was the pivotal even that prompted an official inquiry.

Past outrages in medical research reveal a pattern in which unethical behaviour or abuse perpetrated by a few is ignored, or actively covered by colleagues, administrators, and their institutions. A possible explanation for this pattern is that loyalty to colleagues has led to a reluctance to speak out against others within the institution. Loyalty to coworkers is an accepted precept that is enshrined in some professional codes of ethics. Another possible explanation is that those accused of wrong-doing react defensively in order to protect themselves. Whatever the mechanism, the pattern is commonplace. When concern for oneself or one's colleagues takes priority over an honest appraisal of actions, which may be leading to (or have led to) harm to others, that pattern must be challenged.

The importance of accepting and responding openly to critical reports from members of research teams is now recognised by professional and regulatory bodies. Counsel for the General Medical Council in London (GMC) said that it is "of 'supreme importance' that those involved in trials could represent their honestly held views without fear."[11] She made this statement at the trial of Robert Davies who was struck off the medical register for bullying and threatening junior colleagues, and for misleading investigators who were looking into allegations that he had tried to cover up blunders in a clinical trial of a new asthma drug. Davies was professor of respiratory medicine at St Bartholomew's and at the Royal London School of Medicine and one-time chair of a research ethics committee. His research registrar had raised concerns about the research with him and Davies had threatened to ruin his career. On advice from a medical defence organisation, the registrar secretly taped their conversation. This evidence contributed to the GMC's finding that Davies was guilty of serious misconduct.[12] Fortunately, in this case, the whistleblower's complaints were effective in stopping the abuse. In general, however, unless there is an adequate mechanism to investigate complaints properly and a commitment to following these procedures fairly, whistleblowers are responded to defensively, the matters complained of are not addressed or investigated, and the whistleblowers themselves are treated badly.[13] Swazey and Scher have said that the "almost universal experience of whistleblowers … is that their actions generate a vehement, angry, and often punitive response by colleagues and superordinates."[14]

REPORTING ON STANDARDS IN RESEARCH

Independent audits of compliance with good clinical practice guidelines (GCP) and regulatory requirements continue to raise questions about the ethics of investigations. Although gross abuse is rarely found, in every country where audits have been undertaken, there is evidence of neglect of common standards designed to safeguard research participants. Most often the research falls short of standards for informed consent.[15] For example, audits have shown that consent is often sought on the same day as the study commences. This indicates that subjects have inadequate time to consider their participation.[15] Cutting "ethical corners" may save investigators' time and expense. The cumulative effect of shortcuts, however, potentially compromises the welfare of patients and research participants, and may undermine the validity of studies into the effectiveness of new drugs or treatment modalities.[16]

Although one purpose of GCP guidelines is to protect research subjects during clinical trials and patients who might receive approved products in the future, auditors' findings are revealed only to sponsors (mostly within the pharmaceutical industry) and to regulatory bodies. Reports to the industrial sponsors and to regulatory bodies may not lead to corrective action. There is a need for mechanisms to ensure that critical reports are acted upon. Failure to deal adequately with revelations of shortcomings is potentially damaging for the industry and could have disastrous outcomes for individual researchers.

Research subjects have recently been called upon to provide evidence of fraud in drug trials. For example, Medico Legal Investigations (MLI) contacts and interviews research subjects to find out whether or not trialists have complied with protocols.[17] Their investigations have led to several doctors being struck off the register by the GMC. The MLI (set up in 1996) is an independent agency that is well supported by the GMC, the British Medical Association (BMA), the medical Royal Colleges, the Association of the British Pharmaceutical Industry (ABPI), and many health authorities. This kind of support for an agency that will prosecute researchers for failure to follow ethical guidelines may be indicative of changing attitudes and a growing intolerance of unethical research. Ideally researchers will follow ethical guidelines from a genuine concern for patients' and research participants' welfare. Ideally institutions that become aware of unethical research will take corrective action. It has to be recognised, however, that the potential for legal redress may cause the recalcitrant few to be more cautious. In our discussion below, however, we question the value of a punitive approach.

PUBLISHED REPORTS OF UNETHICAL RESEARCH

In this section we consider the vexed question of responsibility when reports of unethical research are published. In some cases, such as in the Tuskegee case of the New Zealand Cervical Cancer case, reports in newspapers were sufficient to prompt an inquiry and some form of redress. In many other cases, however, no effective action has followed, even when there is convincing evidence of harmful research, publication of the outcomes, and (in some cases) inquiries by official bodies. The following cases illustrate the difficulties.

Cancer Research Campaign Counselling Case

On their own, few research subjects are prepared to blow the whistle on unethical research, especially where the investigator is their own doctor and where they have a serious health problem. The few who have tried have had great difficulty in making their voices heard. To take one case, for example: Evelyn Thomas noticed differences between the treatment offered to her and to the woman in the bed next to her following their mastectomy operations for breast cancer at King's College Hospital London. Her room-mate received counselling and was given useful information by a trained nurse, whereas Evelyn Thomas was not.[18] It took her four years to discover that she had been a subject in a research program to compare the effect of postoperative counselling with no counselling. These trials were initiated in 1980 by the Cancer Research Campaign and carried out between 1980 and 1985 at 58 centres. They involved 177 doctors and 2230 women, none of whom had been told she was a research subject.[19]

In an article, which was reported in *The Observer* newspaper in 1988, Mrs Thomas wrote that her trust in the medical profession had been abused by the failure of her doctor to recognise and to grant her right to information, and her right to choose whether or not to participate in a trial. In a response to this letter one of the principal researchers defended the investigation by arguing that Evelyn Thomas's treatment was not compromised by 'my concern to improve the quality of cancer care for future generations of women'.[20] This was an evasion of the central issue of patients' rights and amounted to an argument that research goals were more important. It is tantamount to suggesting researchers could ignore patients' rights if there was a good 'research reason' for doing so. It illustrates a central issue debated between Doyal and Tobias in this book – the moral tension between the public interest in successful clinical research (albeit minimally invasive research) and the right of each individual to know that they have been randomised for the purpose of such research.

This point was made even more poignantly some two years after Evelyn Thomas's death by the revelation that the primary reason for not informing patients and seeking their consent was that it was "upsetting" to do so. The nursing sister and mastectomy counsellor had "found it very upsetting, very

emotional to tell these patients all the facts .... In the light of this, it was an unanimous decision of the research ethics committee that in this particular project we should waive consent."[21] In hindsight, the counsellor's upset could have been taken as a signal that there was a serious flaw in the proposal itself. Instead, the right to informed consent was deemed to be less important than the goals of the research.

Mrs Thomas had complained to the Health Service Commissioner and this complaint was followed up in 1991 (after her death) by the Committee on the Parliamentary Commission for Administration. The Committee was reported to appear "unhappy" with the fact that the relevant health authority had failed to discipline any of the staff involved in the research.[21] In our discussion below we suggest that the emphasis should be on safe systems rather than on punishing individuals.

Manchester Christie Hospital Case

In 1979, a new Selectron afterloading machine was installed at the Christie Hospital, Manchester. It was used in a series of experiments conducted to establish a regimen that would replace the well-established Manchester radium treatment for cancer of the cervix. The accepted radium treatment took three days, whereas the proposed new regimen using caesium was expected to take only one day.[22] It is now clear that the trial went ahead with insufficient safeguards. By early 1982 a large number of women treated with caesium, or with combined caesium and radium, was found to have suffered injuries to the rectum, bowel, and vagina as a direct result of the treatment. The hospital attempted to minimise the damage (to itself) by informing each woman that her injuries were unusual. When a few of these "exceptional" cases were publicised in the local press, however, more cases emerged, and it now transpires that hundreds of women had been similarly damaged. Many of these women died.

Some of the surviving women formed a self-help group which they called RAGE (Radiation Action Group Exposure). When this acronym provoked a defensive response amongst doctors, they changed it to COURAGE. In our view, both names are apt. Their rage could well be understood as a response to discovering that their treatment was experimental, potentially toxic, and life-threatening. They are also courageous in suffering the consequence of injuries from this treatment that have caused pelvic pain, incontinence of bladder and bowel, as well as social and emotional problems. Many have needed bowel, bladder, and vaginal surgery, and some have required repeated operations.[23]

It is clear that inadequate animal studies were undertaken before "pilot" research on women was begun.[24] However, it is questionable whether pilot studies should have been allowed. Given their potential for harm, any preliminary studies needed independent review by an ethics committee. It is also clear that many components in treatment were changed in combination, including changes in radiation technique, dosage, and equipment. This made it much harder to be alert to and to identify those elements of the new treatment that were harmful. A paper published in *Clinical Radiology* in 1985 describes the injuries to these patients. Although this article frankly admits error, it displays a cold insensitivity to the suffering of the women. By way of contrast, it finishes by acknowledging the doctors "whose patients have been included in this investigation" and expresses gratitude for "all those surgeons who have rescued many of our patients from their complications".[25]

There is sufficient evidence of harm and evidence of neglect to warrant a more comprehensive review. Such a review should be empowered to investigate shortcomings in the whole enterprise and to look beyond the mistakes of judgment and errors of particular individuals. Its purpose should be to identify changes and interventions within the system as a whole that might have averted the considerable suffering and death that resulted. A proper review process should demonstrate a compassionate concern for the victims and recommend appropriate recompense for the wrongs experienced by these women. Thus far the researchers, their sponsors, and institutions have not accepted this responsibility or undertaken an impartial review.

RESPONSIBILITIES IN PUBLISHING RESEARCH

There is a related issue to the need for publication and the need for action in response to published reports of unethical research. That is the responsibility of researchers and of academic journals to ensure that the conclusions of published research are valid. This responsibility is even greater when the results themselves are potentially alarming. We argue

in addition that researchers have an obligation to protect these people against unnecessary alarm and to forewarn them of a result, prior to publication, when it is concluded that they may be at greater risk of harm. The following case illustrates both these points.

Bristol Cancer Help Centre Complementary Therapy Case

Publication of results from a study conducted by the Bristol Cancer Help Centre (BCHC) purported to show that complementary therapy (which included a recommended diet of mostly organic fruit and vegetables) led to a very poor outcome for women diagnosed with breast cancer. Understandably, those treated by the BCHC were distressed by the reports. When the study results were discredited, they formed a Bristol Survey Support Group (BSSG) and protested about the conduct of investigators.

The study was designed to compare conventional treatment for breast cancer with "complementary" treatment. The comparison was between survival time (overall survival and relapse-free survival) for women with breast cancer who underwent conventional treatment, and survival time for women who, in addition to conventional treatment, received "complementary therapy" provided by the BCHC. The results suggested that women who were offered complementary therapy (including those receiving complementary treatment for one day) suffered relapses of their breast cancer at nearly three times the rate as those receiving conventional treatment. It also purported to have shown twice as many deaths among women receiving complementary therapy as among those receiving conventional treatment alone. The results of the study were leaked to the press shortly before publication in the *Lancet* and these press articles (and following television reports) suggested that the organic diet was responsible for women's earlier demise. At the very least, this finding was counter-intuitive and should have alerted the researchers to the need for more careful scrutiny of their findings before publication. If the researchers had not been alert to this, then surely the journal had a responsibility to investigate.

Subsequent to publication the study was thoroughly discredited. It was found that the women in the "complementary" treatment group had more severe disease in the first place, that controls were poorly matched, investigators had not followed the approved protocol, and the validity of the statistical analysis was suspect. The *Lancet* acknowledged that the study report had not been reviewed by a statistician in its swift (just six weeks) passage from first receipt to publication.

The BSSG urged the Report be unequivocally and publicly retracted, and that the unspent research funds should be donated to the Bristol Cancer Help Centre (BCHC) to compensate it for financial losses, which were a direct result of the misleading research. They also demanded an independent inquiry. The BSSG complained to the Charity Commission that the CRC and the ICRF had allowed charitable funds to be used to denigrate the work of another charity – the BCHC. Their complaint was upheld. The Charity Commissioners found that the charities had "lent their names to the publication of research without ensuring that it was soundly based."[26] One of these charities (the ICRF) reviewed the study and concluded that there was no significant difference in outcome for those attending the BCHC although that conclusion was not published.[27]

Yet no independent inquiry has been held, even in response to a great deal of criticism and the suicide of one investigator. The study results have never been retracted. Investigators have closed ranks, with some going on the attack and accusing victims of unseemly conduct. The extent of harm caused to the women who underwent experimental radiotherapy at The Christie Hospital has not yet been acknowledged. A motion in the House of Commons, signed by 70 members of Parliament, called on the ICRF and the CRC to compensate the women for their emotional distress and pay the BCHC £1 million in compensation for lost donations.[28]

Setting aside for a moment the *Lancet's* responsibility, there was also a prior responsibility on the researchers. Had the results been valid, the researchers should have forewarned the participants, prior to publication, and explained the implications of the study results for each of them. Failure to acknowledge and act on this responsibility is a clear indication that research outcomes had greater importance to the researchers than the welfare of individual research participants. In the event, women who had participated in the study were given no warning of its gloomy findings.[29] They first heard of the potentially alarming consequences from newspapers or reports on television. Understandably they were both shocked and frightened. When it

became clear that the study was fundamentally flawed, their feelings turned to outrage.[30]

DISCUSSION

There is sufficient evidence of on-going error in research to cause alarm. Some of these mistakes and oversights have led to distress and some to extremes of suffering and death. Whilst the incidence of harm to participants in research may be low, it is still of concern. We agree with Mary Warnock that the major issue is that human beings have been exploited for research goals and imperatives. Their individual rights have not been given the priority they deserve.

Having recognised this as a major problem, it is still not clear how to overcome it. The tendency of most analysts is to focus on the ethics of individual researchers or research teams, and to identify the fault as a failure in their ethics. This is not surprising given the history of research ethics, which had its formulation in the Nuremburg Code, and was the outcome of the horrors of Nazi experimentation. We wish to suggest a different approach, however. In our view, focusing on the culpability of individuals may not be the best preventative measure.

We support Leape's recommendation, drawing on the success of the air transport industry in reducing error, that safety principles (similar to those adopted in commercial aviation) be applied to medical practice.[31] In our view there is room to apply those principles to medical research also. The essence of this approach is that error is treated as a problem of the system rather than as a failure of individuals. We already know that individuals make mistakes. Yet by allowing for those mistakes, it is possible to transport large numbers of people, with very few injuries, in technologically complex machines, flying at enormous speeds and landing on busy and crowded runways. In that industry even a 0.01% error rate could mean two unsafe landings at any busy airport per day. Leape makes the translation to medicine and suggests that a culture with an expectation of error-free performance "creates a strong pressure to intellectual dishonesty, to cover up mistakes rather than to admit to them." This is the pattern we observe in the cases we have discussed in this chapter. It is only under extreme pressure that individuals and their institutions will take responsibility for mistakes and maltreatment of participants in research. We agree with Leape that "most would like to examine their mistakes and learn from them." We suggest that this is only possible when the focus is on creating systems with built-in safeguards and margins for error rather than on punishing individuals. As Leape puts it: "Systems that rely on error-free performance are doomed to fail."[31]

So where does that leave us? A starting point must be one of value. The value which is widely endorsed is that individual lives take priority over research. This is Warnock's principle of "non-exploitation". This principle is not always accepted by individual researchers as is evidenced above. In part there is still a role for education in persuading researchers and research trainees. However, the research industry as a whole must commit to this value and ensure that it is put into practice. What follows is that risks in research must be minimal. Any potential harm should be detected as early as possible and before it causes injury. One of those potentials for harm, in our view, is the psychological tendency for researchers to give a higher value to the importance of their own research than to all other considerations (including participants' welfare, social circumstances and preferences). Another is for researchers to be blinded by a belief in their own hypotheses. Knowing and accepting these all too human tendencies, it follows that there needs to be some form of oversight or scrutiny from independent reviewers. For this reason we support the rationale for current review systems adopted throughout the world, which rely on prospective review by committees composed of members independent of the study and committees that include members independent of the research institution.

However, committee review is not sufficient in our view. There is also a need to create a culture in which reports of problems in research can be received and acted on with a prior concern for safety and wellbeing of participants. In the air transport industry, it has been necessary to create protocols whereby a junior officer can challenge an action by a senior officer. That senior officer is obliged to consider the substance of the challenge and set aside any personal reaction. We conclude that the evidence of failure to deal appropriately with whistle blowers and to properly investigate their claims indicates a need for research institutions to establish processes for the impartial investigation of complaints and to encourage those reports. In some institutions it may be appropriate for complaints of unethical research to be considered within the same procedures as are used for other complaints. Information on who to contact and what protections are in place, should be widely distributed and freely available.

It is also clear that publication of reports of unethical research in the popular press has, in some cases, been instrumental in prompting effective action. There is a role, we believe, for investigative journalists and a need for researchers and research institutions to be open to scrutiny. This is an ideal that may not be realised. We have some faith in the persistence of professional journalists when they meet obstacles, however. In air transport a disaster is very public and sets in train a thorough investigation that seeks to determine underlying causes of accidents. In research also, publicity given to harmful research serves a salutary purpose in prompting review. There is a need for public recognition of harm when it does occur, and a willingness of all to learn from the mistakes and seek correction. This willingness however, is likely to be more forthcoming if the focus is on safe systems rather than on punishing individuals.

Professional bodies, governmental agencies, and politicians should also be alert to their responsibility to act on behalf of the welfare of people harmed in research (or potentially harmed), and to take action to investigate claims properly in the public domain. Whilst there can be no single panacea that will guarantee the protection of research participants, we can and should devise approaches that minimise the harmful effect of errors on those who volunteer. Many elements need to be addressed: education, thorough review, openness of reporting, and willingness to consider complaints impartially. If we are to succeed in creating a safe environment for research, we shall need (in Leape's terms) "to fundamentally change" the way we "think about errors and why they occur."

SECURITY, SECRECY, WARFARE AND HUMAN EXPERIMENTS

The "Discussion" above does not adequately address issues of experimentation on human beings conducted in the name of national security, welfare, and the armed services. This is because of a claim that public welfare and national security take precedence over individual rights in times of war, or when questions of national security arise. This claim has led to an abrogation of individual rights within the USA, England, Australia, and elsewhere. Its value and validity, however, are questionable.

The problem is that this claim is in fundamental opposition to that of the principle of "non-exploitation". It has been assumed that the rules are different when it comes to the military, that rights to autonomy and choice in the military are more limited and have to be surrendered to military discipline, and that the need for national security takes precedence over individual welfare. These notions have received support from the Supreme Court of the USA, out of concern that concessions to individual choice would undermine military discipline.[32 (p. 682)]

Yet in the USA, the Army, Air Force, and Navy had all adopted regulations in 1953 that were ostensibly for the protection of human beings in experiments.[33 (p.309)] These regulations followed closely the provisions of the Nuremberg Code and included the provision that "voluntary consent … is absolutely essential".[34] It has been observed that, whilst the regulations were well known at the upper echelons of the military, many researchers and research agencies were unaware of them. They were "Top Secret" for most of the cold war period and only declassified in 1973. The Pentagon had an ambivalent attitude to its own policy. Its policy was designed to protect researchers and the armed forces from legal and political attack without any commitment to protecting human beings on whom the research was conducted.[35] Given this attitude, it is not surprising that some research conducted by armed forces and security agencies since World War II was an outright exploitation of sometimes unwitting participants.[10 (pp. 22–32)]

Experiments with LSD

In perhaps one of the most frightening and blatant cases of the abrogation of rights and the exploitation of individuals in the name of national security was research by the Central Intelligence Agency (CIA) and US armed forces into the effects of mind-altering drugs and, in particular, lysergic acid dethylamide (LSD).[36, 37] These experiments were conducted by the Army on armed force personnel and civilians and by various contractors. The studies were to gain information about the effects of LSD, to see how it would affect combat functions and abilities, and to test the drug's effectiveness in obtaining information.[33 (pp. 305–6)] Several hundred people are estimated to have been experimented on and many of these with no consent or knowledge that a

drug had been administered to them. Some of the lives of individuals who were given LSD during these trials, were devastated by mental and physical illness.[37] James Stanley, a sergeant in the US Army, was administered LSD in 1958 and suffered hallucinations, loss of memory, times of incoherence, and violent outbursts against his wife and children, which led to the breakdown of his marriage. He only learned in 1978 that he had been given LSD when he received a letter from the Army asking him to join a follow-up study. The Supreme Court, however, ruled (by a majority of five to four) that he could not claim damages against the Army because to allow such a claim would "call into question military discipline and decision-making.[32 (p.682)] In an opinion dissenting on this point, Justice O'Connor denounced the conduct of the Army as "so far beyond the bounds of human decency that as a matter of law it simply cannot be considered a part of the military mission."[32 (p.709), 38]

Radiation experiments on US citizens

Radiation experiments were conducted in the USA from the mid-1940s through to the 1980s in experiments designed to test the effects of nuclear radiation on human beings. Information on these experiments was withheld from the public in the name of national security. However, when information did become available, the American Congress authorised a Subcommittee investigation. This Committee wrote a Report (known as the *Markey Report*) that described experiments including one in which patients were injected with plutonium in an experiment to determine the concentration that would cause kidney damage. In another study seven people were left unprotected in a field while a curie of radioactive iodine was released, in order to measure their intake of radiation through inhalation. There were deliberate releases of radioactive iodine into the open air; people were asked to drink milk taken from cows that had fed on iodine-contaminated fields; to eat food contaminated with fall-out material taken from the Nevada Test Site; and to drink solutions containing radioactive caesium and strontium. Prisoners had their testicles exposed to doses of X-rays, at levels which far exceeded safe occupational limits, to determine the effect on their fertility and testicular function.[39]

The *Markey Report* "went virtually unnoticed in the

field".[40] It took a Presidential Commission, reporting nine years later, to bring American and international attention to these experiments.[41] The Commission had been given much greater powers to investigate, to expose classified material. It reported on further unethical studies. In one of these an unconscious trauma victim, arrived at a hospital and was used in a radiation study with no apparent opportunity for consent. In other studies, duplicitous language was used to hide the fact that radioactive substances were being used on patients and school children.[41 (pp. 266, 343)] In its struggle to understand such blatantly unethical behaviour, the Commission observed that some researchers regarded their subjects as "second class citizens"[41 (p.348)]

Gulf War

In the period proceeding the Gulf War in 1990, the US Department of Defense, requested exemption from a Food and Drug Administration requirement (Rule 23 [d]) which requires informed consent in the use of "investigational new drugs". The Assistant Secretary argued that in peace time, "we believe strongly in informed consent and its ethical foundations" but that "military combat is different" in that a preventive or therapeutic treatment might safe a soldier's life, avoid endangering other personnel, and accomplish the mission.[42] This request was granted on the grounds that it was "not feasible" to offer informed consent. As a result almost 700 000 personnel in the Gulf (approximately two-thirds) were administered pyridostigmine bromide and a further 8000 personnel were given a botulims toxoid vaccination. There have been many claims that ill-health in Gulf war personnel since the war was a direct result of the use of these substances.[38, 43]

As Annas has argued, the basis for waiving the requirement for consent for both of these substances was that the drugs were for therapeutic use. Yet both were investigational drugs with known problems. This amounted to a blurring of the distinction between treatment and research. In effect therefore, armed force personnel were experimented on with substances that had not been established to be either safe (in terms of minimal harmful effects) or effective.[44] These substances were used in combination with other substances, and in circumstances in which combatants were potentially more susceptible to the harmful effects of the many chemicals to which they were exposed in the Gulf.

Research in the Armed Forces

What is of great concern is that a whole sector of society (which includes armed forces personnel) is deprived of legal and ethical protection. Given the lack of care shown by the upper echelons of the armed forces and security agencies for their own personnel and for the wider public, it is evident that any research that they conduct should be constrained by the normal requirements, which have been designed to protect human participants. Scandals in radiation experimentation, LSD research, and the Gulf war (amongst others[10 (pp. 22–32)]), make it obvious that decision-makers in the armed forces and security departments give little regard to the welfare of their own personnel or to citizens in pursuing their strategic aims. Therefore there is little to support the supposition that concessions to individual choice would undermine military discipline. We argue strongly that there should be no exception to the principle of "non-exploitation" of participants in research even when that research is sanctioned by the security or armed forces.

There should be a public commitment to this principle from the armed forces or a legislative requirement that any research conducted by, or on behalf of, security or armed forces be governed by the same requirements for review as any other research on human subjects. In addition: all the suggestions we made for research in the Discussion above should apply. There should be no experimentation on human subjects beyond minimal risk and a public commitment to applying principles of safety to security and armed forces research.

CONCLUSION

We have reviewed many cases in which participants have been maltreated in research programs. It is reasonable to assume that these cases represent a small minority. However, given these occurrences (and others not reported here), and the extent of harm caused, it is pragmatic to recognise a pattern that they establish and to adopt preventative measures. This is to recognise that safety requires a thorough understanding of those factors that are precursors to harm, and a systematic response to overcome their injurious effects.

The initial step requires a commitment (and a continual recommitment) to the principle of non-exploitation of research participants. The subsequent steps are all concerned with recognising potentials for harm and adopting preventative practices. Many of these practices are those already relied on. A common feature of many of these practices is independent review. There is a need for independent review to ensure that accepted standards of research and treatment are applied. Independent review includes mechanisms to protect those at risk, to support individuals who complain and those complained about, until the substance of the concern is properly investigated. Independent review includes the formation of investigative teams from government departments or specialist colleges to respond quickly to problems when they become known. Independent review also includes publication of results, regular audits, and quality assurance programs. Possible outcomes of reviews may include establishing bench marks for minimal standards, and requirements for training or retraining. The media also functions as another form of independent review. In many of the cases described in this chapter, the press has played a significant role in bringing an end to harm. The essential ingredient, however, and the highest priority, must be a concern and commitment to averting potential harm to patients. If we are to "build a better present and a better future" we must learn from our own foibles as human beings, foster attitudes and values that give priority to the welfare of research participants, and install systems to support safe practices that will avert future harm.

REFERENCES

1. Jones JH. *Bad blood: the Tuskegee Syphilis experiment*. New York: The Free Press, 1981.
2. President William J. Clinton, Office of the Press Secretary, The White House, May 16, 1997, www1.whitehouse.gov/New/Remarks/Fri/19970516-898.html
3. Warnock M. Informed consent – a publisher's duty *BMJ* 1998; **316**: 1000–5.
4. World Medical Association. *Declaration of Helsinki: Recommendations guiding medical doctors in biomedical research involving human subjects*, adopted by the 18th World Medical Assembly, Helsinki, Finland, 1964; revised by the World Medical Assembly in Tokyo, Japan in 1975, in Venice, Italy in 1983, and in Hong Kong in 1989.
5. Coney S. *The unfortunate experiment*. New Zealand, London, New York: Penguin Books, 1988.
6. Cartwright SR. *The report of the committee of inquiry into allegations concerning the treatment of cervical cancer at National Women's Hospital and related matters*.
   Auckland, New Zealand: Government Printing Office, 1988.
7. Rosier P. The speculum bites back: feminists spark an inquiry into the treatment of carcinoma *in situ* at Auckland's National Women's Hospital. *Reprod Genetic Eng* 1989; **2**: 121–32.
8. McNeill PM. The implications for Australia of the New Zealand Report of the Cervical Cancer Inquiry: no cause for complacency. *Med J Aust* 1989; **150**: 264–71.
9. Mastroianni AC, Faden R, Federman D, eds. *Women and health research; ethical and legal issues of including women in clinical studies. Volume 1*. Washington: National Academy Press, 1994.
10. McNeill PM. *The Ethics and Politics of Human Experimentation*. 1993: Melbourne and Cambridge: Cambridge University Press.
11. Dyer C. London professor struck off for bullying and dishonesty. *BMJ* 1999; **319**: 938.
12. Dyer C. Professor accused of threatening staff. *BMJ* 1999; **319**: 871.
13. Mellor B. Integrity and ruined lives. *Aust Time Mag*, 1991; Oct 21: 51.
14. Swazey JP, Scher SR. The whistleblower as a deviant professional: professional norms and responses to fraud in clinical research. In: *Whistleblowing in biomedical research: policies and procedures for responding to reports of misconduct*. Proceedings of a Workshop Sept 1981, President's Commission for the Study of Ethical Problems in Medicine and Biomedical and Behavioural Research, American Association for the Advancement of Science, Committee on Scientific Freedom and Responsibility. Washington DC: US Government Printing Office, 1982, p. 187.
15. Bohaychuk W, Ball G, Lawrence G, Sotirov K. A qualitative view of international compliance. *Appl Clin Trials* 1998; September 32–41.
16. Boseley S. Trial and error puts patients at risk. *The Guardian* 1999; 27 July: 8.
17. Jay P. Fraud in medical research. *CERES News* 1999; **27**: 1–2.
18. Walker M. *Dirty medicine: science, big business and the assault on natural health care*. London: Slingshot Publications, 1993.
19. Anonymous. Research without consent continues in the UK. *IME Bull* 1988; **40**: 13–15.
20. Nicholson RJ. More questions on the Evelyn Thomas case. *IME Bull* 1988; November; 18–20.
21. Quoted in Nicholson RJ. Final act in the Evelyn Thomas case. *Bull Med Ethics* 1992; **75**: 3–4.
22. Wilkinson JM, Moore CJ, Notley HM, Hunter RD. The use of Selectron after loading equipment to stimulate and extend the Manchester System for intracavity therapy of the cervix uteri. *Br J Radiother* 1983; **56**: 409–14.
23. RAGE. All treatment and trials must have informed consent. *BMJ* 1997; **314**: 1134–5.

24. Wilkinson JM, Hendry JH, Hunter RD. Dose-rate considerations in the introduction of low-dose rate after loading intracavity techniques for radiotherapy. *Br J Radiother* 1980; **54**: 890–3.

25. Sherrah-Davies E. Morbidity following low-dose-rate Selectron therapy for cervical cancer. *Clin Radiol* 1985; **36** 131–9.

26. Charity Commission. *Findings of inquiry under section 8 Charities Act 1993. 1. Cancer Research Campaign. 2. Imperial Cancer Research Fund*. London: Charity Commission, 1994.

27. Nicholson R. Editorial. *Bull Med Ethics* 1994; March: 1.

28. Nicholson R. Bristol study continues to cause debate. *Bull Med Ethics* 1995; May: 3–5.

29. Goodare H, Smith R. The rights of patients in research. *BMJ* 1995; **310**: 1277–8.

30. Nicholson R. Bristol study should be retracted. *Bull Med Ethics* 1991; **74**: 3–6.

31. Leape LL. Error in medicine. *JAMA*, 1994; **272**: 1851–7.

32. *United States* v. *Stanley*, 483, US 669.

33. Annas GJ, Glantz LH, Katz BF. *Informed consent to human experimentation: the subject's dilemma*. Cambridge, Massachusetts: Ballinger, 1977.

34. Annas GJ, Grodin MA, eds. *The Nazi doctors and the Nuremberg Code: human rights in human experimentation*. New York and Oxford: Oxford University Press, 1992; Appendix 4.

35. Moreno JD. The only feasible means: the Pentagon's ambivalent relationship with the Nuremberg Code. *Hastings Center Rep* 1996; **26**(5): 11–19.

36. Thomas G. *Journey into madness: the true story of the CIA mind control and mental abuse*. New York, Toronto, London, Sydney, Auckland: Bantam Books, 1989.

37. Baker R. The acid test. *Sydney Morning Herald, The Good Weekend* 1999; Feb 20: 14–18.

38. Milner CA. Gulf war guinea pigs: is informed consent optional during war? *J Contemp Hlth Law Policy* 1996; **13**: 199–232.

39. US House of Representatives, Committee on Energy and Commerce, Subcommittee on Energy Conservation and Power. *American nuclear guinea pigs: three decades of radiation experiments on U.S. citizens* (ACHRE No. Con-050594-A-1), November 1986.

40. Faden R. The Advisory Committee on human radiation experiments: reflections on a presidential commission. *Hastings Center Rep* 1996; **26**(5): 5–10.

41. The final report of the Advisory Committee on human radiation experiments. Pittsburgh: US Government Printing Office, 1995 (Also published by Oxford University Press, 1996).

42. Department of Defense. Request for exemption from informed consent. 55 Federal Register, 52813–17, Dec. 21, 1990 (reprinted in Annas & Grodin, ref. 34 pp. 346–348).

43. Cotton P. Veterans seeking answers to syndrome suspect they were goats in Gulf war. *JAMA* 1994: **271**: 1559–61.

44. Annas GJ. Changing the consent rules for desert storm. *New Engl J Med* 1992: **236** 770–3.

Part 2

The *BMJ* debate: informed consent in medical research

7 · Informed consent: the intricacies*

Should the *BMJ* reject all studies that do not include informed consent?

Richard Smith

Should the *BMJ* reject all studies that do not include informed consent? That's a simple question, and surely the answer should be equally simple – "Yes". Unfortunately, ethical questions rarely allow simple answers.

ETHICAL PROBLEMS FOR MEDICAL JOURNALS

Medical journals must consider the ethical aspects of all the material they publish, and medical editors are presented with ethical issues just as often as doctors – that is, every day. Almost everything that doctors and editors do has an ethical aspect. However, a paper published in *JAMA* in 1997 shows that many journals do not give their authors clear ethical guidance.[1] A survey of the published instructions to authors of the 102 major English language biomedical journals showed that a quarter did not give authors any guidance on human research ethics, and only half required approval by an ethics committee or institutional review board before publication.

An accompanying editorial looked at 53 consecutive research papers published in *Annals of Internal Medicine, BMJ, Lancet, JAMA, and New England Journal of Medicine*.[2] The authors found that 47% did not record informed consent and 58% did not record approval by an ethics committee or institutional review board. Importantly, they found six papers in which they judged there was a compelling need for informed consent or approval by an ethics committee or institutional review board, and yet where there was no mention of either. These data are supported by a study that found that, of 586 interventional studies published in four geriatrics journals, only 54%

included informed consent, and 40% included approval by an ethics committee or institutional review board.[3] The *JAMA* editorial recommends that journals explicitly ask authors to state that their research complies with the World Medical Association's Declaration of Helsinki.[2]

DECLARATION OF HELSINKI

The Declaration of Helsinki includes four paragraphs specifically on informed consent and does allow physicians sometimes to do without informed consent in the context of "medical research combined with professional care (clinical research)."[4] The first paragraph states: "In any research on human beings, each potential subject must be adequately informed of the aims, methods, anticipated benefits and potential hazards of the study and the discomfort it may entail. He or she should be informed that he or she is at liberty to abstain from participation in the study and that he or she is free to withdraw his or her consent to participation at any time. The physician should then obtain the subject's freely given informed consent, preferably in writing." The next two paragraphs consider patients in a dependent relationship with physicians or who are not legally competent. The "let out" paragraph says: "If the physician considers it essential not to obtain informed consent, the specific reasons for this proposal should be stated in the experimental protocol for transmission to the independent committee."

STUDIES IN THE *BMJ*

Both the studies below comply with the Declaration

BMJ 1997; **314**: 1059–60.

of Helsinki. Both were approved by ethics committees. Those committees agonised over the studies, and both papers include a detailed account of why the researchers did not obtain fully informed consent. But should the *BMJ* set a higher – or at least more explicit–standard than the Declaration of Helsinki?

One of the studies, from Edinburgh, is a randomised controlled trial of whether stroke family care workers improve outcomes for patients with stroke and their families.[5] (p. 1071) The authors decided against seeking consent for randomisation primarily on the grounds that a detailed knowledge of the trial and its exact purpose would bias outcomes, which were essentially subjective. In addition, they did not expect the intervention to be harmful, and patients and their families could decline to see the stroke family care worker.[6] (p. 1077) Sheila McLean, a professor of law and ethics in medicine, argues that their reasons are insufficient to justify deviation from the general rule that good research must at all times respect the subject.[7] (p. 1076) "Any failure", she writes, "to offer this respect is in itself a harm, even if its consequences are not physical."

The second study, from South Africa, was a prospective double blinded study of whether infection with HIV affected the outcome of patients admitted to an intensive care unit.[8] (p. 1077) This is an important question because, when resources are tight, there is a tendency not to admit patients infected with HIV to intensive care units. Patients did not give consent to be in the study or to have their blood tested for HIV. The authors argue that consent could not be obtained from most cases because they were too sick and that the research was of such importance that the patients' right to informed consent could be waived.[9] (p. 1082) The chairman of the ethics committee explains why the committee supported the research after its immediate reaction that it would not be possible to give ethical approval.[10] (p. 1083) The explanations included the facts that the study entailed no interventions of any sort different from those that are necessary and are carried out in standard intensive care, and that the injury done to the patients would be small. Rajendra Kale, an Indian neurologist, argues that the ethics committee was wrong to approve the research and that the *BMJ* is wrong to publish it.[11] (p. 1081) He thinks that such research would not have been allowed in a fully developed country and worries that it may be too easy to flout fundamental human rights in the developing world.

Views on the Studies

The editors of the *BMJ* and our reviewers were divided on whether we should publish these papers. In the end we decided – and I as editor must accept full responsibility – that, rather than restrict the debate to ourselves, we would do better to invite our readers to join in. The papers were thus published together with their commentaries and with an argument from Len Doyal, a professor of medical ethics, that the *BMJ* should not in future publish papers like these.[12] (p. 1107) He proposed a policy that all medical journals might follow.

Professor Doyal wrote: "Our abilities to deliberate, to choose, and to plan for the future are the focus of dignity and respect that we associate with being an autonomous person capable of participation in civic life." To deny patients participating in research full information on that research is, he argued a clear breach of their moral rights. Professor Doyal then examined the arguments against fully informed consent: patients may be distressed by detailed information; it may not be necessary when the risks of the research are negligible; and the interests of the public in medical progress will be undermined by too much emphasis on the rights of individual patients. He found all these arguments unconvincing.

He does, however, identify three sets of circumstances in which informed consent may not be necessary. So long as a set of conditions are not met then research may be allowed without consent on patients not competent to give consent – including children, patients with learning difficulties, and unconscious or semiconscious patients. Otherwise, such patients will be denied the benefits of research. Secondly, epidemiological research on medical records may be acceptable in certain strict circumstances when, for practical reasons, consent cannot be obtained. Thirdly, research without informed consent may sometimes be acceptable on stored tissue from anonymous donors.

Jeffrey Tobias, an oncologist argued that the *BMJ* is right sometimes to publish studies where patients have not given informed consent.[13] (p. 1111) His argument revolved around the facts that patients trust their doctors, and that what is clear in "fine and lofty places", like the letters pages of medical journals, is much less clear in the "real world" where "the doctor must somehow juggle the multiple responsibilities of expert, humane, and above all respectful support for the patient ... with the wider healthcare concerns and requirements of society as a whole."

The patient's voice was heard in this debate from an anonymous patient who was included in 1987 in a British trial of a new radiotherapy protocol for cervical cancer without being asked for fully informed consent.[14 (p. 1134)] She suffered severe consequences from the treatment and later discovered that she was one of many patients who had been included in trials without consent. She felt abused and quoted another patient who wrote: "Somewhere, somehow, I have to expose this abuse of power. The doctors never got my informed consent. This is abuse of society's most vulnerable people. Where is there a platform for my voice to be heard, to make the public aware and the establishment accountable?" Our anonymous patient is against the *BMJ* publishing any trials that do not include informed consent.

A news report from India described how the Indian Council of Medical Research approved research that, without written informed consent, left women with precancerous uterine cervical lesions without treatment to study the natural course of the condition.[15 (p. 1065)] A second news report described how the Council of Europe is developing a legally binding set of rules on bioethics. These stipulate that research can be carried out only if subjects have given informed consent.[16 (p. 1066)] The rules do not have a "let out" clause to waive informed consent in people able to give consent, but they do allow research without consent in some circumstances in those who do not have the capacity to consent.

These are not easy issues, but we cannot avoid them. Researchers are likely to continue to want to do trials that do not include fully informed consent, ethics committees will be asked for their opinion, and medical journals will be offered the results to publish. The Declaration of Helsinki does not provide sufficient guidance, and the *BMJ* needs your help. Should we adopt the policy proposed by Professor Doyal or a version of it? Or should we continue sometimes to publish papers that do not include consent?

REFERENCES

1. Amdur RJ, Biddle C. Institutional review board approval and publication of human research results. *JAMA* 1997; **277**: 903–14.
2. Rennie D, Yank V. Disclosure to the reader of institutional review board approval and informed consent. *JAMA* 1997; **277**: 922–3.
3. Rikkert M, ten Have H, Hoefnagels W. Informed consent in biomedical studies on aging: survey of four medical journals. *BMJ* 1996; **313**: 1117–20.
4. Declaration of Helsinki, *BMJ* 1996; **313**: 1448–9.
5. Dennis M, O'Rourke S, Slattery J, Staniforth T, Warlow C. Evaluation of a stroke family care worker: results of a randomised controlled trial. *BMJ* 1997; **314**: 1071–6.
6. Dennis M, O'Rourke S, Slattery J, Staniforth T, Warlow C. Commentary: evaluation of a stroke family care worker: why we didn't ask patients for their consent to be randomised. *BMJ* 1997: **314**: 1077.
7. McLean S. Commentary: not seeking consent means not treating the patient with respect. *BMJ* 1997; **314**: 1076.
8. Bhagwanjee S, Muckart D, Jenna PM, Moodley P. HIV status does not influence outcomes of patients admitted to a surgical intensive care unit. *BMJ* 1997; **314**: 1077–81.
9. Bhagwanjee S, Muckart D, Jenna PM, Moodley P. Commentary: why we did not seek informed consent before testing for HIV. *BMJ* 1997; **314**: 1082–3.
10. Seedat YK. Commentary: no simple and absolute ethical rule exists for every conceivable situation. *BMJ* 1997; **314**: 1083–4.
11. Kale R. Commentary: failing to seek patients' consent to research is always wrong. *BMJ* 1997; **314**: 1082–2.
12. Doyal L. Journals should not publish research to which patients have not given fully informed research – with three exceptions. *BMJ* 1997; **314**: 1107–11.
13. Tobias JS. *BMJ*'s present policy (sometimes approving research in which patients have not given fully informed consent) is wholly correct. *BMJ* 1997: **314**: 1111–4.
14. Editorial: All treatments and trials must have informed consent. *BMJ* 1997; **314**: 1134–5.
15. Mudur G. Indian study of women with cervical lesions called unethical. *BMJ* 1997; **314**: 1065.
16. Waston R. European bioethics convention signed. *BMJ* 1997; **314**: 1066.

8 · Evaluation of a stroke family care worker: results of a randomised controlled trial*

Martin Dennis, Suzanne O'Rourke, Jim Slattery, Trish Staniforth, and Charles Warlow

Stroke has long been recognised as common, frequently fatal, and disabling. In recent years there has been increasing awareness of the psychosocial problems experienced by stroke patients and their carers.[1-3] Though the traditional medical model of care, including hospital-based rehabilitation in stroke units, may reduce case fatality and institutionalisation,[4] it often fails to identify or adequately address these psychosocial problems. In 1992 we established a "stroke family care worker." As we were uncertain of the effectiveness of this post and which patients and carers might gain most, we evaluated the service in a randomised controlled trial.

PATIENTS AND METHODS

All patients who attended our hospital as an inpatient or outpatient with a diagnosis of recent possible stroke (first and recurrent) were seen and assessed by a stroke physician. Details of patients in whom the diagnosis was confirmed according to World Health Organization criteria[5] were entered into our stroke register. Patients with subarachnoid haemorrhage were excluded. Baseline data were collected before randomisation and as part of the routine registration of patients in our register.

Because we were uncertain about which patients and carers might gain most from intervention by a stroke family care worker we set broad eligibility criteria. Any patient with a confirmed stroke within the past 30 days could be randomised unless.

- they were very likely to die within a few days;
- they lived more than 25 miles (40 km) from the hospital, or

*BMJ 1997; **314**: 1071–6.

- the stroke occurred on a background of another major illness that was likely to dominate the pattern of care, e.g. advanced cancer or renal failure.

Randomisation

Randomisation was balanced in blocks of six within strata defined by age, sex, living alone before the stroke, and stroke severity. Those responsible for randomising patients were unaware of the block size. Stroke severity depended on the prediction by the stroke physician at the time of assessment. Patients with severe strokes were defined as those expected to score over 2 on the Oxford handicap scale 1 year after the stroke. A table with random patient allocation was stored on a personal computer so that nobody concerned in randomising patients could discover to which intervention the next patient would be allocated.

Setting and Consent

The intervention was tested in the setting of a large teaching hospital with a well organised stroke service. Patients were not required to consent to randomisation but consented to follow-up. This approach was approved by our local ethics committee.

Intervention

The stroke family care worker (TS) came from a social work background and had considerable experience in working with voluntary agencies for disabled people. Patients or carers, or both, who were randomised to active intervention were contacted by the stroke

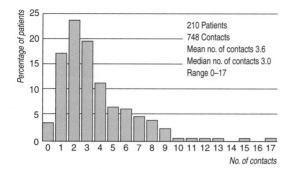

Figure 8.1 *Number of stroke family care worker contacts per patient (or family) in first 6 months after randomisation. Data include face-to-face and telephone contacts.*

family care worker within a week of randomisation. She tried to identify unmet needs and aimed at fulfilling these using any available resources. She would access health services, social services, and voluntary agencies as well as offering some counselling herself. Figure 8.1 shows the considerable variation in number of contacts she had with patients in the first 6 months after randomisation. We did not prescribe how many contacts she would have with families; this was left for her to decide and depended on her assessment of their needs. Patients randomised to the control group had no contact with the stroke family care worker for 6 months, until after our final follow-up assessment had been completed.

Follow-up

We aimed at following up all patients six months after randomisation. A research psychologist (SO'R), who was blind to the treatment allocation, asked the patients to identify a carer and arrange for him or her to be present at the follow-up visit. We followed up only informal carers – that is, spouse or family members – and not, for example, nursing home staff or home helps. Patients and carers were told that we wished to know how they had fared. No reference was made to any assessment of the stroke family care worker.

Follow-up comprised several questionnaires aimed at measuring outcome in various domains. The psychologist helped patients complete the Barthel index,[6] Oxford handicap scale,[7] Frenchay activities index,[8] general health questionnaire (30 item),[9] and social adjustment scale[10] during the follow-up visit.

Meanwhile any carer was asked to complete independently the Frenchay activities index, general health questionnaire, social adjustment scale (on the carer's behalf rather than the patient's), and caregiving hassles scale.[11] Patient and carer were than each left a further questionnaire to return to the psychologist by post. The patient's questionnaire comprised several measures, including the hospital anxiety and depression scale,[12] the mental adjustment to stroke scale,[13] and a patient satisfaction scale.[14] The carer's questionnaire comprised the hospital anxiety and depression scale and a carer satisfaction questionnaire. We modified the mental adjustment to cancer scale[13] for use in stroke patients simply by substituting the word stroke for cancer. In addition, we added further questions to a standard questionnaire to determine the patients' satisfaction[14] with aspects of their care that we thought might be influenced by input from the storke family care worker. We adjusted the wording of this questionnaire slightly for use with carers (see Fig. 8.4).

When patients had cognitive or communication problems that prevented them completing the follow-up questionnaires, their cognitive status was assessed with the Hodkinson abbreviated mental test,[15] and as much information as possible gathered from carers. At the end of the follow-up visit, the research psychologist guessed which treatment group the patient was in to test the efficacy of our efforts to blind her to the treatment allocation.

Analyses

Results were analysed on an intention to treat basis, i.e. the patient or carer was assessed depending on the intervention to which each was randomised, even if he or she had no direct contact with the stroke family care worker. Dichotomous variables at baseline and follow-up were compared by means of risk ratios with 95% confidence intervals and the χ^2 test. Continuous variables were compared by Student's t test. When comparing outcomes measured on ordinal scales, we calculated 95% confidence intervals for the difference between medians.

RESULTS

Between 1 October 1992 and 30 September 1994 we randomised 417 patients, 210 to receive intervention by the stroke family care worker and 207 to receive

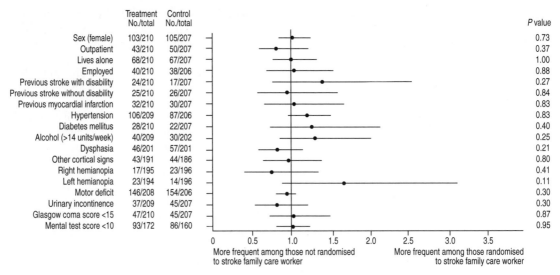

	Treatment No./total	Control No./total		*P* value
Sex (female)	103/210	105/207		0.73
Outpatient	43/210	50/207		0.37
Lives alone	68/210	67/207		1.00
Employed	40/210	38/206		0.88
Previous stroke with disability	24/210	17/207		0.27
Previous stroke without disability	25/210	26/207		0.84
Previous myocardial infarction	32/210	30/207		0.83
Hypertension	106/209	87/206		0.83
Diabetes mellitus	28/210	22/207		0.40
Alcohol (>14 units/week)	40/209	30/202		0.25
Dysphasia	46/201	57/201		0.21
Other cortical signs	43/191	44/186		0.80
Right hemianopia	17/195	23/196		0.41
Left hemianopia	23/194	14/196		0.11
Motor deficit	146/208	154/206		0.30
Urinary incontinence	37/209	45/207		0.30
Glasgow coma score <15	47/210	45/207		0.87
Mental test score <10	93/172	86/160		0.95

0   0.5   1.0   1.5   2.0   2.5   3.0   3.5

More frequent among those not randomised to stroke family care worker   More frequent among those randomised to stroke family care worker

Figure 8.2 *Comparison of baseline characteristics (for dichotomised variables) in patients randomised to treatment and control groups. Points are point estimates of relative risk of characteristic occurring in treatment group compared with control group. Bars are 95% confidence intervals. Denominators vary because some variables were not assessable in a few patients, e.g. hemianopia in unconscious patients.*

standard care (controls). The patients represented 67% of all stroke patients assessed at the hospital. The main reason for non-randomisation was that patients lived more than 25 miles (40 km) away. There were few statistically significant differences between randomised and non-randomised patients with respect to baseline variables. Randomised patients were slightly older (mean age 67.8 years *v* 64.6 years; *P* = 0.006) and more likely to be living alone (relative risk 1.54; 95% confidence interval 1.14–2.08).

There were no substantial or significant differences between patients randomised to the two intervention groups in terms of lesion location, stroke severity, and prestroke function as well as those variables shown in Fig. 8.2. The mean age of the treatment group was 67.1 years and that of the controls 68.4 years (*P* = 0.33).

Outcomes

All randomised patients were accounted for at the end of the study; 19 (9.0%) patients randomised to the stroke family care worker and 22 (10.6%) controls died before follow-up (risk ratio 0.85; 95% confidence interval 0.48–1.53). In four survivors in the treatment group no further follow-up was possible.

One patient had emigrated, another had a brain tumour and was too ill to be followed up, and two patients refused.

Of the patients successfully followed up (187 in the treatment group, 185 controls), 29 (15.5%) in the treatment group and 31 (16.8%) controls had cognitive or communication problems that prevented them completing any questionnaire apart from the Barthel index, Oxford handicap scale, and Hodkinson abbreviated mental test score. Of the 158 patients in the treatment group given the second questionnaire, 145 (91.8%) returned them; and of the 154 patients in the control group given the second questionnaire, 147 (95.5%) returned them. On most measures controls tended to have better outcomes, though the difference was significant only for social adjustment, and was of borderline significance with respect to feelings of helplessness and depression (Table 8.1). Despite this, however, patients in the treatment group were more satisfied with certain aspects of their post-hospital care (Fig. 8.3).

We identified 246 carers. Of these, 119 (48.4%) were carers of patients randomised to the stroke family care worker. Six carers in the treatment group and seven in the control group refused follow-up and two carers in the control group were not assessable. The remaining 231 (93.9%) carers completed the first questionnaire, and 102 (90.3%) in the treatment

Table 8.1 *Comparison of outcomes based on completed questionnaires in patients randomised to treatment and control groups*

		Treatment			Control		Difference between medians (95% confidence interval)†
Measure	No	Median	Interquartile range	No	Median	Interquartile range	
Frenchay activities index	164	37	29–42	164	38	26–45	–1 (–4.0 to 3.0)
General health questionnaire	156	7	2.3–11.8	154	5.5	1–12	–1.5 (–3.0 to 1.0)
Social adjustment scale	164	1.7	1.5–2	160	1.6	1.4–1.8	–0.1 (–0.07 to –0.1)
Hospital depression subscale	128	4.5	3–8	124	3	2–7	–1.5 (–2.0 to 0.0)
Hospital anxiety subscale	128	5	2–8.8	124	5	1.3–7.8	0.0 (–1.0 to 2.0)
Barthel index	187	19	16–20	183	19	15–20	0.0 (–1.0 to 1.0)
Oxford handicap scale	184	3	2–4	184	3	2–4	0.0 (–1.0 to 1.0)
Mental adjustment to stroke scale	113			120			
Fighting spirit – helplessness		60	53–63		57	48–62	–3.0 (–5.0 to 0.0)
Anxious preoccupation		53	48–58		56	48–58	3.0 (–1.3 to 3.0)
Fatalism		54	48–59		54	48–59	0.0 (–5.0 to 0.0)

†Positive value for difference between medians indicates better outcome in treatment group; negative value indicates better outcome in control group.

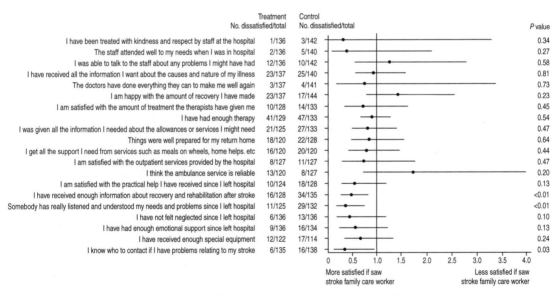

Figure 8.3 *Comparison of responses to individual questions in patient satisfaction questionnaire in treatment and control groups. Points are point estimates of relative risk of patients expressing satisfaction in treatment group compared with control group. Bars are 95% confidence intervals. Difference is significant where confidence interval does not overlap vertical line (relative risk 1.0). Denominators vary because responses were missing in some questionnaires.*

group and 110 (93.2%) in the control group returned the second questionnaire. Carers of patients in the treatment group tended to have bet-ter outcomes than those in the control group. Differences were significant for mood symptoms and of borderline significance for anxiety and hassles

Table 8.2 *Comparison of outcomes based on completed questionnaires in carers of patients randomised to treatment and control groups*

Measure	Treatment			Control			Difference between medians (95% confidence interval)†
	No	Median	Interquartile range	No	Median	Interquartile range	
Frenchay activities index	87	47	42–52	84	48	44–50	−1.0 (−2.4 to 2.0)
General health questionnaire	94	4	0–11	92	7.5	1–13	3.5 (0.7 to 7.0)
Social adjustment scale	112	1.7	1.4–2	116	1.7	1.5–2	0.0 (−0.01 to 0.10)
Caregiving hassles scale	70	4	1–13	69	8	1–21	4.0 (0.0 to 9.0)
Hospital depression subscale	89	4	1–7	96	4.5	1–7	0.5 (−1.0 to 2.0)
Hospital anxiety subscale	89	7	3–10	96	7.5	4.3–11	0.5 (0.0 to 3.0)

†Positive value for difference between medians indicates better outcome in treatment group; negative value indicates better outcome in control group.

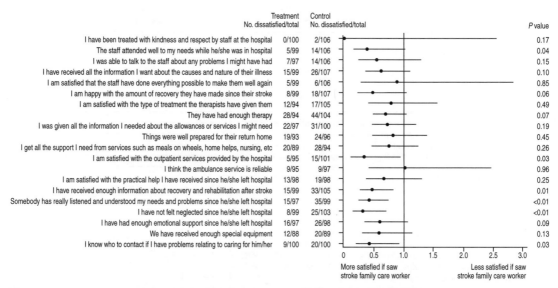

Figure 8.4 *Comparison of responses to individual questions in carer satisfaction questionnaire in treatment and control groups. Points are point estimates of relative risk of patients expressing satisfaction in treament group compared with control group. Bars are 95% confidence intervals. Difference is significant where confidence interval does not overlap vertical line (relative risk 1.0). Denominators vary because responses were missing in some questionnaires.*

(Table 8.2). Carers of patients in the treatment group were also more satisfied with several aspects of their care (Fig. 8.4).

Length of hospital stay was slightly shorter in the treatment group than in the control group (mean 34.7 *v* 38.9 days; median 12 *v* 19 days (*P* = 0.1)). There were no significant differences between the groups in the patients' placement after discharge.

Blinding

After each of 312 consecutive follow-up assessments, the research psychologist was asked to guess whether the patient had been randomised to be seen by the stroke family care worker or not. She guessed correctly in 183 (58.7%) cases, which was more than should have occurred by chance alone (*P* = 0.002), indicating that she was unblinded to some extent. However, the size of any observer bias resulting from this degree of unblinding in a follow-up assessment based mainly on self-report questionnaires was probably small. This is especially so with respect to the carer questionnaires, which were not completed in the presence of the psychologist.

DISCUSSION

Our stroke family care worker and other similar posts were set up with the expectation that they would help patients and their families. However, there is very little evidence from previous randomised trials on which to base this assumption.[16–20] Most of these trials included few patients and were thus prone to type II error, and no systematic review of these trials has been published. We aimed at overcoming this problem by conducting a large trial with greater statistical power and at least partially blinded outcome measurement.

Though we successfully randomised reasonably large numbers of patients, we found few statistically significant differences in outcome between the treatment and control groups. Clearly, it is possible that some bias may have been introduced by patients or carers failing to complete a questionnaire. Theoretically, failure to complete all questions may have been related to the treatment allocation. However, the most common explanations for missing data were patients' cognitive and communication problems and simple omissions – for example, as a result of turning two pages over at once. Similar numbers in each treatment group encountered these sorts of difficulties. Thus significant bias seems unlikely.

The most convincing evidence of benefit of the stroke family care worker was in improving both patients' and carers' satisfaction in respect of various aspects of communication. Intriguingly, patients in the treatment group tended to be more helpless, less well adjusted socially, and possibly more depressed. We could postulate that intervention by the stroke family care worker, by providing support rather than improving patients' coping skills, induced a passive response to their illness, which led to depression and poor social adjustment. Also there was an encouraging trend for carers in the treatment group to be less hassled and to have fewer mood symptoms, especially anxiety, than those in the control group. These moderate effects may, if real, accurately reflect the

effectiveness of our stroke family care worker. There are, however, several possible explanations:

- The post was set up in the context of a well organised stroke service with excellent social work support, and many potential problems for patients and carers were already predicted and averted or managed by the hospital-based team. The post might have had a greater effect in a less well organised service.
- We were concerned that follow up at 6 months might be too early to show the real benefits of the post. Patients and carers may still be adjusting to the stroke and major problems may not yet have developed. At this stage many will still be receiving conventional input from hospital and primary care.
- We may have used measures of outcome that either were not measuring outcomes that might be influenced by our intervention or were insufficiently sensitive to any differences from the intervention.
- Our trial was pragmatic and included 67% of stroke patients. Possibly a subgroup of patients did benefit from the input of the stroke family care worker.
- The stroke family care worker responded to families' needs and wishes and may therefore sometimes have provided too little input to affect outcome.

Though our trial results may be of limited generalisability because we evaluated only a single worker, they suggest that any gain was mainly in satisfaction with aspects of communication and support after hospital discharge, certainly in the setting of a well organised stroke service. Future studies should examine these outcomes as well as psychological ones. Whether purchasers will be willing to fund interventions such as this will depend on the value that they and patients place on such outcomes. Perhaps we need to establish how important patients and their carers regard such outcomes before making any judgments. Pound et al. identified being "cared for" and "cared about" as of value to patients, and they regarded them as important advantages of hospital admission after stroke.[21] We are currently planning a systematic review of previous and ongoing trials of similar interventions, which may go some way in establishing whether stroke family care workers from different backgrounds – that is, working with different intensities for greater durations in different settings – might be more effective.

Key messages

- A stroke family care worker in the context of a well organised hospital based stroke service has no definite beneficial effect on the physical, social, or psychological outcome of patients or their carers.
- A stroke family care worker may reduce carers' hassles and anxiety but render patients more helpless, less well socially adjusted, and more depressed.
- A stroke family care worker may improve patients' and their carers' satisfaction with those aspects of stroke services relating to communication and support.
- Purchasers of health care need to decide the value they and their patients place on satisfaction with health care.

ACKNOWLEDGEMENTS

Funding: TS was supported by the Chest Heart and Stroke Association (Scotland), MD by the Stroke Association, and JS and our stroke register by the Medical Research Council. The trial was funded by the Scottish Office Home and Health Department.

REFERENCES

1. Holbrook M. Stroke: social and emotional outcome. *J R Coll Physicians Lond* 1982; **16**: 100–4.
2. House A, Dennis M, Mogridge L, Warlow C, Hawton K, Jones L. Mood disorders in the first year after first stroke. *Br J Psychiatry* 1991; **158**: 83–92.
3. Anderson CS, Linto J, Stewart-Wynne EG. A population-based assessment of the impact and burden of caregiving for long-term stroke survivors. *Stroke* 1995; **26**: 843–9.
4. Stroke Unit Trialists' Collaboration. A systematic overview of specialist multidisciplinary team (stroke unit) care for stroke inpatients. Revised 27 February 1995. In: Warlow C, Van Gijn J, Sandercock P, eds. *Stroke module. Cochrane database of systematic reviews. Cochrane Collaboration. Issue 2.* Oxford: Update Software, 1995. (Database on disk and CD-ROM.)
5. Hatano S. Experience from a multicentre stroke register: a preliminary report. *Bull World Health Organ* 1976; **54**: 541–53.
6. Mahoney FI, Barthel DW. Functional evaluation: the Barthel index. *Md State Med J* 1965; **14**: 62–5.
7. Bamford J, Sandercock P, Warlow C, Slattery J. Inter-observer agreement for the assessment of handicap in stroke patients. *Stroke* 1989; **20**: 828.
8. Holbrook M, Skibeck C. An activities index for use with stroke patients. *Age Ageing* 1983; **12**: 166–70.
9. Goldberg D. *The detection of psychiatric illness by questionnaire*. Oxford: Oxford University Press, 1972.
10. Weissman MM, Bothwell S. Assessment of social adjustment by patient self-report. *Arch Gen Psychiatry* 1976; **33**: 1111–5.
11. Kinney JM, Stephens MAP. Caregiving hassles scale: assessing the daily hassles of caring for a family member with dementia. *Gerontologist* 1989; **29**: 328–32.
12. Zigmond AS, Snaith RP. The hospital anxiety and depression scale. *Acta Psychiatr Scand* 1983; **67**: 361–70.
13. Watson M, Greer S, Young J, Inayat Q, Burgess C, Robertson B. Development of a questionnaire measure of adjustment to cancer: the MAC scale. *Psychol Med* 1988; **18**: 203–9.
14. Pound P, Gompertz P, Ebrahim S. Patients' satisfaction with stroke services. *Clin Rehabil* 1994; **8**: 7–17.
15. Hodkinson H. Evaluation of a mental test score for the assessment of mental impairment in the elderly. *Age Ageing* 1972; **1**: 233–8.
16. Christie D, Weigall D. Social work effectiveness in two-year stroke survivors: a randomised controlled trial. *Community Health Stud* 1984; **8**: 26–32.
17. Towle D, Lincoln NB, Mayfield LM. Service provision and functional independence in depressed stroke patients and the effect of social intervention on these. *J Neurol Neurosurg Psychiatry* 1989; **52**: 519–22.
18. Evans RL, Matlock AL, Bishop DS, Stranahan S, Pederson C. Family intervention after stroke: does counseling or education help. *Stroke* 1988; **19**: 1243–9.
19. Friedland JF, McColl M. Social support intervention after stroke: results of a randomised trial. *Arch Phys Med Rehabil* 1992; **73**: 573–81.
20. Forster A, Young J. A randomised trial of specialist nurse support for community stroke patients. *BMJ* 1996; **313**: 1642–6.
21. Pound P, Bury M, Gompertz P, Ebrahim S. Stroke patients' views on their admission to hospital. *BMJ* 1995; **311**: 18–22.

No consent means not treating the patient with respect (commentary)*

Sheila AM McLean

It is presumably often difficult for researchers to commit themselves wholeheartedly to the notion that before consent (or refusal) is obtained for research it is necessary that the person concerned should be given the fullest information about the project for which his or her agreement is wanted. The concerns expressed by the researchers – not least the possibility of biasing results – are intelligible. However, they are also insufficient to justify deviation from the general rule.

Researchers in many topics face the same problems about possibly influencing results, and seek to minimise the possible impact this may have. Many kinds of research – clinical and non-clinical – must and do tackle similar problems while still turning out high quality work. However, this and the other rationales cited by Dennis *et al.* disguise a deeper problem. The researchers claim they did not think that failure to provide the fullest possible information would harm their patients. Though this is probably true in a physical sense, it omits to consider the underlying rationale for providing full information – namely, that good research should not only be scientifically sound but must also at all times respect the subject. Any failure to offer this respect is in itself a harm, even if its consequences are not physical. Indeed, it could plausibly be argued that omitting any substantial factor in the research protocol is enough to render the research unethical, no matter how important the postulated outcome. This is particularly true given that no researcher can know in advance that his or her results will be important.

Everyone starting a project believes that there is value in knowing the answer to the question being asked. But it is only when the answer is found that the truth or falsehood of that assumption can be known. Thus there is an inbuilt intellectual bias in any project that presumes the answer is important enough to ignore a fundamental tenet of research method and respect for people.

We must also accept that, had people been asked and then regretted their decision, this would be unfortunate. It is difficult, however, to see how this differs from other projects. Moreover, that the person in question was rendered vulnerable by the nature of the condition argues for more rather than less information. There are always concerns about including in studies people whose condition is precarious. That this research was not directly physical does not remove those concerns or minimise obligations. In addition, I am puzzled by the argument that, as patients and their families would be included, it was "unclear" who might give consent. The answer is clear: anyone who is to be studied must be given the fullest possible information.

We can agree that the conclusions of the study are of considerable interest and that no physical harm was done to patients whose agreement to participate was based on partial rather than full information. It is, however, also dangerous to believe that this is enough. Nor are possible feelings of disappointment on the part of those, who might not have agreed to randomisation, different from findings in other research settings.

In sum, the arguments against providing full information are frankly unconvincing, however well intentioned. If certain research cannot be undertaken to the maximum standards of scientific inquiry, the question is not how much information can be withheld, it is whether the research should be done in the first place. Otherwise we embark on a slippery slope away from one of our most fundamental ethical principles. In the long run the critical issue is not the consequential one; what matters is that people have not been treated with enough respect.

BMJ 1997; **314**: 1076.

Why we didn't ask patients for their consent (commentary)*

Martin Dennis

In our trial we asked patients to consent to follow-up but not to consent to randomisation itself. There were several reasons for adopting this approach, which was approved by our local ethics committee. Firstly, we did not expect our intervention to be harmful, though whether this expectation was fulfilled must be judged from our results. Secondly, patients and their carers could refuse to see our stroke family care worker or follow-up psychologist whenever they wished. Thus half the patients and their carers were asked to consent to the intervention and all were asked to consent to follow-up after randomisation. Thirdly, we were concerned that, if we tried to obtain informed consent, this might bias our results. For instance, if we made patients and their families aware of the help they might receive from the stroke family care worker, and then randomised them to the control group, this might have had a detrimental effect on their morale. This could have led to a false positive result simply by having an adverse effect on the controls.

In addition, as our patients and their carers were not aware that they were in a randomised trial to assess our stroke family care worker, and that our follow-up was attempting to assess her effectiveness, they were in effect partially blinded. We might imagine that loyalty to the care worker might have biased their responses had they known the precise purpose of our follow-up. Fourthly, our approach allowed patients or carers to decide to see the stroke family care worker when it was relevant to them. Some patients might not consent to randomisation shortly after their stroke, when they are unlikely to foresee the possible psychosocial impact of the stroke on them and their families. They might then regret the decision not to be randomised when the potential benefits of the intervention become more evident. Lastly, as our intervention was applied to patients and their families, it was unclear who might most appropriately give consent.

Increasingly, purchasers and providers of health care are looking for evidence from methodologically sound randomised controlled trials and systematic reviews to guide their practice. In a trial where outcome measures reflect the feelings or opinions of the subjects, a detailed knowledge of the trial and its exact purpose are likely to influence or bias responses. Thus responses may reflect either a control subject's disappointment or dissatisfaction with not receiving a potentially beneficial treatment or a treated patient's appreciation or loyalty to those providing the treatment. Those who review such studies will be unable to judge whether this source of bias might account for any difference in outcomes between treated and control groups. Thus no studies would be regarded as methodologically watertight. Is it ethical to randomise patients into trials which, because of an inherent methodological weakness, cannot provide a definite answer to the main question?

BMJ 1997; **314**: 1077.

9 · Does HIV status influence the outcome of patients admitted to a surgical intensive care unit? A prospective double blind study*

Satish Bhagwanjee, David JJ Muckart, Prakash M Jeena, Prushini Moodley

Extensive data are available on the outcome of patients with AIDS admitted to intensive care units.[1,2] The survival rate of these patients has greatly improved over the past 15 years, and refusal to provide intensive care to these patients on the basis of medical futility is therefore deemed unjust.[1] In Africa the pattern of HIV disease is different from that in the developed world, more patients manifesting early HIV disease and fewer progressing to AIDS.[3] This pattern is reflected in our intensive care unit, where most patients are admitted with diseases unrelated to their HIV status. To our knowledge the outcome of patients with HIV infection admitted to intensive care for other reasons has not been described. Our clinical impression was that their outcome was poor.

Limited resources and the high cost of intensive care have compelled clinicians to rationalise the allocation of resources.[1] For example, in our unit it is policy not to admit patients with incurable malignant disease, end stage liver disease, and patients with multiple organ failure who are deemed non-salvageable. The lack of objective data made it unclear whether patients with HIV infection should be treated similarly. To allow rationalisation of the admissions policy with respect to these patients, we conducted a prospective study to determine the prevalence of HIV infection among patients admitted to the unit and assess the impact of HIV status (HIV positive, HIV negative, AIDS) on outcome.

The study embraced a major ethical dilemma. On the one hand, the clinician has an obligation of non-

maleficence – that is, patients must not be harmed by the actions of the doctor. On the other hand, the doctor has an obligation to society to ensure that available resources are appropriated fairly, based on objective evidence. Though the basic ethical tenets of patient autonomy, justice, beneficence, and non-maleficence[4] are useful, they are only the starting points for ethical decision-making.

SUBJECTS AND METHODS

The study was conducted in the 16 bed surgical intensive care unit at King Edward VIII Hospital, a large teaching hospital in Durban. All patients admitted to the unit over 6 months (September 1993 to February 1994) were included. There were no exclusions. Informed consent was not sought. The study protocol was approved by the ethics committee of the University of Natal.

A screening enzyme immunoassay for HIV (Abbott HIV-1/HIV-2 third generation plus kit; Abbott Laboratories, Chicago) was performed on all patients at admission. Positive results were confirmed by the department of virology using an immunofluorescence assay (SEROFLUOR; Virion, Switzerland) and western blotting (HIV western blot 1/2; Diagnostic Biotechnology, Singapore). Patients with positive results in the confirmatory tests were considered HIV positive. The department of haematology was informed of these results and requested a specimen of blood for flow cytometry from three patients, one of whom was HIV positive. Staff were thereby blinded to which patients were HIV positive. Flow cytometry was performed on whole blood

BMJ 1997; **314**: 1077–81.

samples from all HIV positive patients with Coulter's Q-prep method (commercially produced antibodies from the Coulter Corporation, Miami). Samples were analysed on an Epics Profile II Coulter flow cytometer.

In addition to the intensive care unit staff, patients also were blinded to the results of the HIV tests. The protocol permitted disclosure of HIV status to staff in two instances:

- if a staff member sustained a needle-stick injury when the injured staff member, the consultant in charge of the patient, and the matron in charge would be informed of the result;
- if a patient required haemodialysis – when the nurse undertaking haemodialysis and the consultant in charge would be informed of the result.

On discharge all patients were advised that they had been tested for HIV and of the reason for testing, and given the option of knowing the result. Post-test counselling was offered to patients when HIV results were disclosed. Results of HIV testing were made available to the research team only after the patient had been discharged and all other data had been collated. On conclusion of the study, results of HIV testing were permanently removed from laboratory records.

Three groups of patients were defined. HIV positive and HIV negative patients were identified by HIV testing; patients with AIDS were identified by Centers for Disease Control criteria.[5] The following data were recorded in all patients:

- demographic details;
- admission diagnosis and referring discipline; APACHE II score (acute physiological, age, and chronic health evaluation) in the first 24 hours after admission[6];
- incidence of organ failure as defined by Knaus et al[7];
- incidence of sepsis and septic shock as defined by the American College of Chest Physicians and the Society of Critical Care Medicine[8];
- incidence of nosocomial sepsis as defined by our intensive care unit protocol;
- durations of intensive care unit and hospital stay (duration of hospital stay did not include intensive care unit stay);
- intensive care unit and hospital mortality (hospital mortality did not include intensive care unit mortality).

Admission to the unit and treatment offered were not influenced by HIV status. All patients were treated according to standard intensive care unit protocols.

Statistics

HIV positive and HIV negative patients were compared by Student's t test and the χ^2 test for continuous and discrete variables respectively. A probability value of less than 0.05 was considered significant. Associations between HIV status and outcome variables were adjusted for differences in age and analysed by logistic regression. Kaplan–Meier estimates were used to compute the survival distribution function estimates within the HIV positive and HIV negative groups (non-survivors) and the equality of the distributions tested by the Wilcoxon rank sum test. Age was added as a covariate.

RESULTS

No patient had AIDS. The rest of the data therefore refer to HIV positive and HIV negative patients only. Of the 402 patients admitted to the unit during the 6 months, 52 (13%) tested positive for HIV. Though the male to female distribution in the two groups was similar, they differed significantly in age ($P < 0.002$; Table 9.1).

Table 9.1 *Age and sex distribution of HIV negative and HIV positive patients*

	No. (%) HIV negative (350)	No. (%) HIV positive (52)
No. (%) male	228 (65)	39 (75)
No. (%) female	122 (35)	13 (25)
Mean age in years (SD)	33 (18)	28 (9)*

*$P = 0.0018$

Most patients in both groups were admitted after trauma (Table 9.2). HIV infection was more common in patients referred from orthopaedic surgery and obstetrics and gynaecology. There was no significant difference in intensive care unit or hospital mortality or in the duration of intensive care unit or hospital stay (Tables 9.3 and 9.4). Intensive care unit mortality in HIV negative patients was 24% (84/350) compared with 29% (15/52) in HIV positive patients

Table 9.2   *Interdisciplinary distribution of patients*

Discipline	No. (%) HIV negative	No. (%) HIV positive	Overall % HIV positive in discipline
Trauma	188 (54)	30 (57)	14
Obstetrics and gynaecology	40 (11)	8 (15)	17
Paediatrics	30 (9)	2 (4)	6
Vascular surgery	27 (8)	3 (6)	10
General surgery	24 (7)	4 (8)	14
Internal medicine	17 (5)	3 (6)	15
Ear, nose, and throat/maxillofacial	11 (3)	0	0
Orthopaedic surgery	9 (3)	2 (4)	18
Urology	4 (1)	0	0
Total	350 (100)	52 (100)	13

Table 9.3   *Comparison of mortality between HIV negative and HIV positive patients*

	No. (%) HIV negative	No. (%) HIV positive	*P* value	Odds ratio	Age adjusted odds ratio (95% confidence interval)
Intensive care unit	84/350 (24)	15/52 (29)	0.558	1.28	1.45 (0.75 to 2.80)
Hospital	16/247 (6)	1/37 (3)	0.308	0.16	†

†Data on hospital mortality for HIV negative patients were available for only 247 patients; therefore maximum likelihood ratios could not be calculated.

Table 9.4   *Mean and median (range) number of days' stay in intensive care unit and hospital for HIV positive and HIV negative patients*

	HIV negative*		HIV positive		
	Mean	Median	Mean	Median	*P value*
Intensive care unit	6	4 (1–44)	7	5 (1–41)	0.1
Hospital	10	7 (1–50)	8	6 (2–42)	0.08

*Data were available for only 247 HIV negative patients.

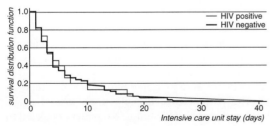

Figure 9.1   *Survival distribution function versus duration of stay in intensive care unit.*

(odds ratio 1.45; 95% confidence interval 0.75 to 2.80); hospital mortality was 6% (16/247) and 3% (1/37) in the two groups respectively. There was no significant difference in survival distribution between the groups (mean survival time 7.3 (SE 2.6) days in the HIV positive group, 6.9 (0.78) days in the HIV negative group; P=0.88) (Fig. 9.1). Information regarding hospital mortality and duration of hospital stay could not be retrieved for 19 HIV negative patients. There was no significant difference in mean APACHE II score between HIV negative and HIV positive patients (scores 9 and 8 respectively).

Table 9.5   *Comparison of total and individual organ failures between HIV negative and HIV positive patients*

	No. (%) HIV negative (350)	No. (%) HIV positive (52)	P value	Odds ratio	Age adjusted odds ratio (95% confidence interval)
Total	171 (49)	37 (71)	< 0.003	2.58	2.87 (1.51 to 5.46)
Cardiac	84 (24)	21 (40)	< 0.014	2.11	2.38 (1.28 to 4.42)
Respiratory	150 (43)	33 (63)	< 0.005	2.32	2.60 (1.41 to 4.78)
Haematological	31 (9)	11 (21)	< 0.007	2.76	3.22 (1.47 to 7.09)
Renal	47 (13)	9 (17)	0.45	1.35	1.75 (0.78 to 3.92)
Neurological	19 (5)	5 (10)	0.23	1.85	1.72 (0.61 to 4.85)

Table 9.6   *Incidence of sepsis in HIV negative and HIV positive patients*

	No. (%) HIV negative (350)	No. (%) HIV positive (52)	P value	Odds ratio	Age adjusted odds ratio (95% confidence interval)
Septic shock	54 (15)	20 (38)	< 0.001	3.43	3.64 (1.91 to 6.89)
Severe sepsis	71 (20)	9 (17)	0.62	0.82	0.84 (0.39 to 1.81)
Nosocomial sepsis	83 (24)	13 (25)	0.84	1.07	1.16 (0.59 to 2.31)

Table 9.7   *Flow cytometry results in HIV positive patients. Cell counts are means (SE)*

	Cell count ($\times 10^6$/litre)		
	HIV positive patients (24)	Normal	P value
T3	949 (86)	800–2800	>0.05
T4	425 (41)	550–1955	0.011
T8	549 (74)	250–1200	> 0.05
T4:T8 ratio	1.2 (0.2)	≥ 2.0	< 0.001
B4	186 (18)	245–850	0.001
NKH-1	170 (24)	25–360	> 0.05

Organ failure was more prevalent in HIV positive patients. Significant differences were found when cardiac, respiratory, and haematological system failures were compared (Table 9.5). Though there was no difference in the incidence of severe sepsis and nosocomial sepsis, septic shock was significantly more common in HIV positive patients (Table 9.6).

It was not possible to perform flow cytometry on all HIV positive patients. This was because either the patient died soon after admission or the request for testing came after the patient was discharged from the unit and could not be reached. Compared with normal values there was significant differences in T4 count, T4:T8 ratio, and B4 count (Table 9.7). The T4:T8 ratio was reversed and B4 count reduced in HIV positive patients.

Accidental disclosure of HIV status occurred in one instance as a result of a laboratory error. The researcher who became aware of the result did not divulge it to other staff and did not participate in management decisions regarding the patient. Data for this patient were collated by another member of the team, who was unaware of the result. As permitted by the protocol, the HIV status of five other patients became known to relevant staff members before patient discharge. One case involved a needle-stick injury to a staff member, and the remaining disclosures were in preparation for haemodialysis. In all instances management decisions and collation of patient data were by other, blinded researchers. Of all 402 patients tested, only three wished to be informed of their HIV status. No patient objected to having been included in the study without prior informed consent.

DISCUSSION

Mortality is the best measure of outcome of patients treated in an intensive care unit. Markers of morbidity may be subjective and are therefore less reliable end points. In this study there was no difference in intensive care unit or hospital mortality between HIV positive and HIV negative patients when results were adjusted for age (Table 9.3).

HIV positive patients were more prone to septic shock and organ failure, and we were therefore surprised that the duration of hospital stay and mortality were not increased. This finding is unlikely to have been the result of observer error because, except for one inadvertent disclosure, HIV results were not available until all other data were collated. Abnormalities in flow cytometry results may have been an important factor. HIV positive patients had low T4 counts whereas T8 counts were comparatively high. As a consequence the T4:T8 ratio was reduced but the total (T3) was not affected. The B4 count was also low. All these features are consistent with the latent phase of HIV infection.[9] Though the behaviour of these cell populations predicts clinical progression of HIV disease to AIDS,[10] to our knowledge its impact on intensive care unit patients admitted for non-HIV related disease has not been described. Conceivably the immune response to major trauma and sepsis is altered. The observation by Munoz et al. that HIV negative patients with sepsis and impaired macrophage responsiveness are more prone to subsequent sepsis[11] lends credence.

Immunological mechanisms have been postulated to play a major part in the pathogenesis of septic shock and multiple organ failure.[12,13] The immune response is complex and paradoxical, pro-inflammatory and anti-inflammatory responses occurring simultaneously and both being mediated by cytokines.[14] This has prompted the use of new drugs which alter the immune response in sepsis.[15,16] We therefore postulate that, though HIV positive patients have disturbances in immune function which make them more susceptible to septic shock and multiple organ failure, the inflammatory response is also altered such that there is no increase in mortality. The patients in this study were young, predominantly male, and admitted primarily after trauma or surgery. That no patient had AIDS concurs with Gilks's observation that the pattern of HIV infection in Africa differs from that in the developed world.[3] Non-HIV disease is far more prevalent in Africa, with rapid progression from seroconversion to HIV to

death from an AIDS defining condition.[3] Data relating to outcome in patients with AIDS cannot therefore be extrapolated to our patients. This emphasises the importance of describing the outcome in patients admitted to intensive care with non-HIV related disease.

Issue of Informed Consent

Decisions on initiating and terminating care for critically ill patients are difficult.[17] The unique nature of the AIDS epidemic in Africa,[3] the tremendous costs associated with advanced life support,[1] as well as the particular ethical considerations in patients with HIV infection[18] are compelling reasons for these decisions to be based on sound ethical principles and objective evidence of disease outcome. In view of the lack of clinical information in our patient population, the acquisition of objective data was imperative. A major ethical dilemma arose when the decision was made not to seek informed consent. This was thought to be essential, as patients who were likely to be at risk for HIV infection would also be inclined to refuse the study, which would seriously limit its value.

There were two consequences of the study. Firstly, patients were denied the option of being excluded and, secondly, they were at risk of having their HIV status disclosed. The first consideration was evaluated in terms of the potential benefit of the study to society as a whole. The consensus of the research team and the ethics committee was that the clinical implications of the study were enough to warrant denying patients the right of refusal. With respect to the second consequence, every effort was made in the design and execution of the study to ensure that indiscriminate disclosure of HIV results did not occur. To our knowledge HIV results were not disclosed except for study purposes and, furthermore, patient care was not influenced by HIV status.

There was no reason to suspect that the racial background of our patients would have any bearing on their outcome. Race as a demographic variable is considered only rarely in South Africa.[19] Our main criterion for denying patients admission to intensive care is futility. This study showed no significant difference in mortality between HIV positive and HIV negative patients. Though the incidence rates of septic shock and organ failure were higher, this did not influence mortality or duration of stay. We therefore conclude that, in our patient population, HIV sta-

> **Key messages**
>
> - HIV positive patients admitted to intensive care for diseases unrelated to their HIV status have a similar mortality and duration of stay when compared with HIV seronegative patients
> - The incidence of septic shock and multiple organ dysfunction is higher in HIV seropositive patients and needs further investigation
> - HIV status cannot be used to deny critically ill patients admission to intensive care
> - The HIV and AIDS epidemic raises unique ethical considerations that must be carefully addressed during clinical studies.

tus cannot be used as a criterion for denying patients admission to the intensive care unit. Our observations regarding septic shock and organ failure require regarding septic shock and organ failure require further evaluation.

ACKNOWLEDGEMENTS

Part of this study was presented at the 12th Annual Critical Care Congress of the South African Critical Care Society (1995) and at the 8th European Congress of Intensive Care Medicine. We thank Mrs QA Karim, Dr SSA Karim, Professor HM Coovadia, Dr EM Barker, Professor DJ Pudifin, Professor AN Smith, Professor J Lipman, and the Ethics Committee for Advice and Miss E Gouws for statistical analysis. We also thank Mr T Doorasamy, technicians in the Department of Virology, Mr H Benimadho, Mr N Bhimsan, and Mr R Loykisoonlal for technical help and Mrs A Pillay for secretarial work.

Funding: The University of Natal's research and travel committee and the Medical Research Council of South Africa.

REFERENCES

1. Cheng EY. Aids patients in the intensive care unit. *Curr Opin Anesthesiol* 1993; **6**: 309–14.
2. Rosen MJ, De Palo VA. Outcome of intensive care for patients with AIDS. *Crit Care Clin* 1993; **9**: 107–14.
3. Gilks CF. The clinical challenge of the HIV epidemic in the developing world. *Lancet* 1993; **342**: 1037–9.
4. Luce JM. Conflict over ethical principles in the intensive care unit. *Crit Care Med* 1992; **20**: 313–15.
5. 1993 revised classification system for HIV infection and expanded surveillance case definition for AIDS among adolescents and adults. *MMWR* 1992; **41**: 1–19.
6. Knaus WA, Draper EA, Wagner DP, Zimmerman JE. APACHE II: a severity of disease classification system. *Crit. Care Med* 1985; **13**: 818–29.
7. Kanus WA, Draper EA, Wagner DP, Zimmerman JE. Prognosis in acute organ-system failure. *Ann Surg* 1985; **202**: 685–93.
8. Members of the American College of Chest Physicians/Society of Critical Care Medicine Consensus Conference Committee. American College of Chest Physicians/Society of Critical Care Medicine consensus conference. Definitions for sepsis and organ failure and guidelines for the use of innovative therapies in sepsis. *Crit Care Med* 1992; **20**: 864–74.
9. Pantaleo G, Graziosi C, Fauci AS. The Immunopathogenesis of human immunodeficiency virus infection. *N Engl J Med* 1993; **328**: 327–34.
10. Stein DS, Korvick JA, Vermund SH. CD4+ lymphocyte cell enumeration for prediction of clinical course of human immunodeficiency virus disease: a review. *J Infect Dis* 1992; **165**: 352–63.
11. Munoz C, Carlet J, Fitting C, Misset B, Blériot J-P, Cavaillon J-M. Dysregulation of in vitro cytokine production by monocytes during sepsis. *J Clin Invest* 1991; **88**: 1747–54.
12. Baue AE. The horror autotoxicus and multiple-organ failure. *Arch Surg* 1992; **127**: 1451–62.
13. Goris RJ, te Boekhorst TP, Nuytinck JK, Gimbrère JS. Multiple organ failure: generalised autodestructive inflammation? *Arch Surg* 1985; **120**: 1109–15.
14. Lin RY, Astiz ME, Saxon JC, Saha DC, Rackow EC. Relationships between plasma cytokine concentrations and leukocyte functional antigen expression in patients with sepsis. *Crit Care Med* 1994; **22**: 1595–602.
15. Knaus WA, Harrell FE, Fisher CJ Jr, Wagner DP, Opal SM, Sadoff JC, et al. The clinical evaluation of new drugs for sepsis. A prospective study design based on survival analysis. *JAMA* 1993; **270**: 1233–41.
16. Dhainaut J-F, Tenaillon A, Le Tulzo Y, Schlemmer B, Solet JP, Wolff M, et al, Platelet-activating factor receptor antagonist BN 52021 in the treatment of severe sepsis: a randomized, double-blind, placebo-controlled, multicenter clinical trial. *Crit Care Med* 1994; **22**: 1720–8.
17. Ruark JE, Raffin TA. Initiating and withdrawing life support. Principles and practice in adult medicine. *N Engl J Med* 1988; **318**: 25–30.
18. Brown J, Sprung CL. Ethical considerations in the treatment of AIDS patients in the intensive care unit. *Crit Care Clin* 1993; **9**: 115–23.
19. Ellison GTH, De Wet T, Ijsselmuiden CB, Richter LM. Desegregating health statistics and health research in South Africa. *S Afr Med J* 1996; **86**: 1257–62.

Failing to seek patient consent to research is always wrong (commentary)*

Rajendra Kale and Laxmi-Kunj

Doing research without the patient's consent is unethical in any part of the world because it violates the fundamental right of the patient to autonomy and self determination. Bhagwanjee *et al.* violated that right because they feared that seeking consent of patients might jeopardise the scientific rigour of their study. They feared that patients at risk of HIV infection would be inclined to refuse the study, so limiting its value.

On what evidence did they base those fears? A separate study designed to find out the willingness of patients admitted to their unit to consent to HIV testing should have been their first step. Such a study might well have shown that their fears were unfounded and that a significant number of patients would have agreed to give informed consent. This would have allayed their fears and obviated their perceived need to do a study without consent. That such a result was likely is suggested by the findings of the "consent after the event" exercise that the authors carried out. The results of that exercise are difficult to interpret but, if true, suggest that most patients did not object to being forced into the study. They might well have consented to the study beforehand.

Were these patients at all aware of their right to informed consent before being included in research? The study was done in a large and busy hospital in South Africa that mainly looks after non-white, poor patients under developing country conditions – a legacy of apartheid. The question of informed consent is not uppermost in the minds of patients and their relatives who attend surgical emergencies in these hospitals. This places even greater responsibility on the researchers to make sure that their patients know their rights.

How many of the patients were white? The possibility that different ethical standards might still prevail in South Africa for patients of different races needs to be discussed. I wonder if such a study would have been done or even considered in a hospital serving a predominantly white population in South Africa.

The arguments that medical resources are limited and that the findings of the study would help to use resources better are valid – but only in justifying the need for the study. They are not enough to permit a study without informed consent.

Such a study would not have been allowed in Britain and other developed countries. But can ethical standards vary from one country to another? Ethical relativism argues that they can and do. But I think that doing research without consent is unethical everywhere. This is possibly more so in a developing county, where patients are likely to be ignorant of their rights.

The *BMJ* was wrong to accept this paper, with or without a commentary. Refusing to publish would not have amounted to ethical imperialism, and any fears that one group was imposing its ethical norms on others are unforced.

BMJ 1997; **314**: 1081–2.

Why we did not seek informed consent before testing patients for HIV (commentary)*

Satish Bhagwanjee, David JJ Muckart, Prakash M Jeena, Prushini Moodley

We agree completely with the Nuremberg code and the Helsinki declaration that informed consent is an essential prerequisite for medical research. However, we believe that there may be extraordinary circumstances when this right may be waived. We identify four crucial requirements that must be fulfilled before research without informed consent may be permitted.

REQUIREMENTS THAT MUST BE SATISFIED BEFORE RESEARCH WITHOUT CONSENT

1. It is impossible to obtain informed consent

Eighty five per cent of admissions to our unit are emergency cases. These patients cannot give informed consent because they are critically ill. A second option is to obtain consent from a relative. In our study this would have resulted in two possible scenarios. Firstly, if the patient survived, he or she could choose to be informed about the result of HIV testing and maintain the right to limited disclosure. But if the patient died the relative would have the right to know the result. This would be a serious breach of patient autonomy. Furthermore, such disclosure of results obtained in the course of research, when there was no risk of infection to the relative, would represent an unacceptable breach of patient confidentiality.[1] It was therefore not appropriate to seek consent from relatives. The third option was to obtain consent on discharge. This would have excluded all patients who died, which would have profoundly limited the value of the study.

2. The research is of sufficient importance that patients' right to informed consent may be waived

The problem of HIV and AIDS in South Africa has reached epidemic proportions.[2-4] By the end of 1992 over 300 000 people were infected.[5] In 1994 the figure was estimated to be 1.2 million.[6] Seroprevalence in the antenatal clinic at our hospital was 12% in 1992 and 23% in 1996 (AN Smith, personal communication). If the worst case scenario materialises, by 2010 it is estimated that 28–52% of all deaths will be related to HIV infection.[7] The impact of the epidemic on scarce intensive care resources is likely to be profound. Our 2000 bed hospital is served by 25 intensive care beds (16 in the surgical unit). Furthermore, our unit is the primary referral intensive care unit for the province of Kwazulu-Natal. As a consequence of excessive demand and our limited resources one fifth of all patients referred to our unit are denied admission. Hence given the extent of the HIV epidemic it was essential that any decisions regarding allocation of resources should be based on objective data and not subjective impression (the ethical principle of social justice). The study was therefore deemed to be of sufficient importance to waive patients' right to informed consent.

3. There must be unanimous agreement among appropriate individuals and groups that the aforementioned conclusions are valid

The exhaustive procedure followed in verifying the suitability of the protocol shows that we satisfied the third prerequisite – namely, that there must be unanimous agreement among appropriate individuals and groups about the importance of the research and the impracticability of obtaining consent. In order to pre-empt prejudice against HIV positive patients (and therefore prevent breach of two other principles of medical ethics – namely, beneficence and non-maleficence), and in view of the above considerations, it was deemed essential that a prospective blinded trial should be conducted. We consulted three clinical departments, two laboratory depart-

BMJ 1997; **314**: 1082–3.

ments, and two international AIDS experts. The institutional ethics committee appointed a subcommittee comprising Dr EM Barker (bioethicist and principal author of the Medical Association of South Africa Guidelines), Professor DJ Pudifin (clinician and AIDS expert), and one of us (SB) to investigate the most suitable approach. Eighteen months after initiation and deliberation among the various parties concerned the protocol was finally approved by the ethics committee.

4. Every attempt must be made to protect patients' interests after enrolment

Every effort was made to protect patients after enrolment. Their HIV status was not disclosed to staff members lest disclosure might result in discrimination. Patient care was never influenced by knowledge of HIV status. HIV status of patients was not disclosed to relatives, and the results were used exclusively for the study. On completion of the study patients' HIV test results were permanently removed from the hospital records.

CONCLUSION

HIV and AIDS raise unique ethical considerations, which are not limited to patient autonomy, but encompass the three other principles of medical ethics (beneficence, non-maleficence, and social justice). In adhering to these three principles we breached the first principle. Our decision to embark on this study was not taken lightly. On the contrary, every attempt was made to ensure that the decision was correct in the light of our unique circumstances.

REFERENCES

1. Medical Association of South Africa. Guidelines for the management of HIV/AIDS. *S Afr Med J* 1992; **82**(Suppl.): 1–16.
2. Ncayiyana DJ. HIV/AIDS – nagging questions. *S Afr Med J* 1995; **85**: 7.
3. McIntyre J. HIV/AIDS in South Africa – a relentless progression? *S Afr Med J* 1996; **86**: 27–8.
4. Gilks CF, Haran D. Coping with the impact of the HIV epidemic – the Hlabisa-Liverpool link. *S Afr Med J* 1996; **86**: 1077–88.
5. Kustner HGV, Swanevelder JP, Van Middelkoop A. National HIV surveillance – South Africa, 1990–1992. *S Afr Med J* 1994; **84**: 195–200.
6. Latest figures on HIV pregnancies. *S Afr Med J* 1995; **85**: 610–11.
7. Lee T, Esterhuyse T, Steinberg M, Schneider H. Demographic modelling of the HIV/AIDS epidemic on the Soweto population – results and health policy implications. *S Afr Med J* 1996; **86**: 60–3.

No simple and absolute ethical rule exists for every conceivable situation (commentary)*

YK Seedat

The obvious ethical problems posed by this study concern (a) the fact that all patients admitted to the intensive care unit over a 6-month period were included in the study without their knowledge or consent, and (b) the fact that blood samples obtained from all patients were tested for HIV infec-

*BMJ 1997; **314**: 1083–4.

tion without the consent of the patients, with the information that blood samples had been tested for the infection being given to patients only after the test had been done.

At first sight the decision to override the patients' right to full information, and to give or to refuse consent to inclusion and testing, seemed to all members of the research ethics committee to be so fundamentally at variance with the ethical principles governing research involving patients that it seemed impossible to give ethical approval for the study. However, during lengthy discussions with the investigators several considerations emerged.

Firstly, the information being sought by the investigators was clearly going to be of crucial importance to the community, not only in South Africa or in Africa as a whole but also worldwide. The importance of the study was perceived to be twofold. If it showed that a patient's HIV status significantly worsened his or her chances of a favourable outcome from intensive care – to a degree comparable to the poor prognosis associated with criteria already established for non-acceptance for admission to an intensive care unit – then the clinicians who have to make decisions on allocating the community's scarce intensive care resources would have to include HIV positivity among the criteria for non-acceptance. If, on the other hand, the study showed that HIV positivity *per se* did not adversely affect a patient's likelihood of a favourable outcome, then the current widespread tendency to include HIV positivity among the criteria for non-acceptance into intensive care facilities would become manifestly unjust. Such information gained from the study would be of life and death importance to the large and increasing numbers of people who are HIV positive.

Secondly, the study entailed no interventions of any sort different from those that are necessary and are carried out in standard intensive care. The blood samples that would be tested for HIV infection would be aliquots of samples taken for other necessary clinical purposes. Apart from the HIV testing, the study did not depart from normal standard of care and consisted essentially of analysis of data that would be recorded even if the study were not undertaken.

Thirdly, apart from the HIV testing, the "injury" that would be done to the patients as a result of not being given the opportunity to consent to or to refuse inclusion in the study was considered to be so small as to be virtually not appreciable and entirely analogous to the "injury" to patients whose hospital records are reviewed for retrospective research projects. Given the importance of the study, the failure to ask patients for permission to analyse data necessarily generated during their clinical care did not seem to be material.

Fourthly, testing the patients' blood for HIV infection without their consent and only informing them afterwards posed an important ethical dilemma. In considering this aspect of the study, the committee took into account several considerations. It agreed that there is no such thing in ethics – and particularly in the increasingly complex field of bioethics – as a simple and absolute ethical rule that must be observed in every conceivable situation. Virtually every ethical dilemma necessarily poses the problem of competing and conflicting ethical obligations. There are no absolutely satisfactory resolutions of ethical dilemmas, and the best that one can hope to achieve is to accord, with justice, preference to those ethical considerations (or "rules") that seem in the particular circumstances to be of preponderant weight.

The committee was also at pains to satisfy itself that the effective performance of the proposed study could not be achieved if any of the subjects were not to have their blood tested for HIV infection. Unless it could be shown, scientifically, that it was absolutely essential to include all admitted patients in the study, the committee would not have considered the proposed testing of blood without consent as ethical.

The committee was also strongly influenced by the fact that the results of the HIV tests would remain strictly confidential to only one investigator and that all potential linkage of the results of the tests to identifiable individuals was to be destroyed at the end of the study. The situation, as the committee saw it, was analogous to the anonymous and unlinked testing of attenders at antenatal and sexually transmitted disease clinics, for epidemiological purposes. This testing, to be of value, has to include all attenders, and for this reason consent to testing of aliquots of attenders' blood samples taken for other purposes is not obtained. This practice has ethical approval throughout the world, on the basis that the community's need for reliable epidemiological data outweighs by far the almost imperceptible injury done to the patient's autonomy. From a practical point of view, the clinic attender is in the same situation as he or she would have been if HIV testing had not been done at all. Similarly, for the patients in this study the end result was the same as it would have been if their blood samples had never been tested, with the sole difference that, if they so wished, they would be informed of the outcome of the test. Weighing the importance of the study in terms of the welfare of the community against the almost imperceptible injury that would be inflicted on patients, the committee was satisfied that the proposed method of obtaining complete data regarding the patients' HIV status was ethically acceptable.

In the outcome, it seems that the committee's view on the ethics of this study was vindicated by the fact that no patient expressed any objection to the fact that his or her blood had been tested in this fashion. Furthermore, the fact that only two patients elected to be informed of the result of the test is in keeping with the general reluctance of well people to undergo HIV testing and suggests that, if inclusion in the study depended on a patient's consent to HIV testing (even if effectively performed anonymously), then it is quite likely that the study would not have produced a reliable outcome.

10 · Journals should not publish research to which patients have not given fully informed consent – with three exceptions*

Len Doyal

Fifty years ago, the immorality of which clinicians are capable in the name of medical research was made clear at Nuremberg.[1] The code of research ethics which was articulated to judge them was uncompromising about the importance of informed consent in preventing such outrages against humanity from occurring again.[2] Volunteers competent to do so should choose whether or nor to participate in medical research after being given correct information about the

> "nature, purpose, and duration of the experiment; the method and means by which it is to be conducted; all inconveniences and hazards reasonably to be expected; and the effects upon his health or person which may possibly come from his participation in the experiment." Participants should not be subject to "force, fraud, deceit, duress … or coercion."[3]

It took almost 30 years for many medical researchers to accept the full implications of this doctrine of informed consent. The prevailing attitude during this period was that the Nuremberg code primarily applied to Nazis and similar fanatics.[4] Such optimism became quickly tarnished in the late 1960s and 1970s with the recognition that in the United States and the United Kingdom, for example, horrors continued to be inflicted on vulnerable groups in the name of medical progress. By the late 1980s it was obvious that this problem knew no national boundaries.[5]

As a result, the professional and legal regulation of medical research has been made more rigorous, with the right of volunteers to informed consent remaining at its heart.[5] Yet some now argue that

things have gone too far and that full disclosure of information to research subjects who are competent may not always be warranted.[6] Local research ethics committees have allowed research to proceed with variable standards of informed consent, and journals have published the results of studies where no consent was obtained.[7–10]

In this paper I oppose such moves through arguing that, with three exceptions, the principle of informed consent to participate in medical research should remain inviolate. The focus of discussion will be on competent patients who volunteer for either therapeutic or non-therapeutic research. No-one questions the strict right of healthy volunteers to informed consent. I will outline a draft editorial policy for medical journals for the rejection of research where informed consent has not been appropriately obtained. Interestingly, had it been adopted at least three papers would not have appeared in the *BMJ*.[8–10]

THE MORAL AND LEGAL IMPORTANCE OF INFORMED CONSENT

Patients who volunteer for medical research can face risks over and above those normally encountered in their everyday lives. The degree of such risks can often be known only after the research has been completed. Professional pressure can lead researchers to under-estimate inconvenience and hazard, misleading volunteers in the process.[11] Volunteers must have accurate and detailed information about potential risks in order to protect themselves. Equally, for them to weigh up their personal willingness to face such hazards against whatever motivations they might

*BMJ 1997; **314**: 1107–11.

have for participation, volunteers must also have adequate information about goals, methods, and possible benefits of the research.

To deny volunteers such information is a clear breach of their moral rights. Our abilities to deliberate, to choose, and to plan for the future are the focus of the dignity and respect that we associate with being an autonomous person capable of participation in civic life. Such respect is now widely regarded as essential for good medical care and should dominate the practice of medical research.[12] This is especially important in the case of volunteers who are patients and who, despite their vulnerability, often accept extra inconvenience and risk in the public interest, sometimes with no potential benefit to themselves.

This moral emphasis on informed consent is reflected by the law.[13] Legally, a battery is committed if volunteers who participate in medical research are touched without being provided with adequate information about what the researchers propose to do and why. The specific circumstances under which different interventions under investigation will be offered should also be communicated (for example, whether the participants will be randomised). Researchers will be negligent if they do not adhere to their professional duty to communicate adequate information about risks. Here the standard of disclosure is stronger than for ordinary treatment. Prudent researchers should warn volunteers of risks in the detail that any "reasonable person" would want, and researchers should recognise and attempt to satisfy specific informational needs of individual volunteers (such as those relating to language or employment).

In short, unless they respect the right of volunteers to informed consent, researchers should be morally and, where possible, legally censured.

ARGUMENTS AGAINST INFORMED CONSENT

Despite the preceding arguments, some researchers maintain that there is now too much emphasis on informed consent for patient volunteers for medical research. Three reasons are usually given, although in practice they are often combined.

Firstly, patient volunteers might be distressed by detailed information about aims, methods, and risks.[14] To weigh up the balance of potential benefits over risks will entail a good understanding of both, and patients may discover for the first time how poor their prognosis really is. Further, patients may realise the full implications of randomisation – that neither they nor their doctor will know which intervention they will receive and that their doctor does not know what the best treatment is. Such patients may not want full disclosure of information but still wish to be included in trials thought by their clinicians to be in their best interests. To force unwanted information on them is needlessly cruel, may compromise recovery, and may keep patients from entering trials in sufficient numbers to make such trials possible.[15] Clinical researchers, therefore, should have more discretion about how much detail to communicate.

Secondly, while informed consent may be necessary for studies where there are considerable risks, it does not follow that it should be obtained for research where invasiveness and risks are negligible. This is especially so if the requirement for informed consent might jeopardise methodological rigour.[16] For example, knowledge of the aims of some research might bias responses to related therapies or questionnaires. Awareness of randomisation – including the possibility of inclusion in the placebo arm of an investigation – can equally confound results through biasing the attitudes and behaviour of volunteers.[17] If the research is worth doing and the risks are minimal, then it is surely being obsessive to continue to insist on full disclosure of information.

Thirdly, the interests of the public in medical progress will be undermined by too much emphasis on the rights of individuals. Existing effective clinical interventions are based on the willingness of previous patient volunteers to participate in medical research. Thus it can be argued that patients receiving such care have a duty to promote further research for future generations. Yet we know that in the face of full disclosure of aims, methods, and risks of research, patients might not do their duty to serve the public interest – sometimes making the research impossible.[18] A more limited disclosure of information about the research might encourage more patients to volunteer.

It follows from these reasons that local research ethics committees should implement the clause in the Helsinki Declaration that states that there may be circumstances in which informed consent is not required.[19] Similarly, journals should publish the results of medical research approved by committees adopting this lower standard of disclosure.

WHY THESE ARGUMENTS SHOULD BE REJECTED

Each of these arguments is flawed. Potential for distress is not a sufficient reason to deny patient volunteers full disclosure of information. Such arguments are extensions of a tired and discredited paternalism. If volunteers discover that information has been withheld, their distress and sense of betrayal may be far greater than that engendered by learning the truth.[20] This will particularly be so if participation has interfered with the achievement of other personal goals about which the researchers knew nothing. In any case, surveys have indicated that in ordinary therapeutic situations patients – even those who are terminally ill – want accurate information and are not necessarily upset by it. There is no reason to believe that this same desire does not apply all the more so to participants in medical research.[21–23]

Anticipated negligibility of risks does nothing to abate the right of patient volunteers to information about them. An acceptable hazard for one may be rejected by another.[24] Even minimally risky interventions (venepuncture and questionnaires, for example) can have unwanted side effects (bruising and depression). Equally, it is sometimes argued that minimal risks might justify the randomisation of patient volunteers without their consent (for example, in studies where one group is unknowingly used as a control). Yet some patients have been outraged to discover that they were used in a trial without their knowledge.[25] The fact that they faced small risks in the process was not the point. Aside from the potential distress to volunteers who discover that they were denied informed consent, such denial also jeopardises the reputation of the researcher, along with the enterprise of medical research. If patients feel that they might be inadequately informed, this fact in itself may dissuade them from participating in research.[26] The moral price of keeping volunteers in ignorance is too high and against the public interest.

It is unlikely that any of these arguments against informed consent would be taken seriously unless they were linked to the further belief that it is acceptable to compromise individual rights if the public interest demands it. Such arguments amount to justifying exploitation of individuals and ignore the objective harm that is inflicted upon them by disrespect for their autonomy. Harm of this kind should not be equated with physical damage or emotional distress, and is therefore not affected by the level of risk of either. Rather it is an attack on human dignity: the harm is to the moral integrity of the uninformed volunteer.[27] Accepting the unconscionability of inflicting such harm in the public interest may well mean that some potentially fruitful medical research cannot be done because of the problem of under-recruitment. So be it; this is the price we pay for living in a society that is morally worth preserving, one where we treat each other with respect and where we take human rights seriously.

Despite the discretion offered by the Helsinki Declaration to do otherwise, research ethics committees should be rigid in their application of the principle of informed consent to competent patients asked to participate actively in research.[19] They should not approve research proposals that breach it, and journals should not publish the results of such research, even if it has been so approved.

WHEN INFORMED CONSENT IS NOT NECESSARY

The demand thus far has been that competent patients should be protected from exploitation by being allowed to evaluate for themselves whether or not participation is consistent with their best interests. Sometimes, however, research that is of potential importance should be permitted without the requirement of informed consent. Generally speaking, this will be either when patients are unable to provide consent because of their incompetence or when, for practical reasons, consent is difficult or impossible to obtain. Research without informed consent should be allowed to proceed and be published only in three circumstances.

Incompetence to Give Informed Consent

Firstly, some categories of patient volunteers will be incompetent to give informed consent, e.g. young and immature children, patients with learning disabilities, and unconscious or semiconscious patients in intensive care or accident and emergency.[28–31] To exclude them from participation in research specific to their conditions and treatments might deprive both them and others of potential benefit. To allow such research is not an affront to their human dignity, if they really are incompetent to provide informed consent. We have no moral obligation to respect others in ways that are practically impossible. However, the levels of autonomy that patients who are thus incompetent do possess should still be respected (for example, if they resist participation, then it should not be forced), and their vulnerability demands that they should be protected from harm (for example, if the research can be done on a less vulnerable group then it should be). Local research ethics committees should have the discretion to approve both therapeutic and non-therapeutic research involving incompetent patients, and journals should have the discretion to publish the results under certain conditions[32]:

- There are important potential benefits from the research.
- The research cannot be completed with patients or healthy volunteers who are able to provide informed consent.
- Participation in therapeutic research will entail risks which are minimal in relation to the standard available treatment. For non-therapeutic research, this level should not exceed that associated with everyday life or minimally invasive therapeutic interventions.
- Informed consent in research with incompetent children will always be obtained from someone with parental authority.
- Informed "assent" for incompetent adults will ordinarily be sought from appropriate advocates (such as relatives), provided with the same information that would have been given to the patient if competent.
- Such "assent" may not be required for therapeutic research with adults when it is impossible to obtain and when there is minimal risk, again, by comparison with standard available treatment (for example, research in intensive care and in accident and emergency medicine).
- The purpose and methods of the research are explained after its completion to participants who were unable to consent to it but then regained their competence to do so. This does not amount to retrospective consent.

Conditions on Use of Medical Records

Secondly, we have seen that informed consent should always be obtained from competent patients who are actively involved in medical research, where they either receive or are denied some form of intervention under investigation. However, some research occurs without such involvement and entails only the use of medical records. Normally, patients should give their explicit consent for their records to be accessed for this purpose; they should have received appropriate information about who will use them and why and about how confidentiality will be maintained. Yet suppose the research is epidemiological, patients might benefit from it in the long term, but for practical reasons informed consent cannot be obtained. Also assume that no further consequences should follow for such patients, e.g. that there is no intent to ask the patient to receive or be denied any intervention as a result of the research. In spite of the arguments already outlined in favour of informed consent, should we allow this kind of research to proceed without it?[33]

The moral balance here is a fine one. If such research proceeds, there is little doubt that, through not obtaining consent, a moral wrong is being done. The issue is the degree of this wrong in light of the potential benefit which can follow for the patient, provided that confidentiality is maintained and no further active involvement is expected. Clearly, the public interest will also be served. This moral tension will be minimised through better informing patients about the importance of medical research and the desirability at times for their records to be accessed by researchers.[34] They should also be reassured about confidentiality and given the opportunity to decline. Yet these steps have not widely been taken. The most that can be said for now is that the moral balance favours local research ethics committees having the discretion to approve such research, and journals to publish the findings. There are minimal conditions.[35–36]

- Access to the clinical record is essential for the completion of the research and consent is not practicable.
- The research is of sufficient merit.
- The research pertains to some future planning, preventive, or therapeutic initiative that may benefit the patients whose records are studied.
- Where possible, identifiers have been removed from the parts of the record to which researchers have access; where not, patients will not be identifiable when the results are made public.
- It is not anticipated that contact will be made with the patients as a result of research finding.
- Access is restricted to specific categories of information that have been approved by the local research ethics committee.

- Permission is obtained from the clinician responsible for the patient's care and, depending on the type of record and access concerned, the person responsible for its administration.
- Researchers who are non-clinicians are formally instructed about their duty of confidentiality. They must also have a clinical supervisor, who formally accepts professional responsibility for any breach of confidentiality that may occur.

Stored Tissue from Anonymous Donors

The third exception where research is permissible without informed consent concerns the use of human tissue that is the byproduct of surgical intervention or other stored clinical material (for example, frozen serum). Such tissue or materials may have been recently removed and stored, or archived for considerable time. Where the link between the identity of patients and their stored material is broken, research may be conducted without further explicit consent, always assuming that it conforms to other moral principles governing good research.[37] Where the identity of the patient might become known to the researcher, the local research ethics committee must review and agree the research. Here again, the moral balance is a delicate one.[38] Consent need not necessarily be obtained, provided that the committee is satisfied that patients (if alive) might at some time derive benefit from the research under consideration, that there is no intent to further involve them in the research, and that adequate standards of confidentiality will be maintained. In general, similar rules apply as have been outlined above on the use of clinical records without consent, and journals should only publish accordingly.

This third exception does not apply to research into the genetic causes of or predispositions to disease, where research materials have not been strictly anonymised and where there is any possibility of further patient contact. Here informed consent should always be obtained and counselling offered to people who are potential sources of such materials. If not, the results of such studies should not be published.[39]

CONCLUSION

The suffering and indignity that some medical research has visited upon unsuspecting and vulnerable patients must never be allowed to happen again. To ignore the lessons of the past through not taking the right of informed consent seriously is to insult the memory of those who paid such an unacceptably high price in the name of medical progress. This paper has argued that local research ethics committees and professional and academic journals like the *BMJ* should not approve or publish research which violates this right. Three exceptions have been outlined. Further work is required, however, to clarify the moral foundations of these exceptions, including the nature and scope of the duty of individuals to act in the public interest. For now, the reasonably strict interpretation of the principle of informed consent developed here should be seen to be consistent with such interest even if this means that some potentially worthwhile research is not allowed to proceed or be published. In the words of Hans Jonas:

> Society would indeed be threatened by the erosion of those moral values whose loss, possibly caused by too ruthless a pursuit of scientific progress, would make its most dazzling triumphs not worth having.[30, 40]

ACKNOWLEDGEMENTS

I thank Lesley Doyal, Claire Foster, Richard Nicholson, Daniel Wilsher, and Jennian Geddes.

REFERENCES

1. Leaning J. War crimes and medical science. *BMJ* 1996; **313**: 1413–15.
2. Appelbaum PS, Lidz CW, Meisel A. *Informed consent: legal theory and clinical practice*. New York: Oxford University Press, 1987, p. 212.
3. Nuremberg Code. *BMJ* 1996; **313**: 1448.
4. Rothman DJ. Ethics and human experimentation: Henry Beecher revisited. *N Engl J Med* 1987; **317**: 1195–9.
5. McNeill PM. *The ethics and politics of human experimentation*. Cambridge: Cambridge University Press, 1993, pp. 17–36, 53–115.
6. Tobias JS, Houghton J. Is informed consent essential for all chemotherapy studies? *Eur J Cancer* 1994; **30A**: 907–10.
7. Harries HJ, Fentem PGH, Tuxworth W, Hoinville GW. Local research ethics committees. *J R Coll Physicians* 1994; **28**:150–4.
8. McArdle JMC, George WD, McArdle CS, *et al.* Psychological support for patients undergoing breast cancer surgery: a randomised study. *BMJ* 1996; **312**: 813–17.

9. Dennis M, O'Rourke S, Slattery J, Staniforth T, Warlow C. Evaluation of a stroke family care worker: results of a randomised controlled trial. *BMJ* 1997; **314**: 1071–6.

10. Bhagwanjee S, Muckart D, Jenna PM, Moodley P. Does HIV status influence the outcome of patients admitted to a surgical intensive care unit? *BMJ* 1997; **314**: 1077–81.

11. Evans D, Evans M. *A decent proposal–ethical review of clinical research*. Chichester: Wiley, 1996, pp. 62–7.

12. Doyal L. Needs, rights and the moral duties of clinicians. In: Gillon R, ed. *Principles of health care ethics*. Chichester: Wiley, 1994, pp. 217–30.

13. Kennedy I, Grubb A. *Medical law – texts and materials*. London: Butterworths, 1994, pp. 1042–67.

14. Tobias J, Souhami R. Fully informed consent can be needlessly cruel. *BMJ* 1993; **307**: 1199–201.

15. Collins R, Doll R, Peto R. Ethics of clinical trials. In: Williams CJ, ed. *Introducing new treatments for cancer: practical, ethical and legal problems*. New York: Wiley, 1992, pp. 49–65.

16. Kanis J, Bergmann J. Full consent may bias outcome of trials. *BMJ* 1993; **307**: 1497.

17. Barer D. Patients' preferences and randomised trials. *Lancet* 1994; **344**: 688.

18. Baum M. The ethics of randomised controlled trials. *Eur J Surg Oncol* 1995; **21**: 136–7.

19. Helsinki Declaraction. *BMJ* 1996; **313**: 1448.

20. Bok S. *Lying*. Brighton, Sussex: Harvester, 1978.

21. Fallowfield L, Ford S. Lewis S. Information preferences of patients with cancer. *Lancet* 1994; **344**: 1576.

22. Kerrigan DD, Thevasagayam RS, Woods TO *et al.* Who's afraid of informed consent. *BMJ* 1993; **306**: 298–300.

23. Deber R. Physicians in health care management. 7. The patient-physician partnership: changing roles and the desire for information. *Can Med Assoc J* 1994; **151**: 171–6.

24. Martin D, Meslin E, Kohut N, Singer P. The incommensurability of research risks and benefits: practical help for research ethics committees. *IRB* 1995 March-April, pp. 8–10.

25. Research without consent continues in the UK. *Bull Inst Med Ethics* 1988; **40**: 1315.

26. Thornton HM. Breast cancer trials: a patient's viewpoint. *Lancet* 1992; **339**: 44–5.

27. Crisp R. Medical negligence, assault, informed consent and autonomy. *J Law Society* 1990; **17**: 77–89.

28. Mason JK, McCall Smith RA. *Law and medical ethics*. London: Butterworths, 1994, pp. 369–74.

29. Fulford K, Howse K. Ethics of research with psychiatric patients: principles, problems and the primary responsibilities of researchers. *J Med Ethics* 1993; **19**: 85–91.

30. Dresser R. Mentally disabled research subjects: the enduring policy issues. *JAMA* 1996; **276**: 67–72.

31. Biros M, Lewis R, Olson CM, Runge JW, Cummins RO, Fost N. Informed consent in emergency research: consensus statement from the coalition conference of acute resuscitation and critical care researchers. *JAMA* 1995; **273** 1283–7.

32. Royal College of Physicians. *Guidelines on the practice of ethics committees in medical research involving ethics committees*. London: RCP, 1996.

33. Wald N, Law M, Meade T, Miller G, Alberman E, Dickenson J. User of personal medical records for research purposes. *BMJ* 1994; **309**: 1422–4.

34. Baum M. New approach for recruitment into randomised controlled trials. *Lancet* 1993; **341**: 812–14.

35. East London and City Health Authority. *Guidelines for the completion of application forms–research ethics committee*. London: ELCHA, 1996.

36. Working Group to the Royal College of Physicians Committee on Ethical Issues in Medicine. Independent ethical review of studies involving medical records. *J R Coll Physicians* 1994; **28**: 439–43.

37. Nuffield Council on Bioethics. *Human tissue–ethical and legal issues*. London: Nuffield Foundation, 1995, pp. 23–9. 39–54.

38. Clayton EW, Steinberg KW, Khoury MJ, Thomson E, Andrews L, Ellis Khan MJ, *et al.* Informed consent for genetic research on stored tissue sample. *JAMA* 1995; **242**: 1786–92.

39. Nuffield Council on Bioethics. *Genetic screening–ethical issues*. London: Nuffield Foundation, 1993, pp. 29–40.

40. Jonas H. Philosophical reflections on experimenting with human subjects. In: Freund PA, ed. *Experimentation with human subjects*. New York: George Braziller, 1970, pp. 1–31.

11 · BMJ's present policy (sometimes approving research in which patients have not given fully informed consent) is wholly correct*

Jeffrey S Tobias

Few if any issues engender such passionate – often acrimonious – disagreement among clinicians, ethicists, statisticians, and representatives of patient groups as does the continuing debate about informed consent and clinical research trials. In the blue corner: clinicians and biostatisticians keen to "move the field forward," so to speak, and answer as quickly as possible the research question currently under investigation. In the red corner ... just about everyone else. Anyone left in the centre? Only the hapless referee, in this case the somewhat perplexed journal, whose editorial board – constantly hectored from both sides – somehow has to give all parties a decent airing and ensure fair play.

Those arguing in favour of fully informed consent as an inviolable rule (except, perhaps, in very special circumstances) often point out the essential, non-negotiable nature of a patient's right to autonomy and self-determination. Quite rightly they remind clinicians that patients now wish to participate in decisions concerning their own management, to a far greater degree than ever before. Indeed, over the past decade, the move towards fully informed consent for all participants in clinical trials has become increasingly difficult to resist and is now formalised in various guidelines.[1] However, neither lawyers, ethicists, nor medical scientists have so far agreed precisely what this term actually means, although it is generally held to imply a full declaration of the competing treatment options for any patient participating in a clinical research study particularly one which involves randomisation between two or more treatment options. Together with the full description of treatments, there should be an explanation of the

*BMJ 1997; **314**: 1111–14.

possible side effects of both new and standard therapies, and a clear explanation that the "choice" of treatment is no choice at all – in the conventional sense – but is no more than a computerised flip of the coin.

Most clinicians recognise that the anxious patient sitting opposite them in the consulting room requires both reassurance and a clear exposition of what needs to be done to provide a cure.[2] However, an increasing degree of frankness on the part of the doctor, for the most part laudable and constructive, may also cause considerable distress to patients who would prefer to be directed rather than participate as an equal partner. For clinicians who genuinely believe in evidence-based medicine and recognise the central role of randomised trials, it is the need for explaining the randomisation concept, coupled with a detailed account of the shortcomings of standard treatment, that jointly symbolise the difficulty of the task: how to put these points across to a frightened patient in a highly charged atmosphere, with limited time available yet so much ground to cover and so many questions to answer. As Souhami and I have previously pointed out, many doctors repeatedly faced with this difficult task will not surprisingly decide that for them the game is simply not worth the candle.[2] Hence the lamentable record in Britain of poor patient recruitment even where excellent clinical trials are on offer. British clinicians certainly don't seem to be signed up to the proud Harvard Medical School slogan, "Clinical research is an obligation not an option."

Doctors' concerns about their patients' anxieties in these circumstances were supported by the findings of an Australian study that compared two methods of seeking consent for clinical trials of different standard treatments for cancer: an individual approach at the discretion of each doctor, or a policy of total disclosure of relevant information given both verbally and in writing.[3] This study found that, although patients having total disclosure became more knowledgeable about their illness and treatment, and about the research aspects of what was proposed, these same participants were less willing to enter as subjects for the trial and had a significantly higher anxiety score. As many clinicians had expected, there are clearly trade-offs to be made in the amount of information patients are given before consenting to studies, at least in the field of cancer. Detailed information, given indiscriminately, resulted in a more knowledgeable yet more reluctant and anxious patient. What is more, the ethical position of clinicians who decide, for whatever reason, not to inform patients about appropriate clinical trials for their particular condition, has increasingly – and rightly – been questioned.[4]

CONCERNS FOR PATIENTS' RIGHTS

Although ethicists, counsellors, and other commentators argue their case – as research clinicians do – with the best possible intentions and concerns for patients' rights to information (and retention of as much control as possible in the face of serious illness), an atmosphere of mistrust has clearly developed. For example, the *BMJ* published a randomised study of psychological support for patients undergoing breast cancer, in which they were randomised (without informed consent) to receive routine care from ward staff, or with interventional support from a breast care nurse, a voluntary organisation, or both.[5] Yet after publication of the paper, one distinguished member of the journal's editorial board felt moved to write that "the hospital ethics committee was surely at fault in allowing the research to proceed in contravention of the Nuremberg code" and even complained at the fact that two of the authors of the study were related.[6] The authors of the study were clearly concerned to assess the potential benefits of an expensive and labour-intensive form of intervention, and the journal felt the paper important enough to publish with a commentary regarding the ethics of clinical research without patient consent.[7] The letters to the editor, however, were heated and even produced friction among the trialists, with a published reply from one of them as dissenting author.[8]

In my view, the origins of this mistrust stem largely from a single source of disagreement: the passionate belief of those who insist that the individual patient in the consulting room should be the sole focus of concern for the doctor, and those who feel – and are prepared to say publicly – that they owe a duty not only to the patient sitting opposite but also to society at large, which, with an equally urgent passion, has charged us to get on in all haste and find that cure. No point in pinning one's colour firmly to the fence: I'm for the latter group. This does not in any sense mean that the clinical trial is more important than the patient sitting so anxiously in the waiting room. A kind and caring approach to patients should always be the *sine qua non* of the doctor–patient relationship, as Sally Magnusson reminded us even when (especially when) there is little that can be done.[9]

A proper respect for the patient's individual circumstances inevitably leads the research clinician to a varied set of approaches. The highly informed, articulate 39-year-old journalist with a small but operable node positive breast cancer may be a candidate for several randomised trials, and is likely to need a full, frank discussion with total disclosure of not only all the available treatment choices, but also the limitations of current treatment. In the enthusiasm to engage this intelligent and questioning patient in a proper dialogue, the chief danger generally lies in forgetting that above all she is a patient and, instead, falling into the trap of conducting a two-way research seminar rather than a kindly and courteous consultation. On the other hand, and often at the other extreme of the social spectrum, the patient so characteristic of the clientele in a head and neck cancer clinic is much more likely to be male, older, far less educated, an enthusiastic consumer of cigarettes and alcohol: in short, someone quite unused to being "in control" of his own circumstances. Such patients are often homeless or struggling in an inner city hostel to retain what they can of their dignity and self-respect. A cool and dispassionate discussion about the current research study (at present a trial essentially addressing the question of whether or not to offer chemotherapy in addition to radical surgery or radiotherapy) may be highly inappropriate since it pays no attention to the circumstances and culture – and, dare I say it, the need – of this particular patient. Indeed, as Brewin has pointed out, it may be better to consider that doctors participating in randomised treatment trials should not be thought of as research workers at all (in the normal sense of the word "research") but simply as clinicians with an ethical duty to their patients "not to go on giving them treatments without doing everything possible to assess their true worth."[10]

PRACTICAL DIFFICULTIES WITH INFORMED CONSENT

Quite apart from the difficulty with randomisation – such an elegant, reliable, sophisticated concept to the research clinician, but so brutal and harsh from the patient's viewpoint – it is the nearness of the consent discussion to the diagnosis which causes greatest concern, together with the patient's perception of the intensity of the threat. Imagine yourself (this is often worth doing: after all, we're all of us either patients or potential patients) in the shoes of the thousands of patients taken each year to hospital with severe chest pain and acutely aware that this could be a fatal heart attack. We now know (through well conducted randomised clinical controlled trials, of course) that clotbusting drugs such as streptokinase play a valuable part in recovery; but would you really wish at this moment of crisis to be faced with a medical registrar keen to treat you properly but equally aware of the need to gain your informed consent before randomising you to one or other of the appropriate treatments? It's not that you're no longer competent to take it all in, but simply that there are likely to be other concerns on your mind – to say nothing of the need to feel full confidence both in the judgment and technical competence of those looking after you.

As Collins and others have pointed out, at the time when the key studies addressing this issue were taking place, the differing ethical requirements (relatively low key in the United Kingdom but far tougher and with more constraint in the United States) led to a greatly differing recruitment rate (6000 patients from Britain compared with 400 from the United States despite an approximately equivalent degree of apparent interest by cardiologists in the two countries).[11] In turn this led to a compelling statistic: if the United States had recruited as fast as Britain then the trial would have ended 6 months earlier, and since the eventual results transformed medical practice (improving the treatment of several hundred thousands of patients a year worldwide), that 6-month delay meant about 10 000 unnecessary deaths "directly due to whatever it was that slowed

recruitment" in the United States. It should at least be a matter of some concern when what is judged ethical in one civilised society is dealt with so differently in another.

Ah yes, the proponents of universal informed consent might reply, this is just one of those "special circumstances" that we all agree should be exempt from the usual rules. How then might we go on to define these circumstances further? I have previously tried to divide or classify studies in oncological practice (at least those involving studies of new types of chemotherapy) into those which might or might not require fully informed consent.[12] As others in similar or analogous situations have discovered, it is not always easy to recognise the differing circumstances that might demand full, partial, or non-disclosure when the study in question is randomised.[13]

In the case of cancer trials, highly refined studies investigating technical differences between the two arms of treatment may be reasonably straightforward, in the sense that the patient will realise that the difference between the treatments represents only a relatively minor point of detail – not too alarming. On the other hand, where the treatment options are startlingly different, the situation is altogether more charged. It can be extremely unnerving to discuss, for example, the possible use of chemotherapy in cancers, such as those of the cervix or head and neck, in which we don't yet know for sure whether such treatment is genuinely valuable or simply meddlesome; with full disclosure of options, one finds oneself explaining carefully the pros and cons of the new treatment, then randomising half the patients to the control (the current "best buy") treatment, to be met later with a disappointed patient who often feels "let down" by the loss of perceived benefit from the newer treatment (chemotherapy), which, naturally enough, in previous discussion had been described as "promising." This often leads the doctor towards a rather shabby display of back pedalling in which the possible advantages of the chemotherapy are "talked down" and perhaps the side effects "talked up."[14]

Still more difficult were the studies undertaken a few years ago to try to establish whether or not mastectomy for breast cancer – the traditional treatment during the first half of this century, hallowed by tradition but never validated by science – was tested for the first time against less mutilating surgical alternatives. The outcome of these studies, showing no clear superiority for the traditional approach,[15] has proved hugely influential; yet it is hard to envisage how a strict and honest adherence to principles of fully informed consent could have been possible. I don't know about the American studies, but it certainly proved impossible in Britain. Although it was described as "the breast cancer trial that everybody needs but nobody wants,"[16] the Cancer Research Campaign, which supported and paid for the study, had to accept that recruitment was impossibly slow as a result of the disinclination of even the most committed trialists to put their patients through the rigours of informed consent.

Yet partial disclosure[17] or disclosure of the facts of the randomised study only to some (usually half: those in the "new treatment" arm) of the participants, is clearly regarded as an ethical minefield, making it unattractive to many clinical researchers and almost all health ethicists. Although it protects the right of patients not to be allocated novel treatments that are not yet fully established (and might never be), and ensures reasonable recruitment for clinical studies, it is generally rejected by hardliners as unethical since it denies the right to autonomy and self determination to each and every patient in the study – even though carrying the obvious and humane advantage of sparing all the patients treated to the best of current standards (the control arm) the anxiety of knowing that further improvements or refinements in their treatment are still urgently required. In my view, these benefits represent substantial gains for the individuals concerned and for any group of patients with the same illness, since valuable academic information might well flow from the study.

Perhaps a still more helpful approach would be for patients to be informed at the outset of their treatment that several clinical and laboratory studies (some randomised, some not) might be in progress during their illness; might they be prepared to offer "blanket" approval here and now, accepting that the doctor would always act in good faith and be prepared to explain further any unconventional or novel treatment, if required, at any future point? In childhood leukaemia, for example, it is already commonplace for pretreatment blood samples to be stored and used later for laboratory tests not available when the sample was obtained. I greatly dislike the current trend towards ownership and commercial exploitation of medical samples – blood, tissues, cell lines – and admire the altruism behind this type of donorship. Shouldn't medical material be treated just as a personal letter might be after it has been posted through the letterbox slot – no longer strict-

ly yours, even though you created its content in the first place? The posting is best viewed as a consignment to a higher authority. Once again, Brewin has provided an elegant and clear-headed argument designed to protect patients and at the same time allow sensible research studies to be conducted without unnecessary constraint:

"The idea that the mere fact of randomisation always requires special informed consent – with all its disadvantages and potential for causing misconception and anxiety – is surely illogical. A doctor in his normal practice, giving treatment without randomisation, is trusted to choose from several options, even though there may be no way that he can be sure which is best. Why should we not also trust a doctor who submits such options to randomisation, while taking full responsibility for the suitability of each? Are the two situations really so different?"[18]

Buried in the quotation is that small but compelling word "trust." Not really a word at all: a concept, a philosophy. Somewhat outmoded, certainly unfashionable. Yet most patients, it seems, still trust their doctors; and for their part, most doctors are well aware of the responsibilities that the trusting patient-as-supplicant brings to them. The correspondence pages of this journal are fine and lofty places to discuss these issues in a detached and intellectual manner – but do they approximate closely enough to the demands of the real world, in which the doctor must somehow juggle the multiple responsibilities of expert, humane, and above all respectful support for the patient in his consulting room with the wider healthcare concerns and requirements of society as a whole?

REFERENCES

1. Royal College of Physicians. *Guidelines on the practice of ethics committees in medical research involving human subjects*. 2nd edn. London: RCP, 1990.
2. Tobias JS, Souhami RL. Fully informed consent can be needlessly cruel. *BMJ* 1993; **307**: 119–20.
3. Simes RJ, Tattersall MHN, Coates AS, Raghavan D, Solomon HJ, Smartt H. Randomised comparison of procedures for obtaining informed consent in clinical trial of treatment for cancer. *BMJ* 1986; **293**: 1065–8.
4. Segelov E, Tattersall MHN, Coates AS. Redressing the balance – the ethics of not entering an eligible patient on a randomised clinical trial. *Ann Oncol* 1992; **3**: 103–5.
5. McArdle JMC, George WD, McArdle CS, *et al.* Psychological support for patients undergoing breast

cancer surgery: a randomised study. *BMJ* 1996; **312**: 813–17.

6. Goodare H. Patients' consent should have been sought. *BMJ* 1996; **313**: 361.

7. Foster C. Commentary: ethics of clinical research without patients' consent. *BMJ* 1996; **312**: 817.

8. Moodie AR. Reply from dissenting author. *BMJ* 1996; **313**: 362.

9. Magnusson S. Oh, for a little humanity, *BMJ* 1996; **313**: 1601–3.

10. Brewin TB. Truth, trust, paternalism. *Lancet* 1985; **ii**: 490–2.

11. Collins R, Doll R, Peto R. Ethics of clinical trials. In: Williams CJ, ed. *Introducing new treatments of cancer: practical ethical and legal problems*. Chichester: Wiley, 1992, pp. 49–65.

12. Tobias JS, Houghton J. Is informed consent essential for all chemotherapy studies? *Eur J Cancer* 1994; **30A**: 897–9.

13. Bhagwanjee S, Muckart DJJ, Jeena PM, Moodley P. Does HIV status influence the outcome of patients admitted to a surgical intensive care unit? A prospective double blind study. *BMJ* 1997; **314**: 1077–81.

14. Tobias JS. Informed consent and controlled trials. *Lancet* 1988; **ii**: 1194.

15. Fisher B, Bauer M, Margolese R *et al.* Five year results of a randomised clinical trial comparing total mastectomy and segmental mastectomy with or without radiation in the treatment of breast cancer. *N Engl J Med* 1985; **312**: 665–71.

16. Le Fanu J. The breast cancer trial that nobody wants but everybody needs. *Med News* 1983; **12**: 30–1.

17. Zelen M. A new design for randomised clinical trials. *N Engl J Med* 1979; **300**: 1242–5.

18. Brewin TB. Consent to randomised treatment. *Lancet* 1982; **ii**: 919–22.

12 · Responses to Chapters 7–11: letters to the *BMJ*

Informed consent: one standard for research, another for clinical practice*

Richard Smith

The *BMJ* is written for reading now, but we sometimes spare a thought for those who will be reading the current issue of the journal 100 years from now. They may not even be human; in the week that the world chess champion was for the first time beaten by a computer this seems a distinct possibility. Those people, machines, or intergalactic travellers will not doubt conclude that we touched on an important issue with our articles on informed consent (12 April). We have so far had over 50 letters, as many as on natural contraception or obituaries.

We publish today 19 letters on informed consent. Among these, nine think that we should stay with our current policy of sometimes publishing papers that have not included informed consent; four want us to publish papers that do not get informed consent only when they meet the three strict criteria laid down by Len Doyal (12 April, p 1107). Our correspondents are divided almost equally on what we should do. The letters make many different points, but some themes emerge.

One theme is that informed consent is just as important in clinical practice as in research, and some correspondents are worried that lower standards apply in everyday practice. Researchers will have their protocols scrutinised by funding bodies, ethics committees, and editors, whereas clinicians may be questioned only by a bamboozled and fright-

ened patient. Carl Counsell and Peter Sandercock write: "There is a good deal of hypocrisy in clinical medicine about informed consent. Many so-called established treatments have been poorly evaluated so their true risks and benefits remain unclear. These treatments should still be regarded as experimental and yet, because they are accepted, they are widely given without any form of consent being required." Sarah Stewart-Brown agrees: "In Britain, thousands of women receive treatment for cervical dysplasia each year, believing that it is saving them from cancer, when the chances are that they have been subjected to an unnecessary intervention. If the real problem is informed consent in clinical practice, making researchers do things the right way won't solve it."

Dr Stewart-Brown has an answer to our problem. "Ensuring that those who have been abused by the present system are given a public voice … might be a more ethical way to proceed than is a blanket ban on publication of the results of some studies." Hazel Thornton, chairwoman of the Consumers' Advisory Group of Clinical Trials, agrees. Her group wants to advance public understanding of and involvement in clinical trials. "Collaboration is the name of the game. Research is for the benefit of us all: all should be involved in debates about its improvement and promotion."

---

*Editor's choice *BMJ* 1997; **314**: 1059.

Letters*

DOCTORS ARE ARROGANT TO THINK THEY NEED TO DEBATE ISSUE OF PATIENT CONSENT

The editorial by Richard Smith raised the issue of publishing studies in which the researchers did not seek patients' consent.[1] Firstly, I would think that of all the professions, only in medicine would there be any sort of debate about whether people need to be told that they, their bodies, their body fluids, their emotions, or whatever were to be subjects of research. This is arrogance on the part of doctors. Has anyone thought of asking these "patients" what their opinions are?

Secondly, I also think that doctors in developing countries need to be especially careful about obtaining consent from patients for anything, not only research. I would like to know that when I read a paper from a developing country in the *BMJ*, I can be sure that the individuals on whom the research was done had given informed consent.

David E Bratt, *Paediatrician*, Diego Martin, Trinidad and Tobago, West Indies

NO-ONE HAS A MONOPOLY ON DECIDING WHAT IS ETHICAL

Having just come to the end of my term as chairman of our local research ethics committee, I would like to contribute to the debate on informed consent.
I have no doubt that informed consent should be obtained in virtually all research studies. The difficulty comes in those rare instances when the need to obtain informed consent may be waived. Len Doyal has made a thoughtful and useful contribution to the debate,[2] but it is interesting that, whereas I would have said that the study by Satish Bhagwanjee and colleagues qualified under his suggestions,[3] he seems to imply that it would not.

The commentaries of Rajendra Kale and Sheila McLean were critical of the two studies published in the *BMJ*,[3, 4] but they failed to address the specific issues raised by the trials and resorted instead to

BMJ 1997; **314**: 1477–83; **315**: 247–54. References cited within this section are listed on pp. 120–22.

vague generalisations. Neither was prepared to consider seriously the harm that can be done by not performing trials from which bias has been excluded as far as possible.[5] In contrast, Martin Dennis and Bhagwanjee and colleagues, who defended their decision not to obtain informed consent, wrote clearly about the different issues entailed and had obviously agonised about the problem.[3, 4] I believe that it was perfectly reasonable in both studies not to obtain informed consent. In neither case was there any possibility of harming the participants and important information for the care of future patients was obtained. I do not subscribe to the view that not seeking informed consent indicates a failure to respect the subjects in these studies. Indeed, the care with which the issues were considered before starting the studies and the safeguards that were put in place indicate that the reverse was true.

Richard Smith asked whether the *BMJ* should publish papers describing studies in which informed consent was not obtained.[1] There is clearly so much disagreement about the situations in which such trials might be conducted that it would be wrong for the *BMJ* to decline to publish the results of these studies if they have been given the approval of properly constituted research ethics committees. No-one can claim to have a monopoly on deciding what is ethical. By publishing such trials the *BMJ* will provide important material showing what different research ethics committees think. These data may then inform the continuing debate with the decisions taken by a wide range of concerned individuals, dealing with real life issues.

Pat Soutter, *Past Chairman, Research Ethics Committee*, Hammersmith Hospitals NHS Trust, London, UK

LET READERS JUDGE FOR THEMSELVES

I am a medical statistician, not a doctor, so my experience is rather remote from the patient. I think there are two issues here: is it ever right to randomise people without their consent? is it ever right to treat or measure people without their consent? I think it can be right to randomise people without their consent when randomisation is to what the person would have received in the absence of the trial. Thus the stroke worker study seems defensible.[4] I did such a study – the "Know your midwife" study – in which the lead researcher, very committed to the scheme, thought that no woman who knew of the scheme would accept anything else.[6] Women were randomised to be offered the continuity of a midwifery care regimen and then offered a choice of that regimen or standard care. Others were offered standard care only. All were asked to consent to a study of events around birth and interviewed. I thought this was all right and still do. Sometimes we randomise people by general practice. I don't think we could get consent to randomisation. However, we can still obtain consent to treatment.

I think it is rarely acceptable to treat a person without consent. But consider a patient who is unconscious after an overdose. Should we revive the patient? The patient's action suggests that consent is not given, but I think we might do it anyway. I have recently discussed a trial of different methods of treatment for these cases. I think my conclusion would have to be that, if it is ethical outside a trial, it would be ethical inside a trial, too. However, the Durban patients were mostly able to consent, as the HIV test could presumably have been done afterwards with stored blood.[3] I think that study was unethical.

I think it is dangerous to let one moral principle – informed consent – become absolute. Hence I would not banish all such research from the *BMJ* and only if the editor thought the work indefensible, would I keep it out. If the issue was debatable I think I would publish the paper, though I would expect authors to justify their actions. Readers could then judge for themselves.

Martin Bland, *Professor of medical statistics*, St George's Hospital Medical School, London, UK

ETHICS COMMITTEES AND THE *BMJ* SHOULD CONTINUE TO CONSIDER THE OVERALL BENEFIT TO PATIENTS

We support Martin Dennis in his commentary to his and his colleagues' paper that the decision to fully or partially inform consent should take into account the likely effect on important outcome measures, as well as the benefit of good research for all patients.[4]

We made the difficult decision – in consultation with local ethics committees – that patients attending their general practitioner with a sore throat should be asked to consent to the procedures and to the aim of assessing the natural history but, in trying to "mimic" normal practice, doctors were encouraged not to discuss the randomisation to one of three approaches in common clinical use: antibiotics, no antibiotics, or the offer of delayed antibiotics.[7] Randomisation to the three approaches replaced the normal bias or preference of the general practitioner, which the patient is also uninformed about.

We showed that prescribing antibiotics medicalises sore throat and increases intention to consult. We believe that a full discussion of the educational purpose of the research, and of the different management groups – which must be rare in normal practice – would have significantly biased the results so that groups would have been much more similar. High prescribers would then see no benefit from changing their prescribing, with encouragement to waste the £60–120m of NHS money spent annually on sore throat, with disbenefit to all future patients. Similar arguments apply to fully informing the control group of many other important open studies – for example, effect of leaflets on stopping smoking and the Oxcheck study. The technical breach of autonomy – to give complete information for some patients on one occasion – has to be seen in the context of deviancy from routine practice and judged against breaching the same principle the next time the same patient sees their doctor, i.e. not being able to inform the patient fully of correct management, as well as the beneficence to many more patients. This utilitarian argument was made by Len Doyal in condoning the use of medical records,[2] and there is no clear justification of why the ethcal issues for randomised trials should be different.

Adopting an absolute ethical view in open trials ignores the realities of – and would undermine the ability of research to inform – normal practice, and thus could ultimately harm patients, including those who agree to take part in trials. The *BMJ* and ethics committees should continue to judge the overall benefit for patients.

Paul Little, *Wellcome Training Fellow*; and
Ian Williamson, *Senior Lecturer*, University of Southampton, Primary Medical Care, Southampton, UK

RISK OF BIAS MAY BE ANOTHER REASON NOT TO SEEK CONSENT

Reading through the various articles on informed

consent has confirmed the view I already held that there are situations in which informed consent is more trouble than it is worth. Consequently, I am of the view that the *BMJ* was right to publish the papers in question and would be wrong to impose a ban on publishing such papers in future.

The rights of individual patients must, of course, be protected, but not to the exclusion of all other considerations; people have obligations as well as rights. I consider it sufficient that a study is approved by an ethics committee. If the members can be convinced that the study remains ethical without informed consent, then the paper should be considered for publication. It would be unethical not to publish a sound and valuable piece of work, thus denying useful knowledge to the medical community, simply because informed consent was not sought. Presumably the lobby in favour of the ban hopes that such studies would not then be done. This I doubt.

I think any policy adopted by the *BMJ* on this issue should be framed in terms for ethics committee approval. If the *BMJ* decides to follow a policy along the lines proposed by Doyal[2] I would like to see at least one other category of exception – that is, where there is a perceived risk that seeking informed consent might bias the conclusions of the study (as in the stroke family care worker study[4] and the breast cancer study of McArdle *et al.*[8]).

As another example, suppose one wished to set up a study comparing methods of persuading pregnant women to stop smoking during pregnancy. If you tell the patient that you are going to try to stop her from smoking, either by not haranguing her or by haranguing her frequently, her ultimate behaviour might be influenced by this knowledge. This is a testable hypothesis. It would be possible to set up such a study as a two by two factorial, in which one of the treatment factors was informed consent and the other was whatever intervention treatment was of interest. The presence of an interaction between the two factors would support the hypothesis. I am not aware that such a study has ever been done, but it would help to settle the question of whether seeking informed consent can bias the results of a study. If the *BMJ* had already implemented a ban on publishing papers without informed consent, how would the results of such a study see the light of day?

I applaud the *BMJ*'s decision to open this issue to wider debate.

Dennis O Chanter. *Principal Consultant Statistician*, BRI International, Battle, East Sussex, UK

CLINICIANS ARE BEING DISINGENUOUS WITH THEMSELVES

I would like to raise a concern about the relation between the ethics of medical research and the ethics of clinical medicine. Clinicians play a lead role in the great majority of medical research projects, and the framework within which they practice medicine plays a part in their judgement of the ethics of their research. Although the principle of informed consent is widely accepted, the actuality may be different, as illustrated by Ganapati Mudur's report of the condemnation by ethicists of a study in India of the clinical course of cervical dysplasia.[9] The study is necessary because the available evidence is insufficient to quantify the risks of dysplasia, and shows that cervical dysplasia normally resolves spontaneously rather than progressing to cancer. A gynaecologist objecting to the study argued that it was unethical because "the investigators had not informed the study participants that their lesions were known to progress to cancer."[9] While clinicians are being disingenuous with themselves, it is hard to see how they can be truly honest with their patients.

In Britain, thousands of women receive treatment for cervical dysplasia each year, believing that it is saving them from cancer, when the chances are that they have been subjected to an unnecessary intervention. This suggests that they are being treated on false pretenses, rather than on the basis of informed consent.

If, as proposed, the *BMJ* and other journals refused to publish the results of studies in which informed consent had been obtained,[1] the problem of not obtaining informed consent in research would eventually be solved – but, although researchers would be learning the lesson the hard way this would abuse the time, energy, and good will of patients who had volunteered to participate in studies without informed consent, on the grounds that their participation would benefit humankind. If the real problem is informed consent in clinical practice, making researchers do things the right way won't solve it.

It is excellent that the editorial broad of the *BMJ* is concerned to tackle this problem and is opening the debate on the way to proceed. Ensuring that those who have been abused by the present system are given a public voice, as in the anonymous personal view,[10] might be a more ethical way to proceed than a blanket ban on publication of the results of some studies.

Sarah Stewart-Brown, *Director*, Health Services Research Unit, Department of Public Health, University of Oxford, UK

WE ALL HAVE A RESPONSIBILITY TO CONTRIBUTE TO RESEARCH

Jeffrey S Tobias identified an atmosphere of mistrust by patients towards clinical trials.[5] Perhaps we can begin to reverse this atmosphere by involving those groups of thoughtful bystanders who were round the outside of the arena[11] but have now been encouraged to clamber in to join the combat.[12] Collaboration is the name of the game. Research is for the benefit of us all: all should be involved in debates about its improvement and promotion.

The Consumers' Advisory Group for Clinical Trials, a distinctive working group of professionals and patients, sees the need to promote a new image of research as an ongoing process of extreme importance. It works directly with the professions, helping to develop their protocols and to prepare their information leaflets for patients. The group identifies an urgent need to advance public education about clinical trials. Concepts such as randomisation, risk perception, and probability are poorly understood. Educating members of the public when they are well,[13] identifying the importance of language, and educating children and medical students about research concepts are all strategies that would widen appreciation of the need for research while balancing these responsibilities with the right to informed consent, as and when it is appropriate to the particular study.[14]

Such cooperation, shared responsibility, and greater understanding of research concepts will create a different attitude to research, which will be seen not as an imposition but as an activity to which we all have a responsibility to contribute.

Hazel Thornton, *Chairwoman, Consumer's Advisory Group for Clinical Trials*, Rowhedge, Colchester, UK

MINIMUM ETHICAL STANDARDS SHOULD NOT VARY AMONG COUNTRIES

I am glad that you have opened discussion on the important issue of informed consent in medical research, and in such a comprehensive way.[1] I have recently been teaching research methods in different countries. the courses always include a session on ethics in research (including qualitative research – sometimes thought not to need informed consent). Many developing countries, including some Asian countries, have not yet established research ethics committees, although there are individuals keen for this to happen. However, in one country, where members of the medical profession tend to be part of a small elite, some course participants said in a discussion on informed consent: "But if we ask the subjects they might say no."

I agree that there is a danger that researchers from developed countries may undertake certain studies in developing countries where they may believe, or argue, that ethical issues are different. I have heard the argument that informed consent by individuals is not required or appropriate where people tend to have a "group" rather than an "individual" identity, that it is sufficient to obtain consent from, for example, a village chief. I am wary of such arguments. By all means get consent from the chief, but also from every individual concerned. Although cultural differences need to be taken into account in ensuring that a study is carried out in a sensitive and ethical way, minimum ethical standards should not vary among countries.

Although Satish Bhagwanjee and colleagues clearly considered the ethical issues with great care in their study on HIV status,[3] I think that you should not publish such studies. Editorials that remind readers of this policy from time to time, and the reason for it, would be very helpful. A series of articles in simple language on different ethical issues, such as informed consent, privacy, ownership of data, community involvement, dissemination of data, responsibility for publicity, etc. (including how to establish an institutional ethics committee) would be interesting and valuable.

Wendy Holmes, *Lecturer*, International Health Programs, Key Centre for Women's Health, University of Melbourne, Victoria, Australia

SOUTH AFRICAN STUDY RAISES THE GHOSTS OF NUREMBERG AND APARTHEID

I am astonished that the *BMJ* should publish the findings of a research study that failed to seek the consent of the patients.[3] In particular, by tacitly condoning this most unethical practice from a group of researchers from South Africa, the *BMJ* has missed an opportunity to teach them how the civilised world outside the confines of apartheid treats its patients.

The *BMJ* also lost the opportunity to show its local edition partners all over the democratic and emerging democratic world how to stand up for ethics and human rights even in the face of extreme pressure from prospective authors (big and influential) who fail to observe accepted ethical practice.

Even before the Nuremberg code was designed in 1947[15] and then reasserted by the Helsinki declaration of 1964,[16] the inviolability of the right of patients to an unambiguous and informed consent in all forms of experimentation was already standard practice. In 1898 Albert Neisser, the discoverer of the gonococcus and a pre-eminent professor of his generation, was prosecuted and fined for conducting experiments with prostitutes without their consent. The disciplinary court based its judgment not on questionable science but on the lack of patients' consent. It also concluded that intervention without consent fulfilled the criteria for causing physical injury in criminal law.[17]

Bhagwanjee and colleagues state that their study was deemed to be of sufficient importance to waive patients' right to informed consent. The Helsinki declaration prohibits absolutely any human experimentation in dying patients because it recognises that respect for the rights of patients has the same importance for the good of mankind as medical and scientific progress. Would any ethics committee in the United Kingdom, the home of the *BMJ*, approve a study without patients' consent? How many of the South African study victims were black men and women? Considering the recent experience of that country during the apartheid years, how many of such unethical practices were condoned? Who compensates for the injury that these human guinea pigs suffer? This study raises the ghosts of Nuremberg and apartheid, and it is a big shame that the *BMJ* should indirectly encourage it. There is no point in closing the stable door after the horse has escaped.[1] In this case why publish the paper before asking readers for their views on the issue of informed consent in research? I fail to see what new ground this study was going to break for mankind and even then the patient's right to give or withhold consent must not be violated.

Joseph N E Ana, *Private practitioner*, Luton, UK

CONSENT IS NOT ALWAYS PRACTICAL IN EMERGENCY TREATMENTS

Richard Smith asks for readers' views on whether papers should be published only if there has been informed consent for the study.[1]

I agree completely that for the vast majority of clinical research the patient should be fully informed about all aspects of the trial or study and their consent freely and willingly obtained. However, there are occasions when this is not practical. In the main, these are clinical trials related to emergency treatment. Some aspects of care of newborn infants at birth have not been properly investigated and badly need data from good randomised trials – for example, the treatment of meconium aspiration. When meconium aspiration has occurred, there is no time to ask for consent to a trial, and it is rarely possible to predict the problem and ask for consent beforehand. Even with warning signs, the mother is not in a position to give fully informed consent; the father may not be present and, even if he is, he will be worried by what is happening to his wife and child, so that it is inappropriate to try to inform him about a randomised trial and ask for his consent. There are several possible solutions to this problem, although none are ideal.

- Inform every woman entering the maternity hospital about the trial and ask for consent, should her baby has meconium aspiration. However, to obtain such blanket consent in a busy delivery unit would be difficult and probably inappropriate, as meconium aspiration occurs only in a small proportion of babies. Consent would not be obtained from a woman with an acute problem on admission and the baby would not be enrolled. This will bias the trial because such babies would be likely subjects for the trial.
- Enrol only babies for whom consent could be obtained from the parents. This is possible, but it is likely to result in a biased trial because the most difficult acute cases will not be enrolled, and therefore the babies will not represent the full clinical spectrum.
- Conduct a trial with the approval of a professional peer group and the hospital ethics committee that asks for consent when possible but, if this is not possible because of the nature of the emergency, the patient is allowed to be enrolled in the trial. The parents would be informed and asked for their consent as soon as possible, allowing them to withdraw from the trial if they wish.
- Not do a randomised trial and continue to use the unproved treatment.

None of these solutions is ideal and all have

ethical problems. The question is which technique is the most ethical? I suggest that the least unethical solution is to conduct a good, well planned, vetted, and approved trial, even if previous consent cannot be obtained in all cases, and then inform the patients, or in this case parents, afterwards. If such trials are refused publication, it will impede research in emergency procedures, and those that are published will be unsatisfactory because they will not represent the full range of patients.

Colin Morley, *Clinical Director*, Neonatal Intensive Care Unit, Addenbrookes Hospital, Cambridge, UK

CHILDREN FROM THE AGE OF 5 SHOULD BE PRESUMED COMPETENT

When considering informed consent in medical research, Len Doyal states that one of the three circumstances in which research should be allowed to proceed in the absence of informed consent is when subjects are not competent to give consent.[2] One group given as an example was that of young and immature children. Before this statement is accepted, the terms young and immature have to be defined.

Alderson and Montgomery argue that children can and should play a greater part in decisions about their own health care.[18] They recommend that any child who can express a view should be given information, listened to, and have his or her views taken into account when decisions about treatment are being considered. Their suggestions for a statutory description of capacity would be present when a child understands the type and purpose of the proposed treatment, the nature and effects of the treatment in broad terms, the principal benefits and risks, and the consequences of not receiving treatment and, when he or she has the capacity to choose, whether to accept the treatment. When children are competent to take responsibility for a decision the responsibility for that decision would become theirs.

They argue that young people from the age of 5 – that is, of compulsory school age – should be presumed competent. The young age was chosen as the presumption does not exclude parents from discussion. It also encourages recognition that young children may be competent to make certain decisions – for example, whether to take more analgesics, if not more complex ones – and allows for the children to be deemed not competent and for their decisions to be overruled, especially if their decision would result

in serious irreparable harm to their health. Perhaps these criteria could be used as a basis for discussion when how to assess children and young people's competence to consent to participation in research is being considered. This would be in line with Doyal's additional statement that "the levels of autonomy that patients who are thus incompetent do possess should still be respected (for example, if they resist participation then it should not be forced)."[2]

A third point is that, just as in adults, competence in children is not something which is merely present or absent. Its presence may vary in children of the same age, depending on when, where, and how the question is asked, the cognitive capacities of the child at that time, and the level of competence[19] required – for example, the mere ability to assent or a full understanding of the decision and the possible consequences for the individual.

Moli Paul, *Senior Registrar in Child and Adolescent Psychiatry*, Parkview Clinic, Birmingham, UK

RESEARCH IN PATIENTS WITH MENTAL RETARDATION POSES SPECIAL PROBLEMS

In response to the editorial by Richard Smith and the articles on informed consent in biomedical research by Len Doyal and Jeffrey S Tobias,[1, 2, 5] I suggest that the issues surrounding incompetent patients as in cases of mental illness or mental retardation are particularly important. People with mental retardation warrant specific mention, especially because those with severe degrees of disability will never be able to exercise their right to autonomous decision-making. Yet, they as patients have the most intensive needs and have increased rates of challenging behaviour or mental illness, or both, and the treatments for these conditions remain symptomatic and have probably been investigated (originally) only in normal subjects.

The advent of community care for this population and the emphasis on social care[20] has created a resistance to research carried out in children and adults with learning disabilities, further aided by the ever present and gruesome memories of the eugenics movement in the early 20th century and the Nazi experiments. However, time and again, clinicians are faced with intractable disorders in their patients with learning disabilities that compromise the patient's quality of life, may be extremely stressful to manage and cope with, and may put other residents and staff at risk. In addition, self-injurious behaviour may be extremely severe, thus compounding the effects of the disability. Research on the pharmacological treatment of developmental disorders has been mainly based on small scale studies with inadequate methodology, i.e. the use of antipsychotics/antidepressants and opioid antagonists in severe and unremitting aggression and self-injurious behaviour. Evidence is still scant on the advantages and disadvantages of the different types of drugs for controlling challenging behaviour, with serious financial and clinical practice implications. It is a pity that the recent advances in medical technology and non-invasive procedures and improved understanding of the interaction between brain function and environment, which could yield important results for patients with learning disabilities, are not used to their full potential. Doyal's guidelines[2] certainly go some way towards addressing the issue of consent with incompetent patients, although more work, such as canvassing views of service users and carers and promoting advocacy for this client group, will be necessary before the stigma of unethical research stops beneficial treatments from being used.

A Hassiotis, *Honorary Senior Lecturer in Developmental Disorders and Learning Disability*, Department of Psychiatry and Behavioural Sciences, University College London Medical School, London, UK

STUDIES WITH IMPORTANT CONCLUSIONS BUT WITHOUT PATIENT CONSENT SHOULD BE PUBLISHED

Your debate on informed patient consent for medical research made fascinating reading, and the situations where informed consent is, and is not, appropriate were comprehensively discussed by Len Doyal and Jeffrey S Tobias.[2, 5]

That a study is methodologically sound so that meaningful conclusions can be drawn is of paramount importance and is the greatest problem we face in medical research. While those authors who have spent time and effort in designing a study adequate to produce a sound paper will probably also have obtained informed consent in appropriate cases, this will not be a perfect correlation, partly because of varying interpretations of what constitutes an appropriate case. An occasional paper will therefore emerge with valid and important conclusions, but no patient consent. A prohibition on publication of papers without patient consent would cause valuable information to be absent from the literature, a scientifically and morally unacceptable situation. Each paper should be judged on its merits, with the appropriate presence of informed consent representing an important, but not paramount, consideration.

The *BMJ*'s present policy of sometimes publishing research in which patients have not given fully informed consent is indeed wholly correct.

Mark F G Hulbert, *Senior Registrar in Ophthalmology*, Moorfields Eye Hospital, London, UK

FAILURE TO PUBLISH COMPLETED RANDOMISED CONTROLLED TRIALS IS UNETHICAL IN ITSELF

In response to Richard Smith's request for help in deciding the *BMJ*'s policy on informed consent,[1] we would argue strongly in favour of maintaining the journal's present position. Nobody wishes to promote unethical research, but failure to publish completed randomised controlled trials is unethical in its own right: the efforts of all those who participated in the trial are wasted, and both health professionals and patients are deprived of information that they may need to make informed decisions.[21]

There is a good deal of hypocrisy in clinical medicine about informed consent. Many so called established treatments have been poorly evaluated so that their true benefits and risks remain unclear. These treatments should still be regarded as experimental and yet, because they are accepted, they are widely given without any form of consent being required. For example, many treatments are widely used in different countries to treat patients with acute stroke, e.g. aspirin, heparin, glycerol, haemodilution, corticosteroids, ancrod,[22, 23] but none of these has definitely been shown to reduce the risk of death or disability and many could be harming patients; for example, antithrombotic agents could increase the risk of intracranial haemorrhage.[24] Many more patients are exposed to this abuse of consent than in randomised controlled trials but this is rarely questioned. Hardening of the already stringent requirements for informed consent in randomised controlled trials will lead to fewer and smaller randomised trials and continued uncertainty over the risks and benefits of many treatments and hence to continued widescale abuse of patients' consent in clinical practice.

Carl E Counsell, *Clinical Research Fellow*; and **Peter A G Sandercock**, *Reader in Neurology*, Department of Clinical Neurosciences, Western General Hospital, Edinburgh, UK

SUBJECTS MAY BE COERCED INTO PARTICIPATING IN STUDIES

Whether prospective research with no explicit statement about informed consent should be published is an issue avoided by journals for too long.[1] Subjects in some experiments believe that they are receiving standard treatment when there is no evidence of utility.[25–27] Recently I reviewed a prospective multicentre study of myocardial infarction in which the end points included death. There was no statement about ethics approval or informed consent. I suggested that, if this was not an oversight, the journal "would have to decide whether it wants to publish an unethical trial."

When subjects give informed consent the experiments may still be unethical if consent is not given freely. Subjects may be coerced by poverty into participation or find it difficult to refuse a request from an employer, colleague, or teacher. I am aware of recent research involving military staff who were ordered to volunteer.

I have particular concerns about research in diving medicine. Most is performed outside hospitals and without the safeguard of hospital ethics committees. In *Diver* magazine I reported that volume 9 of *Undersea and Hyperbaric Physiology* contained 111 scientific papers, of which 47 described human research.[28] Twelve studies were on patients and 35 on so-called volunteers, who were often military staff or employees of the commercial diving organisations that conducted the research. Only seven papers mentioned that ethics approval was granted, and only 12 mentioned informed consent. Some experiments were highly hazardous and might be best described as adventures in survival for the participants. Many studies failed to mention adverse effects. When they did, it was evident that at least 38 of the so-called volunteers had decompression illness in studies that were often too small or incorrectly designed to give a statistically valid result.

Senior institutions are not above reproach. Eight years ago the Medical Research Council Decompression Sickness Panel proposed introducing "professional diver super medicals." Like the current medical assessments, the super medicals would be performed at intervals during a diver's career, but would include additional expensive investigations such as radionuclide scanning. The results were to be used in a prospective survey of long-term health hazards of diving, but the divers were to be told that it was for individual screening, and that they would be asked to pay for the investigations. Those who refused would lose their licence and livelihood. The plan was abandoned only recently, though I and others expressed concerns about the ethics when it was first proposed.

Peter Wilmshurst, *Consultant Cardiologist*, Royal Shrewsbury Hospital, UK

THE WHOLE POPULATION MUST BE MOBILISED IN THE WAR AGAINST CANCER

Ethicists should carefully avoid absolutism lest they become hostages to fortune. Len Doyal, an ethicist whom I much admire, has fallen into this trap.[2] For example, he states and restates his belief that it is unacceptable to compromise individual rights, even if the public interest demands it. I presume therefore that he is too young to remember the conscription that was necessary to fight a just war against the Nazi powers, the very ones guilty of the worst atrocities committed in the name of medical science.

Cancer commits atrocities on the human body, and the fight against cancer has often been likened to a war: "The war against disease and for health cannot be fought by physicians alone it is a people's war in which the entire population must be mobilsed permanently."[29] If there is to be a war against cancer and if it is considered unethical to conscript patients as the foot soldiers in this war, then it is up to the lay public to recognise their responsibilities to society on a voluntary basis, in addition to demanding their rights of autonomy and progress for the treatment of malignant disease. It was precisely that argument that I described in my paper in the *Lancet* in 1993,[30] which was inappropriately cited by Doyal to support his argument about access to medical records.

I am glad to report that many women with breast cancer have risen to this challenge,[30, 31] and we now have a consumer's advisory group of committed lay women chaired by Hazel Thornton who see themselves as equal stakeholders in the fight against cancer. Until we have permanently mobilised the whole population in this war, the agonising debate about the process and ethics of informed consent will continue to thunder on and on. In the meantime, in a less than perfect world I have to side with Jeffrey S Tobias, who like me, every day of his working life, has to make these tough decisions.[32] It would help the debate if the armchair ethicists got down from their verandas and mixed with the natives – perhaps first-hand experience would dilute their uncompromising zeal.

Michael Baum, *Professor of Surgery*, Department of Surgery, Institute of Surgical Studies, University College London Medical School, London, UK

PATIENTS MAY NOT UNDERSTAND ENOUGH TO GIVE THEIR INFORMED CONSENT

Much debate has focused on the need for informed consent and the ethical difficulties that arise when this is not obtained.[1] Little attention has been paid to what patients understand that they have consented to.

We report preliminary data from a study of 102 patients receiving radiotherapy for cancer: 22% (22/99) had no recollection of consenting to the procedure (all had consented); 36% (29/80) of those who did recall consenting thought that they had consented to "any procedure that the doctor thinks is necessary including chemotherapy, radiotherapy, or surgery." Moreover, 60% (48/80) thought that by consenting they had undertaken to accept "any side effects caused by the treatment," and 44% (42/95) believed that by consenting they would be unable subsequently to complain about side effects.

Clearly, the issue of informed consent implies a sharing of information, yet 24% (24/99) of our sample could not recall being told about any side effects from radiotherapy, not even common effects such as burning skin or tiredness, of which they were informed. These were all patients who had had an appointment with their consultant when treatment options and side effects were discussed followed by a pretreatment meeting with a radiographer. In addition, 60% (54/90) of patients received information leaflets and 47 out of 100 saw a specialist cancer counsellor on at least one occasion. If patients are not retaining the information that they have been provided with or if they are misunderstanding precisely what they are consenting to, they are being ill equipped to make the psychological adjustment that will be necessary throughout their treatment.

Our findings highlight the need for more research

to be conducted into the process for obtaining informed consent and whether patients take in and understand information given to them. If the subject has not taken in the information then their consent is hardly informed. It may be that the timing of information sharing is crucial as to whether it is retained and that this should be viewed as more of a process than a one off event.

Charles Montgomery, *Senior Registrar in Psychiatry*, Wonford House Hospital; **Anna Lydon**, *Senior Registrar in Clinical Oncology*, Royal Devon and Exeter Hospital; and **Keith Lloyd**, *Senior Lecturer*, University of Exeter, Postgraduate Medical School Department of Mental Health, Wonford House, Hospital, Exeter, UK

COMMUNICATION WITH POTENTIAL SUBJECTS NEEDS TO BE EFFECTIVE

As a past chairman of a local research ethics committee and a recently practising clinical oncologist and clinical researcher, I endorse the views of Len Doyal.[2] I would argue that Jeffrey S Tobias's highly reasonable anxieties for the wellbeing of individual research volunteers[5] would be better served by much greater attention being paid to the comparatively neglected area of clinical interpersonal communication. Nowhere in either article is this fundamental issue clearly addressed.

My experience of dealing with research protocols from a wide range of sources, some of them extremely august, leads me to the reluctant conclusion that the last feature to be tackled by a researcher is the means by which the nature of the research will be made comprehensible to potential subjects. It is not uncommon for the local research ethics committee to have to rewrite the patient information and consent literature for the applicant, and this is a common source of delay in obtaining approval.

Even when the written material is deemed acceptable, the diverse nature of the circumstances and abilities of research subjects demands a personal presentation of the information by a senior member of the research team. This is, I suspect, the most vulnerable point in the process, dependent as it is on the range of communication skills available to the informer. The profession places a lower value on having effective abilities in interpersonal communication than it does on having more obviously acceptable concrete medical and scientific skills.

I have seen in my own practice that with the use of effective communication skills most patients can be given an individualised, accurate, and comprehensible paraphrase of the protocol information leaflet, within an acceptable time frame. It is, however, essential to have formally learnt the necessary skills to do so. Is this so different from having had to master any other useful clinical skill?

Those who aspire to undertake clinical research should place as much emphasis on their ability to communicate effectively as on the methodology and statistics considered to be essential to the conduct of a trial. Surely this is a more acceptable means of extending the range of trial opportunities than being forced into the ethical dilemma resulting from denying the fundamental rights of individuals?

Christopher Wiltshire, *Retired Consultant Clinical Oncologist*, Ipswich, UK

IN ROUTINE PRACTICE THE CONSENT FORM IS A REQUEST FORM AND INFORMED CONSENT IS INFORMED CHOICE

We read with interest Richard Smith's editorial on the ethical problems of informed consent in research.[1] However, for the most part, doctors face the issues of informed consent in their daily routine practice of patient care. It is in daily practice that many doctors feel uncertain of their role and may fear litigation, despite the publication of general guidelines. We think that the principle of informed consent implies that it is for the benefit of the doctor and not the patient to provide medical care, and this is especially reflected in the written operative consent form. It is ultimately the patients' decision to opt or not to opt for care and the doctor's duty to provide relevant information. Therefore, we recommend informed consent for routine, non-research care should be renamed informed choice. We also suggest that the consent form be renamed a request form. We believe that this terminology would be more informative to both doctors and patients.

A C Frosh, *Ear, Nose, and Throat Specialist Registrar*, St Mary's Hospital, London, UK; and **J Hanif**, *Ear, Nose, and Throat Registrar*, Charing Cross Hospital, London, UK

The following set of letters subsequently appeared and carried on the debate begun by the first. **These and other related correspondence constituted the largest 'mail box' on a particular topic in the history of the BMJ.**

THE CENTRAL PROBLEM IS OFTEN POOR DESIGN AND CONDUCT OF TRIALS

We are concerned about some aspects of the recent articles on consent.[2, 5] Len Doyal claims that informed consent may not be necessary for three most vulnerable groups: young children, patients with learning difficulties, and unconscious or semiconscious patients. Yet young children (unlike all adult groups) have the protection of their parents' consent, and this should always be respected.[33] The other two groups show the limitations of applying Kantian respect for autonomy, designed for property owning 18th century gentlemen, to vulnerable dependent patients. There is an urgent need to agree new ways of making research decisions with and for these minority groups.

As is usual in arguments against seeking informed consent, there is a tendency to concentrate on dramatic extremes: patients with severe mental impairment and patients receiving heroic cancer treatment. The development of principles from extremes is dangerous and should be discouraged. Difficulties with relatively small groups should not be used to excuse researchers from requesting the consent of the vast majority of the millions of people every year who help with research into mundane pharmaceutical trials of treatments of arthritis or everyday misery.

A deeper problem with the articles is the assumption that consent is the central problem in research. We suggest that, more often, the central problem is the poor design and conduct of trials which alienate or distress people on whose practical support researchers depend. The solution here is not to tinker with consent but to clean up research. Health service users could help at every stage of clinical research: the selection of questions worth investigating; the design and conduct of trials, including the information materials; the interpretation and reporting of the evidence; dissemination; and working with practitioners to put findings into practice. Consumers for Ethics in Research has been working with health service users, researchers, and practitioners on these issues for the past eight years, partly through regular open meetings, during which many practical ideas have been advanced.

Naomi Pfeffer, *Honorary Treasurer*; and **Priscilla Alderson**, *Honorary Secretary*, Consumers for Ethics in Research, London, UK

JOURNALS SHOULD REQUIRE ROUTINE REPORTING OF CONSENT RATES

We wish to contribute to the debate on informed consent.[1] Two of us (HC, SAMS) have recently conducted a review of randomised control trials published in the *Archives of Diseases in Childhood* from 1982 to 1996. We found that 112 (45%) of 249 trials did not report whether informed consent had been obtained. Of the trials that did note that informed consent had been obtained, 111 (81%) of 137 quoted consent rates of 100%. This proportion varied by study setting and paediatric subspecialty and was particularly high in trials in inpatients (90%) and trials in neonates (96%). Two of the trials that reported 100% consent rates included over 500 children.

Some of the trials may have considered obtaining patients' consent to the part of the inclusion criteria for participation. We are concerned, however, that investigators may have been following the letter of the law but not the spirit of the law. The process of obtaining consent should include the elements not only of information, comprehension, and consent but also of voluntariness – which includes absence of persuasion. It is important that investigators understand that patients' dependency can lead to absence of participation and choice, and that non-verbal behaviour and the setting can exert considerable influence.[34]

Beyond our immediate concern about the legitimacy of consent rates of 100% in large trials, we believe that a perceived lack of care in obtaining consent may lead to the imposition of a legalistic approach to gaining consent in paediatric research. Concern exists in several quarters that parental consent may not be sufficient to justify research with children. It could be argued that the individual circumstances of each specific study should be assessed by investigators and local research ethics committees. In law, however, research with children remains a grey area, and a shift towards greater emphasis on individual autonomy could restrict research much more than at present.

Such a shift is made more likely if the process of obtaining consent is perceived to be less than fully empowering to the subjects concerned. In this context, local research ethics committees and editors of medical journals should be alert to the possibility of informed consent that is not freely obtained, should required routine reporting of consent rates, and should challenge investigators to explain or comment on extremely high consent rates. Even more

importantly, however, investigators should be encouraged to regard the process of obtaining informed consent not as an irritating chore but as an opportunity to use their clinical skills to secure the subject's wholehearted cooperation in an important task.

Harry Campbell, *Senior Lecturer in Epidemiology*; **Kenneth M Boyd**, *Senior Lecturer in Medical Ethics*, University of Edinburgh, UK; and **Susan A M Surry**, *Medical Student*, University of Western Ontario, London, Ontario, Canada

OTHER SOCIETIES HAVE DIFFERENT CONCEPTS OF AUTONOMY

There is a disturbing undertone of cultural imperialism in the debate about informed consent. It shows itself most starkly in the tacit assumption that the whole world shares the same philosophical meanings as those that underpin our own shaky Judaeo-Christian-liberal ethic. That this is far from so is vividly illustrated in the very different concepts of autonomy held by different societies. In many traditional African cultures, and certainly in Bantu culture, the individual does not take his or her autonomy from "cogito, ergo sum" ("I think, therefore I am"), as in the West, but from "sumus, ergo sum" ("we are, therefore I am") – membership of an intensely important group that enhances the individual. In many parts of Africa it is simply not possible, especially for women, to make important decisions without reference to the group; any clinician or researcher who believes that a "yes" given by a terrified and lonely patient, in or out of a hospital bed, amounts to anything approaching informed consent is either naive or a knave. Add to this the very real social difficulty in ever saying "no" and thus threatening a relationship, and you have the perfect situation for doing anything you like.

Tim Cullinan, Head of Community Health Department, University of Malawi, Blantyre, Malawi

BRITISH INSTITUTIONS COLLABORATING IN PROJECTS OVERSEAS MAY FACE DILEMMA

We agree with the principle that medical research that does not include informed, individual consent should not be published[1] unless it falls into one of the three categories detailed by Len Doyal.[2] We would, however, argue for an additional guiding principle requiring community consultation over difficult ethical issues. Satish Bhagwanjee and colleagues might have sought opinions about HIV testing without consent from former patients of the intensive care unit in South Africa (and their relatives) before putting the study protocol to the ethics committee.[3] It might also have been more appropriate for a local HIV support group to be consulted instead of the subcommittee of the institutional ethics committee comprising a bioethicist, a clinician, and an AIDS expert.[3]

We would also argue that a properly constituted ethics committee should remain the final arbiter of the extent to which informed consent should be sought for a given study. This committee must be independent, as suggested by the Declaration of Helsinki, and as close to the community involved in the research as possible.

One problem is that, particularly in developing countries, many ethics committees remain to be set up or exist but are not properly constituted to include lay representation. Bhagwanjee and colleagues' study was reviewed by a subcommittee of the postgraduate committee.[3] However carefully that committee agonised over the fact that informed consent was not to be sought, the independence of its judgment must be questioned until its constitution is clarified.

As researchers based in a British institution but collaborating in many projects overseas, we are constantly faced with a dilemma. While it is presumptuous to impose an ethical opinion on research that will take place in circumstances very different to our own, it is unethical to be associated with research that does not come under any independent ethical scrutiny at all. All our research is reviewed by our own ethics committee, which includes independent lay representation from a variety of religious and cultural backgrounds. We emphasise that ethical approval from this committee does not absolve researchers from seeking local ethical approval. We recognise that this situation is not ideal and are building up a database of the ethics processes present in those countries with which we have links.

We hope that the debate on informed consent in the *BMJ* will encourage the development of independent ethics review processes in those places where they currently do not exist. Otherwise, medical journals will continue to have difficulty in judging whether, on ethical grounds, to publish some research.

S B Squire (*Chairman*) and *Members of Research Ethics Committee*, Liverpool School of Tropical Medicine, UK

RESEARCH STUDIES IN DIVING MEDICINE ARE CONSIDERED BY MINISTRY OF DEFENCE RESEARCH ETHICS COMMITTEE

In his letter Peter Wilmshurst made some general comments on the use of human volunteers for medical research; however, he singled out his concern about the adequacy of the ethical control of research in diving medicine, most of which, he asserts, "is performed outside hospitals and without the safeguard of hospital ethics committees" (p. 105). Diving medicine is a highly specialised branch of medicine covering basic physiological, operational, and commercial aspects of the subject. It is appropriate, therefore, that ethical considerations of nonclinical research in diving medicine should be dealt with by committees that are independent of hospital ethics committees but nevertheless conform with the codes of practice outlined by the Royal College of Physicians.[35] Examples are the procedures that are adopted by the Ministry of Defence at its two experimental diving establishments: DERA (Defence Evaluation and Research Agency) Alverstoke and the Institute of Naval Medicine at Alverstoke, where nonclinical aspects of diving are dealt with.

Each research project is first scrutinised from the scientific and ethical points of view by local advisory committees. It is then considered by the Ministry of Defence (navy) personnel research ethics committee for final assessment. The membership of this committee is constituted according to the guidelines recommended by the Royal College of Physicians[35] and consists of nine civilian personnel, all but one being independent of the Ministry of Defence. In addition, Royal Navy personnel and others with a specialist knowledge of diving medicine are coopted.

The volunteers are drawn from Royal Navy or Ministry of Defence personnel, and there is no question of their services being obtained by coercion. Before being invited to sign the consent form, they receive in writing a description of the project and an account of their proposed participation in it, the methods to be used, the benefits likely to accrue from the project and any possible risks to their own health. They are given the opportunity of discussing the project with the project officer and independent medical officer, and it is emphasised to them that they can withdraw from the project at any time, either before it starts or during it, without having to give a reason why. Their decision does not entail any loss of earnings or seniority and does not affect their prospects of promotion. All volunteers are examined for medical fitness by the independent medical officer.

I hope that these details will help to allay any fears that ethical aspects of the use of human volunteers in naval diving medicine in Britain have not been properly addressed.

M de Burgh Daly, *Chairman, Ministry of Defence (Navy) Personnel Research Ethics Committee*, Department of Physiology, Royal Free Hospital School of Medicine, London, UK

SUBJECTS MAY NOT UNDERSTAND CONCEPT OF CLINICAL TRIALS

We agree with Richard Smith that the issue of informed consent is not simple.[1] Even when a paper clearly states that information was given and consent obtained, readers cannot assume that the information given was "full" or that the consent was "fully informed."

We recently conducted a qualitative interview study with the parents of 21 babies enrolled in the United Kingdom collaborative trial of extracorporeal membrane oxygenation.[36, 37] The trial compared two methods of life support in critically ill newborn babies: conventional management (ventilatory support) and oxygenation of the blood through an external circuit.

In the qualitative study the parents were asked about their reactions to the offer to participate in the trial and to randomisation. The findings showed that they often had difficulty with the idea of randomisation and the rationale for its use. An example of a difficulty in explaining the scientific method is the use of the word "trial." The concept of a clinical trial was unfamiliar to most parents and the term did not necessarily convey the crucial information that two treatments (allocated on a random basis) were being compared. The trial was seen by some parents more as "a trial period." There were other areas of difficulty for the parents. For example, where parents did not know that medical uncertainty was the basis for the trial they sought other means to explain the use of randomisation (perhaps as a way for doctors to circumvent a difficult choice between treatments, or to decide between babies competing for scarce beds).

We generated three hypotheses from the data: (*a*) that parents were given accurate information but did not retain the details; (*b*) that parents were given partial information at the discretion of the caregiver, so that if they were perceived to be under too much stress the caregiver withheld or softened certain details; and (*c*) that parents were given inaccurate information, which reflected the caregivers' own beliefs about the trial. These hypotheses are not mutually exclusive.

We are continuing our research in other trials to try to develop strategies to support caregivers and to ease the process of obtaining and giving informed consent. We would be interested to hear from others working in this or related fields.

Diana Elbourne *Senior Lecturer*, Medical Statistics Unit, London School of Hygiene and Tropical Medicine, London, UK; **Claire Snowdon**, *Researcher*; and **Jo Garcia**, *Social Scientist*, National Perinatal Epidemiology Unit, Oxford, UK

INFORMED CONSENT IS NOT ALWAYS OBTAINED IN UNITED STATES

A code of silence and a spirit of denial surround one of the oldest and most perplexing conundrums in medical research: how to recruit large numbers of fully consenting subjects. So it was refreshing to note the *BMJ*'s pioneering willingness to devote space to questions of informed consent. "Rather than restrict the debate to ourselves," as the editor, Richard Smith, put it,[1] the *BMJ* dared to display publicly what institutional review boards and healthcare professionals usually handle with discretion or denial.

Our own analysis, published in *The (Cleveland, Ohio) Plain Dealer* and other American newspapers late last year, suggests the extent to which questions of consent persist.[38] This is despite the American government having apologised formally recently to survivors of a study of the natural course of syphilis in black men in Tuskegee, Alabama.[39] President Clinton has diverted the mandate of the National Bioethics Advisory Commission (which was formed to grapple with issues such as informed consent) to take up the more sensational if speculative topic of human cloning. Headlines have overtaken the issue before: in 1995, on the day that the Advisory Committee on Human Radiation Experiments warned of questions of consent in contemporary medical research, public interest focused on the verdict in the case of O J Simpson. In the past few months, disclosures in Augusta, Georgia, and Orange County, California, raised questions of consent, illustrating that the topic is more than a matter of distant history.[40, 41]

Since 1977 the US Food and Drug Administration (FDA) has conducted 4154 inspections of clinical trials. Our analysis of records of those inspections showed that 53% of the investigators were cited by the FDA for failing clearly to disclose the experimental nature of their work. In 46 trials involving at least 1000 men, women, and children, drugs were tested without any written evidence that subjects had consented.

We also found evidence that the US government, which makes annual payments to survivors of the study in Tuskegee, has sponsored experiments on unsuspecting subjects well into the 1990s. Among our case studies were tests by the Centers for Disease Control and Prevention, begun in 1990 in Los Angeles, of the immunogenicity and efficacy of the Edmonston–Zagreb measles vaccine, which the centres knew had earlier caused excess mortality in Africa; and a study in 1991 of hepatitis A vaccine, conducted on a Sioux reservation, in which the letterhead on the consent form implied an established prevention programme rather than the safety and efficacy trial it was.

Nor does the record overseas appear any better. Foreign and internal FDA documents that we reviewed contained accounts of fraud, concealed side effects, experiments diverging from protocols, and questions of consent. Consent forms were incomplete or inadequate in 65 of 137 inspections by the FDA of trials conducted in countries other than the US. In Canada, consent forms were inadequate in 21 of 36 inspections. Verifiable scientific data were missing from 53% of the international research submitted to support a US new drug application.

Our analysis of FDA data also showed that internal review boards, the front line in protecting test subjects, cannot be counted on to ensure that people know they are being used in medical research. At 942 internal review boards between 1990 and 1996, FDA inspectors found multiple violations: no evidence of continued safety monitoring (at 20% of the review boards); no copies of consent forms, injury reports, or protocols (19%); and that patients were not clearly told when procedures were experimental (16%), not offered proved alternative treatments (13%), not informed of expected risks and pain (10%), and not told of likely benefits (6%).

Some people – among them US senator John Glenn and Gary Ellis, director of the office for protection from research risks at the National Institutes of Health – have argued for stronger controls. Glenn has proposed legislation to close many regulatory gaps. But until more researchers and their publications are willing to come out publicly about what they know and what they believe should be done to better advance medical research without sacrificing – and documenting – consent of the fully informed test subject, prospects appear dim for meaningful reform. Questions of consent can be expected to recur with disturbing frequency.

Keith Epstein, *Investigative Reporter*; and **Bill Sloat** *Investigative Reporter*, *The (Cleveland) Plain Dealer*, Washington Bureau, Washington DC, USA

RESEARCH IN PREGNANCY BRINGS SPECIAL CONSIDERATIONS

The debate on informed consent stimulated by the *BMJ* must be welcomed by anyone interested in the ethics of medicine and research.[1] Subsequent correspondence has highlighted the differences between consent to treatment that benefits only the individual and consent to participation in research that aims to benefit other people. For pregnant women, however, both treatment and research involve third parties, which might influence decision making. When treating pregnant women or offering them the chance to participate in research, we must ensure that consent is truly informed and freely given.

Women feel responsible for the fetus they carry to the extent that they often modify their habits and lifestyle during pregnancy. Pregnancy may affect their ability to make a free choice: they may feel bound to accept interventions that might benefit the fetus that they would rather decline, or they may refuse treatment for themselves in case it should harm the baby. If the risks and benefits to the fetus are not carefully explained they may not give their consent for research to which they feel a personal obligation or in which they are interested.

Research in pregnancy brings special considerations. The "two patient" model of pregnancy disallows the imposition of possible harm on one party for the sake of the other,[42] which is particularly important, for example, in studies on the mode of delivery. The father may have an opinion that will influence whether the mother participates. Previously independent women may be vulnerable and dependent on their doctor, whom they need to trust and whom they may want to please by entering research projects. If they are to forgo the "good" of personal care, they must trust that the trial truly is based on the null hypothesis – that there is no known difference between the proposed treatments or interventions. Some patients will prefer to assume that "[My] doctor knows best [about me and my baby]" and not be happy to enter into the discussion of uncertainty that a trial and the issue of informed consent will raise.

These challenges sometimes lead to the exclusion of pregnant women from clinical trials. For work on drugs such as tocolytic agents, however, only pregnant women can help. Pregnancy does not remove a woman's competence to give informed consent, but it does bring extra considerations that researchers must bear in mind when trying to encourage these women to participate.

These views arose out of interviews with women who had been invited into research projects while pregnant; the work was supported by a grant of £5000 from the NHS Executive (West Midlands) research in primary care initiative.

Kay Mohanna, *General Practitioner*, Lichfield, UK

EXPLICIT GUIDANCE IS REQUIRED ON VALID EXEMPTIONS FOR NEED FOR ETHICAL REVIEW

We welcome the recent attention to the ethical conduct of human experimentation.[1, 43] But we believe that an overzealous interpretation of what are intended to be general guidelines can make it difficult to communicate non-experimental case reports, reviews of case notes, and clinical series. We are often asked for advice on whether studies require review by an ethical committee. To advise that a study does not need ethical review is to make an ethical judgment; that is, of course, the function of the committee. Thus it falls to the investigators to decide whether to seek approval of the ethics committee. We believe that, when an author submits a manuscript for publication, the editor should consider a statement giving valid reasons for exemption from the general need for ethical approval. We find the guidelines issued by the Royal College of Physicians both lucid and helpful.[35] We suggest that editors could adopt these or similar statements making clear what types of report need not be reviewed by a research ethics committee.

In essence, the grounds for exemption could include:

- that the information emerged from clinical practice and so does not constitute research (section 3.1 in the Royal College of Physicians' guidelines);
- that the information concerns innovative treatment applied with the patients' informed consent and so does not constitute research (section 3.2);
- that the investigation was considered to be a quality control or medical audit exercise exempt for the need for ethical review (section 4.8).

The editor should decide whether the claim for exemption is valid and also ensure that the manuscript respects the confidentiality of the patients.

As an example of the difficulties that arise, we are aware of a case in which an editor refused to consider a manuscript because the work had not been reviewed by an ethics committee. The authors were describing five years of clinical experience with a technique generally accepted as a therapeutic option and which they considered to be the method of choice for a life-threatening condition. In our opinion, the authors, who were also the patients' medical practitioners, did not need approval of a research ethics committee to provide what they considered to be the best care for their patients or to refer back to the original case notes in order to aggregate the data. In response to an appeal, the editor concerned asked whether the authors could obtain retrospective approval from the local ethics committee, but it is that committee's policy not to consider retrospective applicaitons.

More explicit guidance on valid exemptions for the need for ethical review would be invaluable in preventing or resolving this type of impasse.

Tom Woodcock, *Honorary Secretary, Joint Research Ethics Committee*; and **John Norman**, *Professor*, General Hospital, Southampton, UK

LACK OF RESPECT FOR PATIENTS IN MEDICAL RESEARCH MAY REFLECT WIDER DISRESPECT IN CLINICAL PRACTICE

I do not think that the *BMJ* should continue to publish papers that do not include informed consent.[4] Martin Dennis and colleagues, who studied the effect of contact with a stroke family care worker, did not ask patients to consent to randomisation.[4] As Sheila McLean points out in her commentary on Dennis and colleagues' study, none of the considerations that the authors faced were unique.[4] I suggest that they are in fact faced by many trialists. Certainly none of them was of such importance as to override fundamental ethical principles. In Dennis and colleagues' study it would have been possible, by using multivariate analysis, to determine whether initial preference (assessed, for example, by a question posed before randomisation) had a significant impact on satisfaction or other variables. This is an approach that colleagues and I used in a randomised controlled trial.[44] I sympathise with the desire to remove as much bias as possible, but we would do well to heed the philosopher Xenophanes (6th century BC), who said: "Through seeking we may learn and know things better, but as for certain truth no man hath known it, for all is but a woven web of guesses."

The situation faced by Satish Bhagwanjee and colleagues was certainly more complex.[3] Nevertheless, Len Doyal rightly suggests that "assent" from relatives of incompetent patients should be sought.[2] Bhagwanjee and colleagues' concern to maintain confidentiality posthumously might have been satisfied by their making clear to the assenting relatives that the result would be destroyed and not disclosed to them if the patient died.

I wonder whether a lack of respect for patients in medical research reflects a wider, subtle, disrespect in clinical practice: how many general practitioners, midwives, or obstetricians, for example, can honestly say that they seek the informed consent of all women for antenatal screening for syphilis? The draft revision of the Hippocratic oath recently circulated by the BMA states: "I will ensure patients receive the information and support they want to make decisions about disease prevention and improvement of their health."[45] Our duty as medical researchers is clear.

Jim Sikorski, *Honorary Research Fellow*, Department of General Practice, UMDS, London, UK

RIGOROUS STUDIES ARE NEEDED TO DETERMINE VALUES OF INTERVENTION

Richard Smith's editorial and the accompanying papers concerning informed consent have considerable implications for research on the "softer" areas of medicine.[1] There are important differences between trials looking at, say, distribution of an information leaflet or provision of a specialist nurse and studies of a new drug or of a surgical procedure.

If offered the choice of receiving an information leaflet or specialist nursing, few patients would opt for the equivalent of no treatment. Results from any such trial requiring informed consent would therefore be extremely unrepresentative and possibly misleading or meaningless.

In her commentary on Martin Dennis and colleagues' study Sheila McLean states: "If certain research cannot be undertaken to the maximum standards of scientific inquiry the question is not how much information should be withheld, it is whether the research should be done in the first place."[4] Many members of the legal profession, whose primary information base is case law, presumably hold this view. Medicine must, in contrast, be based on more than individual case histories.

As well as expecting to be kept informed by their doctors, patients expect their doctors to be informed. If we cannot perform rigorous studies we shall continue to be pressurised to provide interventions of little or no value to patients, and harm may result.

Richard Watson, *General Practitioner*; and **Philip Wilson**, *General Practitioner* Glasgow, UK

TRIALS THAT USE ZELEN'S PROCEDURE SHOULD BE ACCEPTABLE

In his editorial on the ethics of obtaining consent in trials, Richard Smith describes the Edinburgh evaluation of family stroke care workers as one "in which informed consent was not sought," a description taken up in the lay press.[1, 4] In fact, Martin Dennis and colleagues make it clear that they did seek consent, using a variant of Zelen's procedure, the single randomised consent design (Fig. 12.1).[46]

In her commentary criticising the Edinburgh trial, Sheila McLean says: "Anyone who is to be studied must be given the fullest possible information."[4] Len Doyal seems to agree, using the terms informed consent and fully informed consent interchangeably.[2] What is fully informed consent? Does it include details of all the evidence justifying the mounting of a trial and details of the financing of the study, how the sample size was derived, and the methods that will be used to analyse the results? If taken literally, the idea is absurd; consent can never be fully informed. In any case, an attempt at implementation – that is, at ensuring that everybody knows everything – would defeat its purpose. To paraphrase Zelen, what we want is not fully informed subjects but

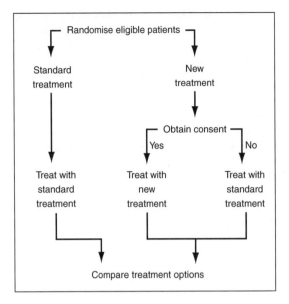

Figure 12.1 *Single randomised consent design.*

fully understanding ones. We must choose what information to impart, or we only confuse. It is adequately informed consent that is the hallmark of ethical research.

In decisions of what constitutes adequately informed consent, the conflict is not simply between researchers' convenience and the moral rights of subjects. Insisting on consent to randomisation in pursuit of one ethical aim may lead to the conduct of an unethical trial for another reason. As willingness to consent to randomisation is a psychological characteristic it may be associated with other characteristics that themselves determine the outcome of treatment. This applies particularly to trials of psychosocial interventions. If refusals are substantial but the trial is completed, sampling bias will be large but uninterpretable. Research that is useless or yields misleading results because of design faults is unethical, just as much as inadequately informed consent is.

It does not help the ethical argument to talk about informed consent, fully informed consent, and consent to randomisation as if they were the same thing. Nor does it help to argue that seeking consent to randomisation is always ethical while not doing so is simply self-serving. A good case has not been made for obligatory adherence to consent to randomisation, and until it has, the *BMJ* should continue to publish trials that use Zelen's procedure.

The authors are conducting a trial of psychological intervention after stroke, funded by the NHS research and development programme, that uses a randomised consent design.

Allan House, *Consultant*, Department of Liaison Psychiatry, Leeds General Infirmary; and **Peter Knapp**, *Research Psychologist*, Research School of Medicine, University of Leeds, UK

NOT SEEKING INFORMED CONSENT BREACHES PATIENT'S CHARTER

The patient's charter has not been mentioned in the recent debate about informed consent.[1] The charter tells patients that they have the right to choose whether or not to take part in medical research.[47] Thus, not to seek patients' informed consent before entering them into research is to breach the charter and to nullify patients' legitimate presumptions. Journals should not publish research whose design depends on avoiding consent or that fails to give particulars of how consent was sought.

Charlotte Williamson, *Vice Chair, York Health Services NHS Trust*, York, UK

ETHICAL PRINCIPLES MAY NEED TO BE ADAPTED WHEN RESEARCH SUBJECT IS NOT AN INDIVIDUAL SUBJECT

Most commentaries on consent have centred on the individual research subject. In public health, however, the "subject" is often a population or unit of service, and both the study design and ethical principles may need adaptation. This gets especially tricky when the style of informing people about a service, and inviting them, is itself the focus of study.

For example, the effect of inviting women aged 65–69 for breast screening is currently being studied in East Sussex, Leeds and Wakefield, and Nottingham. We have argued, and our local research ethics committees have agreed, that the benefit to individual women is already sufficiently proved (and similar to that for women aged 50–64) that the same routine style of invitation to and acceptance of screening are sufficient to achieve informed consent to the procedure. The research question – the area of "therapeutic uncertainty" – is whether those benefits (set against the costs) justify such screening as a national policy. Response to invitation will be one of the key end points; it would be difficult to predict the national response to a standard form of invitation if the trial districts had used a non-standard invitation involving consent.

We could not, in the present state of knowledge, have advanced a similar argument for women aged over 70, and it is a moot point at what stage in the accumulation of evidence our argument became valid for 65–69 year olds. (It is not clear from published accounts how informed consent was secured in previous trials.) The chairman of Wakefield's local research ethics committee thought that one justification for our approach was that the beneficial intervention was being offered to an entire population, with no randomisation or non-intervention group. We hope that journal editors will accept the line taken when the time comes to publish the results.

Graham C Sutton, *Senior Clinical Lecturer*, Nuffield Institute for Health, Leeds; **Linda Garvican**, *Principal Public Health Specialist*, South-East Institute for Public Health, Tunbridge Wells; and **Robin Wilson**, *Clinical Director, Breast Services*, National Breast Screening Training Centre, City Hospital, Nottingham, UK

STUDY IN WHICH PATIENTS HAD HIV TESTS COULD HAVE BEEN DESIGNED DIFFERENTLY

We share Rajendra Kale's view that failing to seek patients' consent to HIV testing is always wrong.[3] In a bronchoscopy study of patients with HIV infection in Harare the patient's consent was sought in every case. It was only rarely declined, and even when this occurred the data were still acceptable for publication.[48]

Satish Bhagwanjee and colleagues' study could have been designed differently. HIV testing could have been done anonymously, with matching of the results of the tests and patient data done by a third party not involved in the patients' care. Alternatively, serum samples from all the patients admitted to the intensive care unit could have been stored and survivors asked for their permission for testing. Serum samples from non-survivors could have been tested and given a number that would render them unidentifiable to anyone outside the study. Testing without consent and then informing the patients can be an unfortunate combination. The fact that only three out of 402 patients wished to know the result of their HIV test suggests some unconscious resistance to being tested, and of course by then they were not in a position to refuse testing. Were all patients asked whether they objected to being included without prior testing, and if so how was this question posed?

We believe that the ethics committee that considered this proposal did the investigators a disservice by not pointing out alternative ways of doing this study while protecting patients' rights.

Adam Malin, *Specialist Registrar in Chest Medicine*, Whittington Hospital NHS Trust; and **Diana Lockwood**, *Senior Lecturer*, London School of Hygiene and Tropical Medicine, London, UK

INFORMED CONSENT IS LIGHT YEARS AWAY FOR BLACK AFRICAN PATIENTS

We wish to cross swords with Y K Seedat over the wild and presumptuous assertions in his commentary about testing subjects without their consent.[3] His piece is apt to mislead and presents a one-sided picture for any doctor who has no idea of South African society.

Seedat is professor of medicine at the University of Natal, an almost exclusively Asian and black medical school. This medical school's main hospital is King Edward VIII Hospital, a black hospital. We find it astounding that no mention is made of the racial breakdown of those tested anonymously for HIV without their consent. We assume that they were almost exclusively black African patients in social classes IV and V (black working class). As black doctors whose medical studies began at the University of Natal, we find Seedat's wild assertions insulting not only to black Africans but to humanity as a whole. His claim that there is no harm or injury to the subjects has never been tested.

The subjects who were tested have never had any rights in South Africa and are forever grateful and indebted to anyone with a white coat and a stethoscope – anyone in authority. Our experience with South Africa during apartheid and since its abolition suggests that true informed consent as part of ethics is light years away for black African patients. Although we are British medical practitioners, we are South African nationals, and we find it unacceptable that black South African patients become subjects of dubious laboratory tests without their knowledge for the benefit of doctors and other races.

S W P Mhlongo, *General Practitioner*, St Raphaels Way Medical Centre; and **G V Mdingi**, *General Practitioner*, Sandringham Practice, London, UK

RESEARCH SUFFERS IF PATIENTS SUSPECT THAT THEIR RIGHTS MAY BE BREACHED

Debate on informed consent has drawn attention to situations in which scientific reliability – specifically, avoiding subjective reporting bias – conflicts with the obligation fully to inform subjects in a clinical trial.[3, 4] When there is a conflict of principles we have to choose which principle will take precedence. The majority opinion both in the medical profession and among ethicists is that the patient's right to choose takes precedence over the researcher's right to seek knowledge, and this involves rights to refuse participation and to request information. Weakening or abandoning the requirement for informed consent on the grounds that bias may result if patients know that they are in a trial is a potentially serious erosion of the protection afforded by the principle of informed consent. It therefore requires careful, and in our view sceptical, review.

In recent years there has been a tendency to argue that badly designed research is inherently unethical. While we have sympathy with this view, the consequence of regarding some methods as carrying moral value is to devalue the patient as the prime source of moral authority. We are approaching a situation in which the requirements of a method may once again take precedence over patients' consent, as, for example, in Dennis and colleagues' study of the introduction of a stroke worker.[4] While the authors argue that the intervention was harmless, we believe that the cost of condoning research that lacks consent will always outweigh any possible benefit.

Even if one ignores the philosophical argument, simply in practical terms research suffers if patients suspect that their rights may be breached. One development that might help patients and researchers is to expand the role that patients have in the research design and reviewing processes. Professional researchers may regard this as unrewarding. We suspect that forms of research other than clinical trials may provide more insight into the effectiveness of interventions than a randomised controlled trial in precisely those cases in which researchers believe that patient subjectivity may confound results.

When consent is a matter of bald choice, it is unsurprising that many patients refuse to participate in trials that seem to be in their own or society's interests, and that the results of trials are hard to apply to non-experimental medical situations. Evidence from trials in breast cancer suggests that good consent processes benefit patients and result in improved outcome measures. Surely this indicates that more and better consent and involvement of patients are needed in research, not less.

Richard Ashcroft, *Lecturer in Medical Ethics*; and **Ben Toth**, *Research Associate*, University of Bristol, Department of Social Medicine, Bristol, UK

PATIENTS' KNOWLEDGE THAT THEY ARE PARTICIPATING IN TRIAL MAY NOT BIAS RESULTS

In his commentary on his and colleagues' study Martin Dennis puts forward arguments as to why patients in a trial of the effect of a stroke family care worker were not asked for their consent before being entered into the trial.[4] We question whether seeking consent would necessarily have biased the results. We are currently involved in a randomised controlled trial in Oxford of a family support organiser for patients with stroke and their families. As in Edinburgh, patients are randomised in our study before consent has been obtained. At the time of randomisation, however, we write to the closest carers of all patients, inviting them to take part. The letter explains the purpose of the study and that whether or not the carers see the family support organiser will be determined by chance. Altogether, 18 of the 179 families contacted so far have elected not to take part, either in response to the letter or when contacted by a researcher 6 months after the stroke. The proportion of families not taking part is the same (10%) in both the intervention and control group. At the following-up visit, the researcher does not specifically remind patients or their family that the purpose of interviewing them is to evaluate the possible effects of a family support organiser. Our study was approved by the Central Oxford Research Ethics Committee.

The theoretical concern is that patients and their families will realise which group they are in and that this might influence the results.[4] Our experience, however, suggests that patients and families do not discriminate between different community services. Prompted by the issues raised by Dennis, we decided to do a limited interim analysis of our (ongoing) study. At the end of the follow-up interview the researcher asks what services have been received since the stroke. Only eight of 80 families in the intervention group have mentioned the family support organiser at this time. The researcher then records which of the two groups she thinks the family was in. She has so far guessed correctly for 102 (64%) out of 159 families (95% confidence interval 57% to 72%). While higher than would be expected by chance, this is not significantly more than the 59% recorded by the researcher in the Edinburgh study. This provides circumstantial evidence that many families were effectively blind to their treatment allocation. Therefore, it would seem that consent can be obtained in trials of this sort without compromising the validity of the results.

Funding: The Oxford family support organiser trial is supported by the Stroke Association.

Jonathan Mant, *Clinical Lecturer in Public Health Medicine, Division of Public Health and Primary Health Care*; **Simon Winner**, *Consultant Physician, Department of Clinical Geratology*, Radcliffe Infirmary; **Judy Carter**, *Research Occupational Therapist*; and **Derick T Wade**, *Consultant in Neurological Disability*, Rivermead Rehabilitation Centre, Oxford, UK

TWO-STAGE RANDOMISATION AND CONSENT WOULD OVERCOME MANY PROBLEMS

We believe that two-stage randomisation procedures potentially provide a solution to the ethical concerns arising from Martin Dennis and colleagues' study evaluating a stroke family care worker.[4, 49] A two-stage randomisation procedure requires that all patients give full consent to their particular role in the trial rather than to a hypothetical scenario. In the first stage of randomisation all patients are asked to give consent for follow-up. Consent for additional (non-standard) treatment is sought only from a random sample selected to be offered the study intervention. Therefore, patients – whether they are in the control or intervention group – consent to the assessments and treatment that they will actually receive. This contrasts with the usual one-stage consent procedure in randomised controlled trials, whereby patients consent to two or more possible forms of care, which they may or may not get. When a one-stage procedure is used patients randomised to standard care may feel disadvantaged as a result of not receiving the intervention, particularly if it is a new clinical service. A two-stage randomisation clearly would be unethical if the control group were receiving non-standard care. In her commentary on the study Sheila McLean argues that patients should consent to the project rather than their role within it.

Surely, however, it is more appropriate that they give personal consent to their assessment and treatment in a project and what will be required of them in the study. We believe that this approach, centred on the patient, is consistent with the highest of ethical standards in medical research.

D J Stott, *Professor of Geriatric Medicine*; **P Langhorne**, *Senior Lecturer in Geriatric Medicine*, University of Glasgow, Royal Infirmary, Glasgow; and **H Rodgers**, *Senior Lecturer in Stroke Medicine*, University of Newcastle upon Tyne, UK

ABILITY TO BE INFORMED IS SEPARATE FROM ABILITY TO GIVE CONSENT

The debate over the need for research subjects' informed consent lacked the patients' perspective. It is true that many people would be reluctant to take part in a randomised controlled trial if they knew that they were doing so. Why is this? It is because they have at best only a 50% chance of being in the group with the most positive outcomes, if there is indeed a difference, and because, by the time the trial has established such distinctions, their own treatment may be compromised. Their reasons are rational; they are just inconvenient for the researcher.

I am concerned by Len Doyal's and others' ready exclusion of consent for people "not competent" to give consent.[2] In the case of a person with a learning difficulty, a juvenile, or a person with a severe mental health problem (my own field of research), what may perhaps be compromised is the ability to be informed. I would argue that this is separate from the ability to give consent, and failure to recognise the distinction allows researchers to take the arrogant view that the only reason why people refuse to cooperate is because they have failed to understand the information offered.

It is easy in practice for researchers to be "economical" with the information, volunteering only those aspects of the study that they suspect are most acceptable to patients. The smaller the potential sample the more likely this subterfuge is, to maximise participation.

Jeffrey S Tobias suggests that there is often a conflict of interests between the best interests of the individual patient and those of society as a whole.[5] But it hardly seems appropriate to leave the research community to decide what the interests of society as a whole are, for we would expect their conclusions to be biased.

It is undeniable that offering truly informed consent will skew outcomes in most cases, though it will not necessarily affect the outcome variables that are being measured. No research design involving human subjects can avoid the human factor. Perhaps we need to accept, as the average sceptical but rational layperson did a long time ago, that scientific research rarely provides unequivocal outcomes. What it does is substantiate reasonable hypotheses, which will help predict outcomes in most cases. Let's not kid ourselves that we work under laboratory conditions; and let's remember that you can't treat people like rats.

Deborah Rutter *Research manager*, Hillingdon Outreach Support Team, Uxbridge, Middlesex UB8 1AR

"BLANKET" CONSENT TO TRIALS WOULD BE A GOOD IDEA

In his editorial on informed consent, Richard Smith discusses the contrasting views of Len Doyal and Jeffrey S Tobias.[1] He highlights Tobias's suggestion that a patient could give "blanket" consent when admitted to a hospital where several randomisation studies are in progress.[5] I supported this idea some years ago, but also suggested that much work would have to be done explaining the need for it and gaining public trust.[50] It could be a useful third option, added to the options of requesting and not requesting informed consent; thorough safeguards and approval of an ethics committee would be necessary.

In all walks of life, when one person seeks help from another, consent based on trust is surely just as valid as consent based on information. There is always a blend of the two, but the proportions vary. Lord Scarman, a judge with liberal views, said, "It may be sensible to trust your doctor and feel that the risks are for him to assess."[51] We all know that "fully informed" consent is often nothing of the kind; there may well be more trust than information. With blanket consent the average amount of trust would have to be even greater, but there would be many advantages.

Those who want the *BMJ* to take a rigid view that might overrule the opinion of ethics committees should spend a day in a ward full of elderly people. They would probably find many who, though far from being mentally incompetent, are at times confused and forgetful. What could be more unrealistic than to refuse to recognise this for fear of being called patronising or paternalistic? Suppose a doc-

tor approaches such a patient, who perhaps feels ill and wants only sensitive care, with a view to gaining his or her fully informed consent to, say, two studies – the randomising of the patient's sleeping tablets and the randomising by the surgeon of a new suture material. Who can be sure that concern or confusion will not follow? Where is the sense in this? Some people underestimate both the danger of not comparing treatments in a reliable way and the harm that can be done to many sick patients when fully informed consent for every trial is sought, no matter how tense or difficult the situation.

There are many grey areas, but we should start thinking seriously about the idea of some general form of consent to the fact that a treatment is being randomised. The result would be fewer misconceptions, less fundamentalism, more trust, less detail, and more time to attend to patients' real needs.

Thurstan Brewin, *Chairman of Health Watch 1993–6*, Oxford, UK

RESPECT FOR AUTONOMY MAY CONFLICT WITH PRINCIPLE OF BENEFICENCE

The argument of Len Doyal and Sheila McLean (in her commentary),[2] that respect for patients' autonomy demands that they should be informed about possible alternative treatments, should be applied not just to clinical trials but to any situation in which there is uncertainty about which treatment is best. As Martin Dennis and colleagues' trial evaluating the introduction of a stroke family care worker shows, any new treatment or care service, no matter how apparently benign, has the potential to do harm, yet many are introduced without formal evaluation.[4] For example, when coronary care units were introduced few people would have questioned their intrinsic benefits in promoting better monitoring and early treatment of complications, yet how many deaths may have been caused by over-enthusiastic use of prophylactic antiarrhythmic drugs?[52] We therefore have a duty to evaluate rigorously not just new practices but many of those that have already come into widespread use.

If uncertainty still exists about the value of coronary care units or about the patients most likely to benefit, should we respect the autonomy of patients with acute chest pain (regardless of age or other commonly applied eligibility criteria) by explaining all the potential advantages and disadvantages of specialised coronary care? Alternatively, should we conduct a randomised trial and explain to patients allocated to care in a general ward exactly what special facilities will not be made available to them? The bias in expectations introduced by such an approach would not only weaken the conclusions of the study, as Dennis points outs in his commentary,[4] but could lead to the wrong conclusions, possibly misleading clinicians for years to come.

Rigid insistence on full disclosure risks undermining the confidence of patients that they are getting the best possible treatment. We know that this can have a substantial adverse effect, so respect for autonomy may thus conflict with the principle of beneficence. Why should one ethical principle take precedence over another, and why should different standards be applied to "normal" clinical practice and research? Could it be because the informed consent procedure is easier to audit, particularly in a clinical trial, and is therefore more susceptible to legal challenge? If we submit to such thinly veiled legalistic threats, then not only will reliable scientific evaluation of health care services be impossible (as Dennis and colleagues have shown) but we will no longer be able to deal with the inevitable uncertainties of clinical practice in a way that protects patients from serious potential harm.

David Barer, *Professor of Clinical Geriatric Medicine*, Department of Medicine (Geriatrics), University of Newcastle, Newcastle upon Tyne, UK

Personal view*

Kulsum Winship

ALL TREATMENT AND TRIALS MUST HAVE INFORMED CONSENT

In 1987 I was diagnosed with late stage cervical cancer, despite three negative smears that year and numerous visits to the doctor. I was told that I was having radiotherapy. I asked many questions, and my consultant explained the treatment as though it was a tried and trusted method, established for years. Eventually I was given the "all clear" and resumed my career. Six months later I returned to the hospital with severe faecal incontinence. I was advised that I might have radiotherapy damage and that I was "unlucky". I was then referred to a bowel specialist. He gave me unstinting support and inexhaustible, honest explanations. I never saw my radiotherapist again.

I was shocked to realise that I had not been informed of any risks before I consented to what turned out to be experimental treatment, only tested on mouse tails. I was admitted for a temporary colostomy and to have my rectum rebuilt. I met other women with radiotherapy injuries on the ward, and we had all been led to believe that we were unique. I was admitted over 100 times and had 24 operations, for adhesion attacks, a hernia operation, a permanent colostomy and urostomy, an operation to remove compacted faeces, formation then removal of both a rebuilt rectum and a mucus fistula, thrombosis, and so on. At present I have a vaginal fistula which intermittently allows faeces to escape through my vagina.

The repeated line of defence to patients who ask for explanations is: "Your injuries are a one-off." A group of damaged patients joined together for mutual support and to prove otherwise. We called ourselves RAGE (Radiotherapy Action Group Exposure). A similar group of patients with breast cancer started in the south of England, so those of us in the north were called RAGE National.†

We discovered that we had been guinea-pigs in a clinical trial of a new radiotherapy protocol. We felt totally betrayed. We trusted the doctors, yet none of us had given our written consent even to treatment (only to the anaesthetic), and we were not given details about possible complications. An investigative journalist found out that we had been involved in trials without our knowledge. We could hardly believe him: this was Britain in the 1980s, not Hitler's Germany.

*BMJ 1997; **314**: 1134–5.
†RAGE National, Tel: 0161 839 2927.

The more we discovered, the worse it became. Hundreds of women had been involved in clinical trials of radiotherapy to the pelvic area, and the morbidity rate rose to 57% in 1982. This was 5 years before I was treated: had nothing been learnt from earlier trials? Worse still, there was an almost complication-free alternative, still being used, but no one gave us a choice.

Most women had no idea that their treatment was so toxic when they consented; not one of the women I have spoken to was told she was in a clinical trial; many have attended the hospital since for corrective or even life-saving surgery. When a friend with early stage cervical cancer died from her treatment, not the cancer (which could have been cured by hysterectomy), we decided to go public and allow our names and photos to be published. Women are angry that others are still not being informed.

Women have tried to commit suicide as their lives have been ruined. Few have been offered counselling, marriages have broken, careers ended, children fostered. Many women cannot have intercourse. Some have developed social phobias, some are housebound through agonising pain and incontinence. RAGE has members from each year of the trials, all receiving different treatment schedules.

A RAGE member wrote: "Somewhere, somehow, I have to expose this abuse of power. The doctors never got my informed consent. This is abuse of society's most vulnerable people. Where is there a platform for my voice to be heard, to make the public aware and the establishment accountable?" Some women only wanted an apology, or more understanding, or psychological support. More than compensation, patients want to protect future generations by ensuring that they are fully informed and do not suffer. Some consultants have shown humanity, by sharing information and giving examples of better practice: despite NHS pressures they have not lost sight of compassion.

Attitudes are slowly changing. Patients now expect to be told the details of the treatment proposed, together with side effects and complications. It is the doctor's duty to state the facts, whether or not they are painful. Reading the Helsinki Declaration, I was troubled to think that clinicians today may even believe that sometimes there is no need for informed consent. We are living proof that nothing should be assumed. Protocols for the trials we were involved in were not even submitted to the local research ethics committee.

Our experience with RAGE tells us that patients are still not involved in their treatment decisions. Clinicians should understand that with new technology, patients can actively access information. If doctors do not provide this information some patients will obtain it anyway. Patients phone us saying that they have read the cancer charity leaflets and spoken to their consultants; now they want "the truth". Patients want to talk to real patients, not those who purport to represent them, and current literature is not specific enough on toxicity. We have found that with careful questioning one can usually provide the level of information each individual wants to receive.

Many people are too shocked at the time of diagnosis to take in details about any treatment proposed. Consent to treatment or research should be sought later, at a second multidisciplinary consultation where the patient is accompanied by a relative or friend. Participants in trials should have easy access to the results of those trials, as a condition of partnership. Joint ownership of the work being done keeps patients involved, instead of isolating them. Psychological morbidity is as significant as physical morbidity; this too goes unrecognised and untreated.

There must be clinicians who genuinely want to learn about the patient's perspective, who are brave enough to accept constructive criticism. When scientists have academic arguments about clinical research they should remember that they are dealing with people's lives. We have feelings and opinions. We don't want to be just another statistic: we're real, we exist, and it is our bodies that you are experimenting with.

REFERENCES

1. Smith R. Informed consent: the intricacies. *BMJ* 1997; **314**: 1059–60.
2. Doyal L. Journals should not publish research to which patients have not given fully informed consent – with three exceptions. *BMJ* 1997; **314**: 1107–11.
3. Bhagwanjee S, Muckart DJJ, Jeena PM, Moodley P. Does HIV status influence the outcome of patients admitted to a surgical intensive care unit? A prospective double blind study (with commentaries by R Kale, S Bhagwanjee *et al.*, and YK Seedat). *BMJ* 1997; **314**: 1077–84.
4. Dennis M, O'Rourke S, Slattery J, Staniforth T, Warlow C. Evaluation of a stroke family care worker: results of a randomised controlled trial. *BMJ* 1997; **314**: 1071–7.

5. Tobias JS. *BMJ*'s present policy (sometimes approving research in which patients have not given fully informed consent) is wholly correct. *BMJ* 1997; **314**: 1111–4.

6. Flint C, Poulengeris P, Grant A. The "Know your midwife" scheme – a randomised trial of continuity of care by a team of midwives. *Midwifery* 1989; **5**: 11–16.

7. Little P, Williamson I, Warner G, Gould G, Gantley M, Kinmonth AL. Open randomised trial of prescribing strategies for sore throat. *BMJ* 1997; **314**: 722–27. (8 March.)

8. McArdle JMC, George WD, McArdle CS, *et al.* Psychological support for patients undergoing breast cancer surgery: a randomised study. *BMJ* 1996; **312**: 813–17.

9. Mudur G. Indian study of women with cervical lesions called unethical. *BMJ* 1997; **314**: 1065. (12 April.)

10. Anonymous. All treatment and trials must have informed consent. *BMJ* 1997; **314**: 1134–5. (12 April.)

11. Thornton HM. Breast cancer trials: a patient's viewpoint. *Lancet* 1992; **339**: 44–5.

12. Baum M. The ethics of randomised controlled trials. *Eur J Surg Oncol* 1995; **21**: 136–9.

13. Thornton H. A "ladyplan" for trial recruitment? Everyone's business! *Lancet* 1993; **341**: 796.

14. Thornton H. What can patients contribute to the design of clinical trials? In: Tobias J, Houghton J, eds. *New horizons in breast cancer: current controversies, future directions*. London: Chapman and Hall (in press).

15. The Nuremberg code (1947). *BMJ* 1996; **313**: 1448.

16. Declaration of Helsinki. *BMJ* 1996; **313**: 1448.

17. Vollmann J, Winau R. Informed consent in human experimentation before the Nuremberg code. *BMJ* 1996; **313**: 1445–7.

18. Alderson P, Montgomery J. *Health care choices: making decisions with children*. London: Institute for Public Policy Research, 1996.

19. Appelbaum PS, Grisso T. Assessing patients' capacities to consent to treatment. *N Engl J Med* 1988; **319**: 1635.

20. Neuroscience Approach to Human Health Initiative Steering Committee. *Mental handicap research: new technologies and approaches. Report of the workshop organised under the initiative of the Neuroscience Approach to Human Health Initiative Steering Committee*. Warwick: University of Warwick, 1993.

21. Chalmers I. Underreporting research is scientific misconduct. *JAMA* 1990; **263**: 1405–8.

22. Lindley RI, Amayo EO, Marshall J, Sanderock PAG, Dennis M, Warlow CP. Acute stroke treatment in UK hospitals: the Stroke Associations survey of consultant opinion. *J R Coll Physicians Lond* 1995; **29**: 479–84.

23. Ricci S, Celani MG, Righetti E, Cantisani AT for the International Stroke Trial Collaborative Group. Between country variations in the use of medical treatments for acute stroke: an update [abstract]. *Cerebrovasc Dis* 1996; **6**(Suppl. 2): 133.

24. Warlow C, Van Gijn J, Sanderock P, eds. *Stroke module of the Cochrane database of systematic reviews* [updated 4 March 1997]. Oxford: Update Software, 1997.

25. Adkisson GH, Macleod MA, Hodgson M, Sykes JJW, Smith F, Strack C, *et al.* Cerebral perfusion deficits in dysbaric illness. *Lancet* 1989; **ii**: 119–22.

26. Wilmshurst PT, Nunan TO. Cerebral perfusion deficits in dysbaric illness. *Lancet* 1989; **ii**: 674–5.

27. Adkisson GH. Cerebral perfusion deficits in dysbaric illness, *Lancet* 1989; **ii**: 675.

28. Wilmshurst P. Ethical or not? *Diver* 1992; **37**(9): 85.

29. Sigerist HE. In: *Human experimentation, a guided step into the unknown* (cited by WA Silverman). Oxford: Oxford University Press, 1985: 161.

30. Baum M. New approach for recruitment into randomised controlled trials. *Lancet* 1993; **341**: 812–14.

31. Baum M. Clinical trials – a brave new partnership: a response to Mrs Thornton. *J Med Ethics* 1994; **20**: 23–5.

32. Harrison JE. Patients should not be discouraged from entering trials. *BMJ* 1996; **313**: 1488.

33. British Paediatric Association. *Guidelines for the conduct of medical research with children*. London: BPA, 1992.

34. English DC. *Bioethics: a clinical guide for medical students*. London: WW Norton, 1994.

35. Royal College of Physicians of London. *Guidelines on the practice of ethics committees in medical research involving human subjects*. 3rd edn. London: RCP, 1996.

36. Snowdon C, Garcia J, Elbourne D. Understanding randomisation: parental responses to the allocation of alternative treatments in a clinical trial involving their critically ill newborn babies. *Soc Sci Med* (in press).

37. UK Collaborative ECMO Trial Group. UK collaborative randomised controlled trial of neonatal extracorporeal membrane oxygenation. *Lancet* 1996; **348**: 75–82.

38. Epstein K, Sloat B. Drug trials: do people know the truth about experiments? *The (Cleveland) Plain Dealer* 1996 Dec 15–18:a1.

39. Harris JF, Fletcher MA. Six decades later, an apology. *Washington Post* 1997 May 17:a1.

40. Teegardin C, Whitt R. FDA inspection finds violations in Augusta studies. *Atlanta Constitution* 1997 May 11:a3.

41. Marsh B, Romney L. Hospital accused of violating consent rules. *Los Angeles Times* 1997 May 30:a3.

42. Tauer C. When pregnant women refuse interventions. *AWHONN's Clinical Issues* 1993; **4.4**: 596–604.
43. Rennie D. Disclosure to the reader of institutional board approval and informed consent. *JAMA* 1997; **277**: 922–3.
44. Clement S, Sikorski J, Wilson J, Das S, Smeeton N. Women's satisfaction with traditional and reduced antenatal visit schedules. *Midwifery* 1996; **12**: 120–8.
45. BMA. Draft revision of the Hippocratic oath. *BMA annual report of council 1996–97*. London: BMA, 1997.
46. Zelen M. Randomised consent designs for clinical trials: an update. *Stat Med* 1990; **9**: 645–56.
47. Department of Health. *The patient's charter*. London: HMSO, 1991.
48. Malin AS, Gwanzura LEC, Klein S, Robertson VJ, Musvaire P, Mason PR. Pneumocystis carinii pneumonia in Zimbabwe. *Lancet* 1995; **346**: 1258–61.
49. Zelen M. A new design for randomised clinical trials. *N Engl J Med* 1979; **300**: 1243–5.
50. Brewin TB. Valid comparison is the key. In: Razis DV, ed. *Medical ethics and/or ethical medicine*. Paris: Elsevier, 1989.
51. Scarman, Lord. Consent, communication and responsibility. *J R Soc Med* 1986; **79**: 697–700.
52. Cardiac Arrhythmia Suppression Trial (CAST) Investigators. Effect of encainide and flecainide on mortality in a randomised trial of arrhythmia suppression after myocardial infarction. *N Engl J Med* 1989; **321**: 406–12.

13 · Other perspectives following the *BMJ* articles and correspondence

Informed consent: edging forwards (and backwards)

Informed consent is an unavoidably complicated issue

Richard Smith

The issue of informed consent within medical practice, research, and publication is coming increasingly to the fore as the balance of power in the doctor-patient relationship tips towards patients. Last week Britain's General Medical Council heard a case in which a paediatric cardiologist was accused of going beyond the consent that he was given to treat a child. The child died, and he was found guilty of serious professional misconduct and erased from the medical register for six months.[1] When, last year, we published a cluster of articles asking whether we should decline to publish studies where patients had not given fully informed consent we prompted a flood of correspondence. We received over 50 letters, most of them argued with unusual care and clarity. Authors split down the middle between those who argued that we should always insist on informed consent (except in very limited circumstances) and those who thought that there were occasions when we need not. Today we try to advance the debate by publishing further responses to last year's debate, including some from patients' representatives. Within the broad context of informed consent we also explore the particular issue of consent for publication of material that emerges from the doctor-patient relationship.

INFORMED CONSENT IN RESEARCH

In our first cluster Len Doyal made the case for insisting on informed consent with only a few narrow exceptions,[2] while Jeff Tobias argued that the *BMJ* should sometimes publish papers that did not include fully informed consent.[3] Both reflect on the subsequent debate, but neither has changed his position (pp. 126–9).[4]

Mary Warnock, a philosopher who chaired Britain's Committee of Inquiry into Human Fertilisation, argues that "the principle of non-exploitation has come to seem to many to be by far the most important moral principle that should govern research using human subjects" (p. 129).[4] She thinks it a "misuse of words" to suggest that not obtaining informed consent in itself constitutes a harm: "sometimes it amounts to exploitation, sometimes it does not." She encourages editors to continue to live in a morally hazardous world, to shun dogma, and to follow a prayer from Hertford College Chapel" to distinguish things that differ." This encouragement is hard to resist because morally hazardous worlds are, I believe, right and proper for journals. Dogma is not only dangerous but also boring. We are in the debate not the certainty business.

We have specifically asked patients' representatives to contribute because patients' voices were not being heard – because the *BMJ* is read mainly by doctors and other health workers. Heather Goodare argues that we should take a strong line and reject all studies that do not include informed consent (pp. 131–3).[4] Lisa Power asks us to consider the broader issue of patients in planning research and thinks that "any hard and fast rule that the *BMJ* made about publication would probably have to be broken at some point" (pp. 130–1).[4]

In a separate article Richard Lindley argues that researchers should be educating the public about trials and that "we introduce a new type of card – the randomised controlled trial card – to be carried by people who understand randomised controlled trials and wish to be considered for future appropriate trials" (p. 135).[5] David and Solly Benatar from South Africa attack both Len Doyal's position and that adopted by the ethics committee in Natal that approved a trial that did not have informed consent (pp. 137–8).[6] In a personal view Josephine Venn-Treloar describes how she felt abused by undergoing an investigation without consent.[7]

None of this provides a simple solution to our dilemma: rather, it complicates it further. For now we are continuing our pragmatic policy of considering each case on its merits, and we have ourselves conducted studies on papers submitted to us without seeking consent from either authors or reviewers (and been criticised for it). Our next steps are to hold a conference in London (see accompanying note) and then to invite a small group of representatives of all views to adivse us on what policy to adopt. If, as seems likely, they cannot agree, then we will decide our own policy and announce it to readers. Any policy we adopt will, of course, be reviewed.

CONSENT AND PUBLICATION

While continuing to swither over the broad question, we have advanced on the particular question of consent for publication of material that emerges from the doctor-patient relationship.[8,9] Now we are proposing to retreat – a little. It used to be, and in many cases still is, that medical journals and books were relaxed about publishing material that emerged from the doctor – patient relationship-pictures, radiographs, case reports, or whatever. Weak attempts were made to anonymise the material, but generally nobody was worried. Then editors and others began to receive complaints, and we realised that annonymity is impossible to guarantee (particularly to the patient himself or herself). The inevitable logic was to move to informed consent for all such material, and that is the position adopted by the International Committee of Medical Journal Editors.[10] Now Britain's General Medical Council is adopting the same line. Proposed guidelines state:

"You must obtain consent from patients before publishing personal information about them as individuals in journals, texbooks, or other media in the public domain, whether or not you believe the patient can be identified. Consent must therefore be sought to the publication of, for example, case histories about, or photographs of, patients."

Catherine Hood and others show in detail how consent can be obtained from patients in 85% of cases.[11] There are, however, a growing list of cases where patients have been distressed by information about them being disclosed without consent, and at least one case led to charges of serious professional misconduct.[12] Those doctors were not found guilty, but under the new guidelines a similar case might result in the charge being sustained. The *BMJ* has recently been embroiled in a further case.[13] We published – without revealing the patients' name and with written consent – a radiograph and photograph of a patient who had been attacked with a machete. Later, when the case came to court, the pictures were reproduced in most of Britain's national newspapers and on television. Journalists had made a link between the case and the *BMJ* pictures. All but one of the newspapers reproduced the pictures without written consent, and we have complained to the press and broadcasting regulatory bodies. Our argument is that by reproducing these pictures without consent the media have invaded the privacy of the patient, undermined the doctor-patient relationship, and made it less likely that patients will consent to have material about them published in medical journals.

David Bullimore accuses us of hypocrisy and naivety in relation to this case[14]: hypocrisy because we placed the pictures on our website and had obtained inadequate consent, and naivety for not recognising that journalists would make the connection between the case and the pictures. Our response is that material on the website is copyright just as in the paper journal and that we published the material without a name attached. This case has, however, prompted us to start asking patients to sign specific consent forms that give information about the *BMJ*. The form is available on our website (www.bmj.com), and we will modify it in the light of readers' and patients's comments.

The GMC's proposed guidelines are brief and clear, but they may oversimplify, be hard to implement, and undermine scientific publishing. Particular – and unresolved – problems arise, for instance, with the publication of family trees. Information, sometimes very sensitive, may be given about large numbers of people, and some of those people may not know that they have a particular genetic trait. Is consent required from everybody? In the process of obtaining consent might people be given information they would rather not have? Series of cases also present a problem. We published a series of cases of patients who had recovered after being diagnosed as being in the persistent vegetative state.[15] In one case permission was denied, causing a critic in *JAMA* to ask whether "a journal that knowingly omits scientific information from a report because of the lack of consent [can] still be called a scientific journal."[16] The implication that science may demand that patients' rights be overridden is perhaps unfortunate, but that author attacks the editors of *JAMA* for declining to publish his paper on an outbreak of drug resistant tuberculosis because patients had not consented. Few if any ethical rules can be absolute, and a case may arise where editors would choose to publish without consent "in the public interest." Certainly there are occasions when doctors break confidentiality in the public interest.

Similar problems arise over confidential inquiries into patient deaths. This methodology began in Britain with maternal deaths and has been extended to surgical and other deaths. The information that arises is extremely valuable but has so far been published withour consent from surviving relatives. Will the GMC allow these to continue? Almost by definition, these are identifiable cases.

RELAXING OUR ABSOLUTISM

We have also been criticised for becoming too absolute in our rules. James Rankine bemoans the fact that a personal view he published in the *BMJ* in 1994 would not now be allowed because of the problem of consent.[17] The fillers that we publish on doctors' interactions with patients are popular with readers, and many make an important point. Yet many describe events that happened years ago and where the patients are almost certainly dead and their relatives untraceable. Should we reject these because we don't have consent? We have been doing so, but we think that we have gone too far. So just as the GMC is introducing clear but strict rules we are proposing to soften ours. The Box contains our proposed guidance, and we welcome readers' comments. In essence, the guidelines ask authors and editors to balance the importance and the interest of the piece against the possibility of harm to patients.

This continuing debate over informed consent illustrates clearly that most ethical conundrums don't submit to simple solutions. Doctors are practical folk who like to get on with things, and many will be frustrated by the expanding complexity of this debate. But doctors will have to learn to inhabit the complicated world in which philosophers feel comfortable. Clearly ethical training is important, which is why our surveys of readers' wants always show ethics second to education. We are trying to oblige.

Box 13.1　Publishing information that emerges from the doctor–patient relationship

Our general policy is that we require written consent from patients to publish material that emerges from the doctor–patient relationship. This is because the doctor–patient relationship must be confidential and because attempts to anonymise information about patients may fail. In papers describing recent experiences with patients consent will thus always be necessary: thus, in almost all scientific papers consent will be needed. Sometimes, however, it may be possible to publish material about patients – particularly general anecdotes – without consent. We cannot produce completely specific guidelines on this subject, but the decision depends on balancing the importance and interest of the information against the likelihood that a patient might be damaged.

Publication without consent may be acceptable in the following cases.

- The patient is long dead and has no living relatives.
- The interaction with the patient was long ago – perhaps more than 15 years.
- Because the interaction was long ago and the patient was elderly or terminally ill, the patient is likely to have died.
- The piece is to be published without the authors' names attached, making it unlikely that anybody could identify the patient.
- All extraneous information that might help identification is excluded. We must be careful about removing information from scientific papers because it is difficult to tell what is important, but these "let outs" will rarely apply to scientific papers. They are more likely to occur with fillers or stories in essays.
- Even if the patient were to identify himself or herself, the events described are unlikely to

Box 13.1 (contd)

cause offence. We must remember, however, that it is difficult to know what will cause offence: some patients will be offended simply by the fact that the information they gave to their doctors was published without consent.

• Sometimes authors – particularly Soundings authors – fictionalise material: they mix stories from different patients together. This is not acceptable in fillers because people read these as true. It may be acceptable in Soundings columns, but the author should make clear that the account is fictionalised.

REFERENCES

1. Dyer C. Consultant suspended for not getting consent for cardiac procedure. *BMJ* 1998; **316**: 955.
2. Doyal L. Journals should not publish research to which patients have not given fully informed consent – with three exceptions. *BMJ* 1997; **314**: 107–11.
3. Tobias J. *BMJ*'s present policy (sometimes approving research in which patients have not given fully informed consent) is wholly correct. *BMJ* 1997; **314**: 1111–13.
4. Doyal L. Tobias JS, Warnock M, Power L., Goodare H. Informed consent in medical research. *BMJ* 1998; **316**: 1000–5.
5. Lindley RI. Thrombolytic treatment for acute ischaemic stroke: consent can be ethical. *BMJ* 1998; **316**: 1005–7.
6. Benatar D. Benatar SR. Informed consent and research. *BMJ* 1998; **316**: 1008.
7. Venn-Treloar J. Nuchal translucency-screening without consent. *BMJ* 1998; **316**: 1027.
8. Smith R. Publishing information about patients. *BMJ* 1995; **311**: 1240–1.
9. Smith R. Commentary: The importance of patients' consent for publication. *BMJ* 1996; **313**: 16.
10. International Committee of Medical Journal Editors. Protection of patients' rights to privacy. *BMJ* 1995; 311: 1272.
11. Hood CA, Hope T. Dove P. Videos, photographs, and patient consent. *BMJ* 1998; **316**: 1009–11.
12. Court C. GMC finds doctors not guilty in consent case. *BMJ* 1995; **311**: 1245–6.
13. Abassi K: *BMJ* to act on media abuse. *BMJ* 1998; **316**: 170.
14. Bullimore D. *BMJ* to act on media abuse. *BMJ* 1998; **316**: 1022.
15. Andrews K. Murphy L, Munday R, Littlewood C. Misdiagnosis of vegetative state: retrospective study in rehabilitation unit. *BMJ* 1996; **313**: 13–16.
16. Snider DE. Patient consent for publication and the health of the public. *JAMA* 1997; **278**: 624–6.
17. Rankine JJ. Most patients don't read the *BMJ*. *BMJ* 1996; **313**: 1026.

Informed consent – a response to recent correspondence*

Len Doyal

The publication of the debate between myself and Jeffrey Tobias about the acceptable limits of informed consent in medical research has generated an immense and varied number of letters to the *BMJ*.[1-4] This in itself is gratifying, whether or not correspondents agree with my arguments. It provides ample evidence of wide-spread and serious deliberation about the moral boundaries of the rights of participants in research.

*BMJ 1998: **316**: 1000–5.

Many correspondents either explicity or implicitly endorse the hard line that I take in my paper on the right of competent people to an acceptable level of information before agreeing to participate in medical research. Other contributions confirm my emphasis on the moral importance of the principle of informed consent but, in light of the highly specific circumstances where I argue that the principle must be qualified, question the degree or clarity of my own commitment to it. What is important here is our shared belief in the moral imperative of respecting human autonomy in almost all circumstances.

I still disagree with those authors who argue that it is not necessary to obtain informed consent if this will lead to the methodological compromise, or possible cancellation, of potentially beneficial studies involving clinical interventions that carry minimal risks. What these correspondents either fail to recognise or to take seriously is that to fail to respect the autonomy of competent people is to inflict harm on them that is just as morally unacceptable as direct physical or mental harm. To do so rejects the letter and spirit of the Helsinki Declaration – the "interests of the subject must always prevail over the interest of science or society." Simply to assert that the declaration is wrong in this regard – without even attempting to rebut counterarguments, which, for example, I outline in my paper – is to embrace the dogma of scientific progress at any price. When human autonomy and dignity are at stake the cost of such progress is too high.

Some correspondents simply misunderstood or misread my paper. For example, Naomi Pfeffer and Priscilla Alderson maintain that I somehow claim that research may be done on children without parental consent (p. 107). In the relevant section I specifically state, "Informed consent should always be obtained from someone with parental authority" (p. 89).[1] Similarly, Pat Soutter (p. 98) suggests that the HIV study of Satish Bhagwanjee and colleagues,[5] which did not obtain informed consent from patients for seropositive testing, conforms to qualifications of the principle of informed consent that I outlined in my paper. It does not. I specifically exclude all studies in which there is an intent to contact subjects in the future, an inevitable consequence of the HIV study in question since it was designed to inform patients later that they had been tested.

This same mistake is made by Paul Little and Ian Williamson (p. 99), who suggest that arguments in my paper are consistent with randomised trials without consent. It is true that I do morally defend some epidemiological research that is based not on direct patient involvement but on medical records – provided, among a long list of other things, that, again, there is no anticipation of further contact with the patients concerned (pp. 89–90).[1] Yet Little and Williamson try to defend their position with reference to the merits of an antibiotic study in which patients were directly involved without obtaining their informed consent. Then, through making this fact clear in their letter, they go on precisely to initiate further potential contact with these patients. We can only speculate about the patients' potential distress and anger when they read or hear about this self-confessed violation of their autonomy. This is the danger: patients may well (and do) find out about such abuse through, among other things, talking to other patients. Then utilitarian justifications can blow up in the face of those who use them to justify disrespect for human rights.

The most puzzling response of all to my paper was that of Michael Baum, a surgeon for whom I have great respect (pp. 105–6). Professor Baum seems to want it both ways. On the one hand, he draws an analogy between the moral appropriateness of conscription in warfare and the "responsibilities" of the lay public to participate as subjects in medical research in the "war against cancer" (and presumably other disease). On the other hand, he never really comes clean about what he proposes to do if members of the public do not live up to his perception of their responsibilities. If, ultimately, he accepts their right to refuse to participate, then he agrees with me that they should be given enough information to do so on an informed basis – and does so despite my "absolutism", "uncompromising zeal", and professional life in an "armchair" on a "veranda". If he rejects this right – as some of his comments and his agreement with Jeffrey Tobias's paper suggest – and really does support the quite extraordinary idea of conscription, then let him say so and try morally to defend himself. It will take more than *ad hominem* arguments to do so successfully.

Changing the *BMJ*'s position on informed consent would be counterproductive

Jeffrey S Tobias

Any author would be gratified by an overwhelming postbag in response to a provocative article – provided, of course, that not all the voices are raised in condemnation. Fortunately, however, it is clear even from the titles of the letters published by the *BMJ* that a wide variety of views persists. On the one hand, titles such as "Doctors are arrogant to think they need to debate [the] issue of patient consent" (p. 98) and "Lack of respect for patients in medical research may reflect wider disrespect in clinical practice" (p. 112) provide a clear and unambiguous view. But on the other hand, "Ethics committees and the *BMJ* should continue to consider the overall benefit to patients" (p. 99), "Consent is not always practical in emergency treatments", (p. 102) and "Let readers judge for themselves" (p. 98) offer a more relaxed view. As Little and Williamson point out, (p. 99) writing from a department of primary medical care, "adopting an absolute ethical view in open trials ignores the realities of – and would undermine the ability of research to inform – normal practice, and thus could ultimately harm patients, including those who agree to take part in trials."

As one of the protagonists of the debate, I am greatly concerned by many of the specific issues raised by correspondents. As well as the problem of, for example, emergency medical situations, the issue of risk of bias raised by a senior statistician (p. 99) is of particular importance since well conducted randomised trials tend to form the most influential basis of today's evidence-based medical practice. Added to this, we have a past chairman of a research ethics committee at one of London's most prestigious research hospitals pointing to the wide disagreement as to which clincial situations require trial without fully informed consent – reminding us that "no-one can claim to have a monopoly on deciding what is ethical (p. 98)."

Equally difficult is the argument – supported by preliminary data – that many patients may not digest information sufficiently well to permit a genuinely informed level of consent (p. 106): at the very least,

it is clear that many patients in this study by Montgomery *et al.* had no recollection whatever of consenting even to a course of radiotherapy – a consent which, we are assured from the article, had most certainly been given. If as I believe, fully informed consent can sometimes be needlessly cruel,[6] what is the point of insisting on it in all cases when about a quarter of patients (judging by Montgomery *et al.*'s study) cannot even recall being told about common side effects of treatment when all had been provided with this information?

As I pointed out when first setting out my stall, one of my chief anxieties concerns the somewhat old fashioned concept of doctoring in its traditional pastoral sense. While applauding the use of evidence-based approaches and recognising the need for powerful trials to generate essential information, I do, nevertheless, feel a responsibility of equal importance – to act as patients' adviser, counsellor, advocate, and support. With many sophisticated patients, well informed and willing to enter into a robust two-way dialogue, the medical scientist occupying a fair portion (I hope) of my brain can take the lead. For the majority, however – less educated, less well informed, and less able to marshal their arguments – a somewhat more directive or (without being pejorative) "paternalistic" approach will often be far more appropriate, and gratefully received. As Dr Thurstan Brewin, past chairman of Health Watch points out (p. 118).

> "Those who want the *BMJ* to take a rigid view … should spend a day in a ward full of elderly people. They would probably find many who, though far from being mentally incompetent, are at times confused and forgetful. What could be more unrealistic than to refuse to recognise this for fear of being called patronising …? … Some people underestimate … the harm that can be done to many sick patients when fully informed consent for every trial is sought, no matter how tense or difficult the situation."

I willingly give Ms Hazel Thornton, chairwoman of the Consumers' Advisory Group for Clinical

Trials, the final word. As she clearly explains (p. 101), her group "works directly with the professions … [and] identifies an urgent need to advance public education about clinical trials. Concepts such as randomisation, risk perception, and probability are poorly understood …. Such cooperation … will create a different attitude to research, which will be seen not as an imposition but as an activity to which we all have a responsibility to contribute." Her letter, entitled "We all have a responsibility to contribute to research," echoes my own view that both doctors and patients have much to gain from this type of partnership and that overzealous directives attempting to monopolise the moral high ground will surely prove counterproductive. The *BMJ* would be unwise to stifle important research by confining too closely the outline, structure, and phraseology of trial consent – details that are far better left to the originators of the studies and their local ethics committees.

Informed consent – a publisher's duty

Mary Warnock

Informed consent has become a shibboleth: you cannot be a respectable member of the medical research world unless you invoke the concept and accede to its demands, nor can you be a respectable publisher of research papers unless you ensure that your authors have clean hands in this regard. Informed consent is also, and perhaps more urgently, required in the case of medical and surgical procedures; but it is in the context of research requirements that the following remarks are offered.

The concept itself is not wholly simple. Questions may be raised about what counts as full consent or sufficiently informed consent, especially in the case of subjects who may find the idea of randomisation difficult to grasp or who have problems, as we all do, with the calculation of risk. I believe, however, that we should not make too much of these difficulties, which are inherent in the nature of medical research and which can be minimised by tactful and sympathetic dialogue with potential subjects. The central moral problem, however, is concerned with the possible exploitation of the subjects of research. For research, including clinical research, is aimed, not at the good of the individual patient, but at the production of medical knowledge, which is for the good of society at large (although the individual patient may benefit from it by chance). This is the difference between research and the use even of innovative treatment for an individual patient.

In a research programme the subjects are being used as a means, not as an end in themselves. To treat someone merely as a means is widely agreed to be a moral evil, a breach of the "categorical imperative", on which the very possibility of morality was held by Kant to depend. Philosophy apart, to make use of people, especially when they are not aware of what is going on, is generally agreed to be wrong. This evil is removed if people offer their services voluntarily. They then become willing partners in a joint enterprise rather than mere tools in it. Since they are free to decline to take part, their power of choice has not been overridden. They are being treated as befits a human as opposed to any other animal. The moral principle involved here is often referred to as the principle of autonomy. I prefer the more precise title of the principle of non-exploitation. Since it is especially easy to exploit the helpless and incompetent – those who, though human, seem to have little power of understanding or making a serious choice – the principle ought to be considered scrupulously in the case of such people. However, if research into the very conditions that produce such incompetence, such as Alzheimer's disease, is to continue, it may be necessary to resort to consent by proxy. It seems morally important that such consent should be sought.

The principle of non-exploitation has come to seem to many to be by far the most important moral principle that should govern research using human subjects. This is understandable on historical grounds: there are far too many cases, in the second world war and, sadly, more recently, of whole populations of people being damaged or destroyed as victims of research programmes about which they were ignorant or had no choice. The relevance of history is that it causes people to deploy the "slippery slope" argument – if once the principle of non-exploitation is allowed to be breached where will it end? To which the answer implied is that it will end in horrors such as were revealed at Nuremberg.

However, the slippery slope is a weak argument (though it exercises an enormous power over the imagination) in that there is no logical connection between allowing the principle to be breached in some cases and allowing it to be totally forgotten. The argument relies on a poor view of human nature: "Give them an inch and they'll take an ell." Biological and medical scientists are especially suspect these days, and this arises from the power of the slippery slope. It is crucial, therefore, that in this context editors should keep their heads and differentiate between different cases in which the principle has been breached.

There is all the difference in the world between, on the one hand, extending the use of anonymous data, collected for a particular study, to a further, previously unthought of, study and, on the other hand, the randomised testing of drugs in the treatment of a specific disease. In the first case there is no question of harm accruing to the subjects, and thus the use of the word "exploitation" is an exaggeration. It seems to me a misuse of words to suggest that not obtaining informed consent in itself constitutes a harm; sometimes it amounts to exploitation, sometimes it does not. Nor does it seem that the use for research purposes of discarded or unwanted tissue is exploitation – though there exists a lack of clarity about the relation between an individual and his or her body parts, which ought to be remedied. The matter becomes critical when a pharmaceutical company may make vast profits from the use of, say, a spleen that has been removed from the body of an individual. Does the person have property rights over something that was once, in some sense, his or her property but is so no longer?

The conclusion is that editors must try, in the words of a prayer much used in Hertford College Chapel, "to distinguish things that differ." This makes the editorial function hazardous, with editors potentially subject to accusations of failing in their duty to ensure the moral respectability of research. Any other policy seems to me to rely on a dogma – that there are no other principles worth considering in the ethics of research except the principle of non-exploitation – and to rely also on an exceptionally wide and unrealistic view of what counts as exploitation.

Trial subjects must be fully involved in design and approval of trials

Lisa Power

Reading the *BMJ* debate about informed consent and publication recently, it seemed to me that there was a basic flaw in the premise. Instead of "Why?" I wanted "How?" If informed consent is about the dignity and empowerment of trial subjects and the genuine participation of patients in our health research, then how can this be maximised throughout the trial process? If we look at the overall issue – the involvement of patients or potential patients – rather than the single aspect of informed consent, we can begin to treat the disease rather than arguing over the symptoms.

I do not believe that you can obtain better practice about informed consent merely by making a rule about publication. There will always be some people prepared to obtain such consent technically without any real commitment to its spirit, because all they see it as is a signature at the bottom of a form and not a partnership. This is not to impugn the motives with which they entered research, but lack of time and money and urgency of need can put pressure upon the best of intentions. Of course, there are trials in which informed consent cannot be obtained, as Len Doyal outlined, and any hard and fast rule that the

BMJ made about publication would probably have to be broken at some point, but the onus of justifying failure to obtain consent should not arise at publication stage for the first time; questions should be being asked far earlier in the process.

To improve the practice of obtaining informed consent wherever possible, there must be a number of changes in attitudes. There needs to be a greater emphasis in doctors' education on interpersonal and communication skills, and a greater willingness on the part of some trial investigators to involve nursing staff in communicating with trial volunteers; doctors are not the only people with a voice and a brain. Secondly, there needs to be an understanding that giving patients or potential patients some say in the design and approval of trials is a positive process and not just a hoop to jump through. This involvement can stretch from trial design to writing information sheets and sitting on ethics committees. Thirdly, the onus should be clearly on those designing trials to show, as part of thier basic data, their process for sub-

ject consent and uptake, rather than on others to challenge them in retrospect.

Placing the subjects of a trial at the centre of the process is not an easy matter. It may need extra finance or education, or other forms of support, and it may take time. Sometimes, I agree, it is not possible because of the nature of the trial, but this should be the exception – the question about informed consent should always be "Why not?" rather than "Why?" In my experience, as a participant in a vaccine trial and as an activist pressing drug companies to talk with us about their trial designs, such involvement is always to the good. I can appreciate that it feels like a nuisance to people who have not had to consider us before, but it leads to better trials with better uptake and, of equal importance, to greater involvement of individuals in their own health.

By fostering debate about informed consent, the *BMJ* has already added more to this process than any simple rule would do. I hope that it continues to do so.

Studies that do not have informed consent from participants should not be published

Heather Goodare

In his editorial of 12 April 1997 the editor asks, "Should the *BMJ* reject all studies that do not include informed consent?"[7] The simple answer is "Yes." This is the stated policy of others that observe the "uniform requirements for manuscripts submitted to biomedical journals."[8] There is no good reason why the *BMJ* should not follow suit.

It is clear that the Declaration of Helsinki is no longer entirely satisfactory as a standard to which medical journals should adhere. The declaration is a watered down version of the Nuremberg Code, formulated after the trials of Nazi doctors who had experimented on concentration camp inmates during the second world war.[9] The code states unequivocally: "The voluntary consent of the human subject is absolutely essential." But the Helsinki Declaration introduced a section on clinical research which says: "If the doctor considers it essential not

to obtain informed consent, the specific reasons for this proposal should be stated in the experimental protocol for transmission to the independent committee" (Clause II.5).

Lack of consent in cancer trials has long been a matter of concern,[10, 11] and this clause could have been used as an excuse for not seeking consent from competent patients in recent examples of clinical research.[12–16] There is some evidence that not seeking consent, far from eliminating bias (which is usually the reason given), actually adds to it. Patients who find that others in the same category are receiving different treatment will want to know why.[17] It is best to come clean at the outset: patients who discover that they have been deceived lose trust in their doctors.

If the present debate leads to a radical rethink of the way clinical research is conducted, matters may improve. Researchers are ignoring a valuable resource if they do not consult patients in designing their trials in the first place. This can save time and money and lead to better outcomes.[18] Also, "joint ownership of the work being done keeps patients involved, instead of isolating them."[15] There should be no more debate about the need to seek consent from competent patients. There are, however, some grey areas that need further consideration.

The Helsinki Declaration makes provision for cases of legal incompetence, or physical or mental incapacity, though national legislation varies, and there is a case for amending legislation when it is deficient, to make proper provision for proxy responsibility where appropriate. We cannot take it for granted that an unconscious person would have consented to a trial had he or she been conscious: indeed, we have a special duty to respect the rights of those who cannot speak for themselves. If a proxy for the patient cannot be found, the research should not proceed. In an emergency the doctor's duty is to do his or her best for the patient in the light of current knowledge. The rights of children, too, need to be respected: in the words of Lisa Hammond, aged 15, "Society should accept people of all types, and respect everyone's right to make their own decisions once they have all the facts, be they adults or children."[19]

There remains the matter of clinical audit and epidemiological research. We cannot assume that patients will not mind their data being used for such purposes. As Doyal observes, "Normally patients should give their explicit consent for their records to be accessed."[1] Moreover, these data must be anonymised: we cannot be sure that patients will not mind if researchers and civil servants (who could well be colleagues in the same office) see their clinical details. Researchers may have overstepped the mark in a recent breast cancer audit,[20] by requiring personal data – including names, dates of birth, and postcodes – not from the patients themselves but from doctors and administrators. This sheds light on the uses to which cancer registries could be put and raises awkward questions.[21] It seems that careful thought needs to be given to this matter, including the possibility of a standard question to patients at the time of treatment asking permission to review their records for research purposes. Some clinicians already follow this procedure.[22] Patients are well aware of the importance of such research, and if it is conducted appropriately they could be enthusiastic participants. However, their consent must not be taken for granted.

A further problem occurs with the use of stored human tissue. Donors of blood, organs, or cadavers usually give explicit consent to the use of their bodies for therapeutic purposes, medical education, or research, but patients who provide tissue specimens during the course of their own treatment normally do not. If any use of this material for other purposes is proposed, patients' permission (or that of a responsible relative) should be sought. There have already been examples of commercial exploitation and even attempts to patent such material: any possible profit should be used in accordance with patients' wishes. A moving story is told by Steingraber of the cell line MCF-7, widely used in medical research. The initials stand for Michigan Cancer Foundation, and the 7 for the seventh attempt to establish a self-perpetuating stock of cells from the body of the patient. The woman was a nun, Sister Catherine Frances, who died in 1970.[23] Would she have wished a donation by way of royalty to be made to her convent every time her cells were used? Was she asked?

A breast cancer patient expressed the dilemma to me as: "In Victorian times they got upset about body snatching. Now they steal bits of your body when you're still alive." These issues need further debate, with members of the public and patients themselves taking a full part in the discussion.

HG experienced breast cancer in 1986 and now works as a counsellor. She chairs the research committee of the UK Breast Cancer Coalition.

The author thanks Clare Dimmer, Carolyn Faulder, Andrew Herxheimer, Pamela Goldberg, Ann Johnson, Margaret King, and Charlotte Williamson for helpful comments on an earlier draft. Responsibility for the final version is, however, the author's alone.

REFERENCES

1. Doyal L. Journals should not publish research to which patients have not given fully informed consent – with three exceptions. *BMJ* 1997; **314**: 1107–11.
2. Tobias J. *BMJ*'s present policy (sometimes approving research in which patients have not given fully informed consent) is wholly correct. *BMJ* 1997; **314**: 111–13.
3. Informed consent in medical research [letters]. *BMJ* 1997; **314**: 1477–83.
4. Informed consent [letters], *BMJ* 1997; **315**: 247–54.

5. Bhagwanjee S, Muckart DJJ, Jenna PM, Moodley P. Does HIV status influence the outcome of patients admitted to a surgical intensive care unit? A prospective double blind study. *BMJ* 1997; **314**: 1077–81.

6. Tobias JS, Souhami RL. Fully informed consent can be needlessly cruel. *BMJ* 1993: **307**: 1199–201.

7. Smith R. Informed consent: the intricacies. *BMJ* 1997; **314**: 1059–60.

8. Writing for the Lancet. *Lancet* 1997; **439**: 1–2.

9. The Nuremberg Code (1947). Declaration of Helsinki (1964). *BMJ* 1996; **313**: 1448–9.

10. Faulder C. *Whose body is it? The troubling issue of informed consent*. London: Virago, 1985.

11. Cancer Link. *Declaration of rights of people with cancer*. London: CancerLink, 1990.

12. Research without consent continues in the UK. *IME Bulletin* 1988; July: 13–15.

13. Burton MV, Parker RW, Farrell A *et al*. A randomized controlled trial of preoperative psychological preparation for mastectomy. *Psycho-oncology* 1995; **4**: 1–19.

14. McArdle JMC, George WD, McArdle C *et al*. Psychological support for patients undergoiing breast cancer surgery: a randomised study. *BMJ* 1996; **312**: 813–17.

15. All treatment and trials must have informed consent. *BMJ* 1997; **314**: 1134–5.

16. Dennis M, O'Rourke S, Slattery J, Staniforth T, Warlow C. Evaluation of a stroke family care worker: results of a randomised controlled trial. *BMJ* 1997; **314**: 1071–6.

17. Moodie A. Psychological support for patients having breast cancer surgery: reply from dissenting author. *BMJ* 1996; **313**: 362.

18. Bradburn J, Maher J, Adewuyi-Dalton R, Grunfeld E, Lancaster T, Mant D. Developing clinical trial protocols: the use of patient focus groups. *Psycho-oncology* 1995; **4**: 107–12.

19. Hammond L. Deciding about leg-lengthening. *Bull Med Ethics* 1993; 92: 36.

20. Scottish Breast Cancer Focus Group, Scottish Cancer Trials Breast Group, Scottish Cancer Therapy Network. *Scottish breast cancer audit 1987 & 1993*. Edinburgh: Scottish Cancer Therapy Network, 1996.

21. Veatch RM. Consent, confidentiality and research. *N Engl J Med* 1997; **336**: 869–70.

22. Pincus I. Analyzing long-term outcomes of clinical care without randomized controlled clinical trials: the consecutive patient questionnaire database. *Advances* 1997; **13**(2): 3–46.

23. Steingraber S. *Living downstream: an ecologist looks at cancer and the environment*. Reading, MA: Addison-Wesley, 1997, p. 121–3.

Thrombolytic treatment for acute ischaemic stroke: consent can be ethical*

Richard I Lindley

According to proposed guidelines by Len Doyal it is unethical to randomise patients who are not competent to give informed consent in a randomised controlled trial when the treatment risks are not "minimal in relation to the standard available treatment."[1] This would rule out trials of many forms of medical and surgical treatment for a wide range of disabling and life-threatening conditions. Is it ethical to condemn millions of "mentally incompetent" patients to no prospect of improving outcome? I

believe a better guideline would be that such a trial is ethical if the treatment is promising but unproved provided that the potential risks are considered acceptable by the public. I illustrate my argument by discussing the role of thrombolytic treatment for acute ischaemic stroke.

ETHICAL REQUIREMENTS FOR TRIALS OF THROMBOLYTIC TREATMENT

The box shows the major requirements that I consider necessary for further randomised controlled

BMJ 1998: **316**: 1005–7.

Box 13.2 Criteria needed to justify trials of thrombolytic treatment for acute stroke

- Treatment promising but unproved
- Patients would be prepared to risk early death in order to avoid the severe consequences of a stroke
- Information overload at randomisation is reduced by local education programmes for those at risk of stroke
- Lay people agree to and contribute to the trial design
- Local ethics committee agrees to the trial design.

---

trials of early thrombolytic treatment for acute ischaemic stroke.

Thrombolytic Treatment Promising but Unproved

This is an absolute ethical requirement for a trial – we must not test unpromising treatments, and we should not withhold proved treatments. Why is thrombolytic treatment for acute ischaemic stroke promising but unproved?

Several small trials have been published, and in a recent overview a consistent picture emerged.[2] There is a definite early risk of death (chiefly due to cerebral haemorrhage), yet those who survive seem to be less disabled. Despite only one of the five trials of recombinant tissue plasminogen activator showing benefits,[3] this has been licensed for use in the United States. In this study of 624 patients, recombinant tissue plasminogen activator was given within 3 hours of onset stroke, and the benefits seemed substantial. For the equivalent of about every 1000 patients treated, about 80–100 avoided a poor outcome (death or dependency), but the net effect of the treatment on mortality was unclear.

Should we base treatment decisions for the next few million people who have strokes in the world on only one positive trial?[4, 5] I suggest not. Indeed, the data from the recent overview suggested that other thrombolytic agents may also be effective if given early.[2] Overall, those randomised to treatment within 3 hours of onset of stroke had a non-significant excess risk of early death of about 9/1000 but a significant increase in long-term independent survival (about 141/1000). So uncertainties remain. Is recombinant tissue plasminogen activator the best

drug? What is the optimal dose? What is the effect of treatment in different patient subgroups? What is the time window of efficacy? Is it safe to use aspirin or heparin after thrombolysis? Is treatment safe when early infarction is visible on a computed tomographic brain scan? Are the impressive results from a few specialist stroke units in the United States generalisable? In view of the uncertainties, thrombolytic treatment seems promising but unproved.

The main problem with further trials is the difficulty of getting consent. Many patients are dysphasic, drowsy, or have anosognosia (no recognition of their stroke deficit), and are therefore mentally incompetent or physically unable to give consent. Doyal has stated that the trial risks must be "minimal" if such patients are to be included into a randomised controlled trial. Some may not consider the risks of early thrombolytic treatment minimal, with an estimated excess of nine deaths for every 1000 patients treated, but may view the potential benefits (more than 100 extra independent survivors per 1000) worth the risk. I would prefer an ethical guideline to be based on the clinicians' uncertainty (i.e. the treatment is promising but unproved).

Patients would Consider Risky Treatments to Avoid Severe Consequences of Stroke

Would patients with acute stroke accept the risk of thrombolytic treatment? Unfortunately, the same problems of obtaining consent apply to any efforts to obtain patients' opinions on this matter. However, some recent studies can help to inform this discussion. Solomon *et al.* asked elderly people for their views on stroke disability, and most respondents rated severe stroke deficits (in language, cognition, and motor weakness) as bad as, if not worse than, death.[6] However, there was no consensus about the impact of minor and moderate deficits. In a similar study Gage *et al.* calculated quality of life for three different stroke scenarios representing mild, moderate, or severe stroke deficit.[7] While most subjects rated the description of a severe disabling stroke as worse than or equal to death, some scored it similar to their current health status. Conversely, some people scored mildly disabling stroke as equally bad as death; the scores for moderate stroke were bimodally distributed.

These studies confirm a widely held belief that many, but not all, people consider severe disabling stroke to be a fate worse than death. Presumably, these people would be prepared to accept a risky treatment. But what about those who do not want to be exposed to such risks? How can we give patients a choice in a thrombolytic trial? One potential solution is to get some of this information across by public education before the patients have a stroke.

Box 13.3   Information needed for informed consent for a thrombolytic trial

- "You have had a stroke"
- After appropriate brain imaging: "Your stroke has been due to a blood clot blocking the blood supply to the brain"
- "Immediate treatment with aspirin may help but it is not a powerful treatment"
- "Clot busting drugs (thrombolytic therapy) can sometimes reverse the stroke and speed recovery"
- "However, these clot busting drugs can sometimes cause massive bleeding in the brain which can make the stroke worse or even kill you"
- "If you are happy to consider the trial, your treatment may, or may not, include the new clot busting drug. This is decided by the study design, a random allocation, a bit like tossing a coin to decide which treatment to use"

(Readability: Flesch Reading Ease 70: Flesch-Kincaid Grade 7; Coleman-Liau 10; Bormuth 9.5 (Microsoft Word 6 Grammar check))

Information Needed for Consent to a Trial of Potentially Risky Treatments

The box shows the sort of information required for consent. This is given in language that has good readability (easy to check with standard computer word processors), but it still represents a substantial amount of information – perhaps too much. Would a public education campaign (based on the box) help? This strategy has been suggested for women with breast cancer,[8, 9] and a similar approach for stroke medicine is worth a try. In these days of evidence-based medicine, surely the purchasers and providers of healthcare (and politicians) have a duty to inform the population on the means to obtain the best evidence? Stroke researchers should "sell" their trial to their "at risk" population. The risk for middle-aged people having a stroke if they live to the age of 85 years is about 20–25%, and about 16% of all

women and 8% of all men die of stroke.[10] It therefore seems reasonable to educate the public about stroke – perhaps adding a bit of preventive medicine along the way (such as stopping smoking, reducing dietary salt, improving diet, etc.).

ENCOURAGING PARTICIPATION IN RANDOMISED CONTROLLED TRIALS

Everyone is a potential subject for a randomised controlled trial. Consent is often considered difficult by doctors and patients,[11] and I suspect this is a reflection of poor understanding. Patients demand the best treatment, and a randomised controlled trial should be evaluating the current "gold standard" with one considered, by all available evidence, to be a more promising treatment. This may or may not prove to be the case, but routine data monitoring of trials in progress will limit any hazard to a minimum. This sort of reassuring information may encourage people to participate.

As a method of educating the public, I suggest we introduce a new type of card – the randomised controlled trial card – to be carried by people who understand randomised controlled trials and wish to be considered for future appropriate trials. The card could be issued to all those who have been randomised into such a trial, and its use could be extended if successful. For example, patients who have just had a transient ischaemic attack could be issued with a randomised controlled trial card if they were happy to carry it. If such a high-risk patient subsequently had a dysphasic stroke, their relatives would be more informed about prior wishes, which should help them give or refuse assent for an appropriate randomised controlled trial. The main drawback to such a scheme would be if some unscrupulous researchers used the card to bypass all consent procedures.

The legal situation in the UK is also unclear. Doctors can proceed with medical treatments without consent (for example, in cases of coma or severe injury) provided that they act in the patient's best interests and the treatment is reasonable as judged by usual medical practice.[12, 13] I consider that randomisation into a well-conducted, randomised controlled trial is "best practice" for many clinical situations, but this particular situation has never been challenged in court. While many ethics committees have allowed (and continue to allow) relatives to assent to randomisation for those who are mentally

---

Key messages

- Recently suggested ethical guidelines would limit inclusion of mentally incompetent patients to trials of treatment that had only "minimal risk".
- Some new treatments may have a substantial risk, but their potential for substantial benefit means that we should not exclude them from further evaluation.
- The criterion of "minimal risk" should be changed to "promising but unproved," provided that the public agrees that the risk is worth taking.
- A new type of card, the randomised controlled trial card, may help educate the public about trials.
- With proper safeguards, it is ethical to randomise mentally incompetent patients into further trials of thrombolytic treatment for acute ischaemic stroke.

---

incompetent, this grey area of the law may need to be clarified for the future protection of patients and to facilitate research.

As I am not sure whether a randomised controlled trial card would work, evaluation would be needed to check that the benefits (more people recruited in trials) outweigh the potential risks (a worried population).

CONCLUSIONS

If we adopt Professor Doyal's ethical guidelines we will not be able to improve the care for many patients with stroke (or other mentally disabling conditions). I suspect the public would disapprove of such a move, and I believe that medical researchers have a duty to inform the public of ethical dilemmas and propose potential solutions.

In the case of a new trial of thrombolytic treatment for acute ischaemic stroke I believe that we need to inform our local, at risk population about stroke, thrombolytic treatment, and the concept of randomised controlled trials, and get a general agreement from our local public that the study is reasonable. The introduction of a randomised controlled trial card may benefit the population by improving participation into clinical trials.

ACKNOWLEDGEMENT

I thank my colleagues at the Department of Clinical Neurosciences, University of Edinburgh, for their comments and helpful suggestions during the preparation of this manuscript, and also members of the British Geriatric Society for their questions and comments after the original presentation of the views expressed in this article.

REFERENCES

1. Doyal L. Informed consent in medical research. *BMJ* 1997; **314**: 1107–11.
2. Wardlaw JM, Warlow CP, Counsell C. Thrombolytic therapy for acute ischaemic stroke: a systematic review of the evidence so far. *Lancet* 1997; **350**: 607–14.
3. National Institute of Neurological Disorders and Stroke rt-PA Stroke Study Group. Tissue plasminogen activator for acute ischemic stroke. *N Engl J Med* 1995; **333**: 1581–7.
4. Murray CJL, Lopez AD. Mortality by cause for eight regions of the world: global burden of disease study. *Lancet* 1997; **349**: 1269–76.
5. Yusuf S, Collins R, Peto R. Why do we need some large, simple randomised trials? *Stat Med* 1984; **3**: 409–20.
6. Solomon NA, Glick HA, Russo CJ, Lee J, Schulman KA. Patient preferences for stroke outcomes. *Stroke* 1994; **25**: 1721–5.
7. Gage BF, Cardinalli AB, Owebs DK. The effect of stroke and stroke prophylaxis with aspirin or warfarin on quality of life. *Arch Intern Med* 1996; **156**: 1829–36.
8. Baum M. New approach for recruitment into randomised controlled trials. *Lancet* 1993; **341**: 812–13.
9. Thornton H. Clinical trials: a "ladyplan" for trial recruitment? – everyone's business. *Lancet* 1993; **341**: 795–6.
10. Bonita R. Epidemiology of stroke. *Lancet* 1992; **339**: 342–4.
11. Toynbee P. Random clinical trials are one of life's biggest gambles. *BMA New Review* 1997; March: 34.
12. Royal College of Physicians of London. *A report of the Royal College of Physicians. Guidelines on the practice of ethics committees in medical research involving human subjects.* London: RCPL, 1990.
13. Royal College of Physicians of London. *A report of the Royal College of Physicians. Research involving patients.* London: RCPL, 1990.

Informed consent and research*

David Benatar and Solomon R Benatar

A full version of this piece is posted on the British Medical Journal website <www.bmj.com/cgi/content/full/316/7136/1008/DC1>.

In the debate opened by the *BMJ* on whether research is ethical if it meets the standards of the Declaration of Helsinki but is conducted without informed consent, Len Doyal provides some powerful arguments for why the request for informed consent should be inviolable.[1]

While vigorously defending the inviolability of informed consent, he concedes that it is not necessary in certain circumstances. An uncontroversial case is that of incompetent patients (although even here other rigorous requirements must be met). However, the other exceptional cases he mentions seem to have some unfortunate implications for his defence of informed consent. He thinks that for epidemiological research on patient records the informed consent requirement may be waived if certain conditions are met:

- that access to the clinical record is essential to the research;
- that consent is not practicable;
- that the research is of sufficient merit;
- that it may benefit the patient whose records are studied;
- that, when possible, the researchers are unable to connect the records with the patient's identity, but that where this is not possible, patients will not be identifiable when the results are made public;
- that it is not anticipated that contact will be made with the patients as a result of research findings; and
- that access is restricted to specific categories of information that have been approved by the local ethics committee. Professor Doyal thinks that similar conditions should apply to research on stored tissue from unconsenting anonymous donors.

The South African HIV study, which Professor Doyal criticised for not obtaining patients' informed consent for HIV tests, involved performing a blood test and not simply viewing records,[2] and

BMJ 1998; **316**: 1008.

thus does not precisely slot into one of his three exceptional categories. However, this point does not seem to be a pivotal issue: one can, after all, have consent to draw blood without having consent to test it for HIV seropositivity. Drawing blood without consent would introduce a problem not permitted by the list of conditions Professor Doyal stipulates, but, assuming that there was consent to draw blood, the anonymous testing of that blood for HIV in the Natal study meets all the conditions enumerated above. Doyal's sixth condition lends itself to variable interpretations, but it seems to us that merely informing patients that they had been subject to an HIV test as part of a study does not constitute contact with patients as a result of research findings. Telling them the result of the test, and counselling for HIV positive status, would constitute such contact, but it would be with the consent of the patients.

It seems then that Professor Doyal gives with one hand what he takes with another. He criticises the South African study for failing to obtain informed consent, yet this study meets the very conditions that he thinks he must obtain in those exceptional cases in which informed consent is not necessary.

The crucial condition is whether the researcher can link the medical record to the identity of the patient. We agree that informed consent is unnecessary in research that involves no withholding or providing of an intervention and which meets the other conditions but where the identity of the patient cannot be linked, even by the researcher, to the medical record. Knowing that there is an unidentified person who has HIV does not inhibit that person's autonomy or violate his or her privacy. By contrast, obtaining the knowledge that an identifiable person has HIV is an invasion of the person's privacy if he or she has not consented to this information being obtained. Thus, the difficult case is when the researcher gains sensitive information about a research subject without consent. In such a case informed consent is important and, if it is to be overridden, a strong argument will have to be made. Professor Doyal's conditions suggest that he may have sympathy for the view that the requirement for informed consent may be overridden in this case, but his arguments suggest that no such exception should be made. We can think of no compelling argument for why an exception should be made in this case.

What are the implications of this for the Natal study? The ethics committee and researchers went to great lengths to ensure that all but one of the researchers were prevented from connecting HIV status with the identity of patients. Moreover, all means of linking the HIV tests with the identity of patients were destroyed at the end of the study. If we are correct that there are no compelling arguments to justify such unauthorised violations of privacy, then the Natal study is ethically defective, even though to only a limited degree. This shortcoming is especially regrettable given that even the limited invasion of privacy could have been avoided by encoding patient identity and thereby ensuring that none of the researchers could have been able to establish a link between a patient's identity and HIV status. Even if one thinks that minor invasions of privacy or other limitations on autonomy are justified if they can bring great benefits, one must agree that it is better if these minor intrusions can be avoided.

REFERENCES

1. Doyal L. Journals should not publish research to which patients have not given fully informed consent – with three exceptions. *BMJ* 1997; **314**: 1107–11.
2. Bhagwanjee S, Muckart D, Jeena P, Moodley P. Does HIV status influence the outcome of patients admitted to a surgical intensive care unit? A prospective double blind study. *BMJ* 1997; **314**: 1077–84.

Part 3

Informed consent and the regulation of medical research

14 • International regulation, informed consent and medical research

The UK Perspective

CM Foster

There is little evidence that research on human beings until World War II in the UK was conducted with the knowledge and consent of its subjects. It would be unfair to conclude that it was never sought; it is the fact that consent can be sought and withheld that distinguishes research on humans from research on animals. Nevertheless, the tendency to paternalism, which predominated earlier this century, lends weight to the assumption that consent was only obtained in a small minority of cases. Rather, the doctors were believed to be acting in their patients' best interests, and if they chose to enrol their patients in research projects, or use them in some other experimental way, that would be a matter for their judgement, rather than their patients'.

Certainly, the views of Sir Austin Bradford-Hill seem to bear this out. Bradford-Hill, a well-respected medical statistician, provided advice on the running of clinical trials which was extremely influential in the days when the concept of the randomised controlled trial was beginning to take firm root in the minds of serious medical practitioners. In his 1963 Marc Daniels lecture, he discussed the forthcoming Declaration of Helsinki, a set of principles to govern medical research on human subjects that had been drawn up by the ethical committee of the World Medical Association. Bradford-Hill expressed concern at trying to codify ethical behaviour in this context, feeling that it unnecessarily constrained doctors who should, anyway, be governed by their own strong sense of moral rectitude. With regard to consent, which the forthcoming declaration was to include as a working principle for research on humans, Bradford-Hill had this to say:

Personally, and speaking as a patient, I have no doubt whatsoever that there are circumstances in which the patient's consent to taking part in a controlled trial should be sought. I have equally no doubt that there are circumstances in which it need not – and even should not – be sought .... Surely it is often quite impossible to tell ill-educated and sick persons the pros and cons of a new and unknown treatment versus the orthodox and known? And in fact, of course, one does not know .... Can you describe that situation to a patient so that he does not lose confidence in you – the essence of the doctor/patient relationship – and in such a way that he fully understands and can therefore give an understanding consent to his inclusion in the trial? In my opinion nothing less is of value. Just to ask the patient does he mind if you try some new tablets on him does nothing, I suggest, to meet the problem .... If the patient cannot really grasp the whole situation, or without upsetting his faith in your judgment cannot be made to grasp it, then in my opinion the ethical decision still lies with the doctor, whether or not it is proper to exhibit, or withhold a treatment.[1]

The *British Medical Journal* responded with outrage at the time, declaring: "If any proof were needed of the necessity for devising a code of ethics on human experimentation it was provided by Sir Austin Bradford-Hill's Marc Daniels Lecture .... No one who conducts experiments on human beings can really free himself from all bias in forming an ethical judgement of what he does. That is why he needs a code."[2]

In an editorial discussing the ethics of controlled trials some years earlier, however, the *British Medical Journal* had acknowledged:

However careful and conscientious the explanation – unfortunately often described as propaganda – there is a limit to the layman's understanding of it. Probably what finally tips the balance in most cases is trust and faith in the doctor, in the wonders of modern medicine.[3]

The widespread lack of reference to an earlier code which required consent to be obtained before using a person as an experimental subject, namely the Nuremberg Code, indicates that more clinicians were of the mind of Bradford-Hill than the later *British Medical Journal* editorial.

Howsoever that may have been, Bradford-Hill's lecture unwittingly led to a speeding up of the imposition of regulations in the UK. Mrs Helen Hodgson, chairman of the Patients' Association, sent a questionnaire to members following the lecture's publication in the *British Medical Journal*. In the questionnaire she said: 'Clinical trials are obviously going on, and on a big scale. Patients are not told if they are receiving new or orthodox treatment. I maintain that they should be told. I think it begs the question to say that it is difficult to explain these things to ignorant and sick people.'[4]

At about the same time, Maurice Pappworth published a damning book entitled *Human Guinea Pigs*, in which he listed hundreds of experiments on unknowing, unconsenting patients, some of which carried considerable risk. It was in this climate that Desmond Laurence, of the Royal College of Physicians, suggested in an open letter to the President of the College that the medical profession should look to self-regulation. He thought committees of doctors should convene on an *ad hoc* basis to scrutinise the research proposals of their colleagues for ethical acceptability.[6] In the late 1960s, these prototype research ethics committees began to be established.

ETHICS COMMITTEES TO REGULATE CONSENT

It would appear that, in their early days, committees were not first and foremost concerned about consent as an ethical issue. A study of a research ethics committee's agenda and minutes during the decade 1970–1979 provides evidences of this.[7] In this survey, the authors found that the primary ethical concern of the research ethics committee at the beginning of the decade under study was the sample size of the research projects the committee considered; in the middle of the decade it had shifted to the risks to which research subjects would be exposed. By the end of the decade the major ethical concern remained that of risks to subjects. Guidelines from the Ministry of Health in the late 1960s asked hospitals to set up ethics committees but do not say what are the ethical issues the committees should be considering.[8] Not until 1975 was the subject of informed consent raised in guidelines.[9]

Today, however, the picture is very different indeed. The most common reason for a research ethics committee not to pass a research proposal on its first scrutiny is that the consent procedures are not adequate.[10] Most research ethics committees require applicant researchers to complete a form that gives the committee information about how the ethical standards of the research are to be upheld. These forms include questions about how consent is to be obtained and by whom, and request copies of all information that is to be given to research subjects to help them to decide whether to participate in the proposed research. It is rare for an information sheet to emerge unscathed from a research ethics committee meeting. In the interests of respecting the autonomy of patients, committee members do their best to ensure that the consent procedures are as adequate as they can be. When I was training members of RECs during the 1990s, I usually found that the one uncontested rule that research applications had to adhere to was that, when research subjects were competent, their consent must be obtained. When I asked why, there was little evidence of any critical examination of the rule. It was "simply right".

GUIDELINES TO REGULATE CONSENT

There are now many guidelines identifying the ethical standards that are expected of researchers in respect, *inter alia*, of consent.[11] The existence of these guidelines reflects the widely-held belief that, without the explicit formulation of ethical requirements, researchers will either not know what they are, or will know but will not meet them – in opposition to Bradford-Hill's view, and in fulfilment of the *British Medical Journal*'s claim that "no one who conducts experiments on human beings can really free himself from all bias in forming an ethical judgement of what he does."

The Nuremberg Code,[12] which is the earliest well-known set of principles for conducting research on humans, identifies the requirement to obtain consent as the first of 10 principles to govern the researcher. The principle is explicit and uncompromising:

> The voluntary consent of the human subject is absolutely essential. This means that the person involved should have legal capacity to give consent; should be so situated as to be able to exercise free power of choice, without the intervention of any element of force, fraud, deceit, duress, overreaching, or other ulterior form of constraint or coercion; and should have sufficient knowledge and comprehension of the elements of the subject matter involved as to enable him to make an understanding and enlightened decision. This latter element requires that before the acceptance of an affirmative decision by the experimental subject there should be made known to him the nature, duration, and purpose of the experiment; the method and means by which it is to be conducted; all inconveniences and hazards reasonably to be expected; and the effects upon his health or person which may possibly come from his participation in the experiment. The duty and responsibility for ascertaining the quality of the consent rests upon each individual who initiates, directs, or engages in the experiment. It is a personal duty and responsibility which may not be delegated to another with impunity.

However, these guidelines referred only to nontherapeutic research on competent subjects. Moreover, they were drawn up following the Nuremberg Trials of the Nazi doctors' experiments in concentration camps and elsewhere, and reflected the deep concern at the time that such atrocities should never be committed again. It is my belief that for that reason, ironically, the guidelines were regarded thereafter as applying only to unethical doctors. Ethical doctors, that is to say, most doctors, did not need guidelines, because they knew what was right and wrong.

The Declaration of Helsinki was first drawn up in 1964.[13] Although it has been the subject of several revisions, and is under consideration yet again at the time of writing, none of these revisions has affected the placing of or emphasis on the principle of informed consent, which remains at number nine thus:

> In any research on human beings, each potential subject must be adequately informed of the aims, methods, anticipated benefits and potential hazards of the study and the discomfort it may entail. He or she should be informed that he or she is at liberty to abstain from participation in the study and that he or she is free to withdraw his or her consent to participation at any time. The physician should then obtain the subject's freely given informed consent, preferably in writing.

In 1991 the Department of Health produced a more substantial booklet of guidelines,[14] than its 1975 brief to Health Authorities. Local Research Ethics Committees includes the following paragraphs on informed consent:

> The procedures for obtaining consent will vary according to the nature of each research proposal. The LREC will want to be satisfied on the level and amount of information to be given to a prospective subject. Some methods of study such as randomised controlled trials need to be explained to subjects with particular care to ensure that valid consent is obtained. The LREC will want to look at such proposals particularly carefully. They will also want to check that all subjects are told that they are free to withdraw without explanation or hindrance at any stage of the procedure with no detriment to their treatment. An information sheet, to be kept by the subject, should be required in the majority of cases.
>
> Written consent should be required for all research (except where the most trivial of procedures is concerned). For therapeutic research consent should be recorded in the patient's medical records. (Paragraphs 3.7, 3.8)

The Royal College of Physicians (RCP) was the earliest professional body to recognise that research ethics committees were not receiving sufficient assistance with the ethical principles of research they were to uphold. In 1984 the RCP produced the first of its guidelines for ethics committees.[15] Still chary of trying to codify what was recognised as an essentially fluid exercise of ethical review, these guidelines nevertheless provided useful early principles for ethics committees, which if they had been more widely known about would have been even more helpful than they in fact were.[16] Informed consent was given an important place in the first edition of these guidelines.

Subsequent editions of the RCP guidelines have been ever more explicit about what is required of the researcher in respect of consent, and how the requirements are to be fulfilled. In the third edition an entire chapter is given over to the issue of giving information and seeking consent. Interestingly, it is recognised that there may be exceptions to the rules. Such occasions are not left to the discretion of the researcher, however:

> Only in exceptional circumstances is there an argument for not telling patients that they are participating in research, for instance, when it would cause more

distress to reveal the nature of the investigation and yet it is in the clinical interest of the patient to participate, or in some emergency medicine, or where the patient cannot understand. Acceptance of such an argument should be a deliberate decision taken as part of the ethical review. Discretionary practice of this sort would deflect the criticism that to obtain consent might be needlessly cruel.

Where it is proposed to withhold from subjects information that would be material to a decision to praticipate, this should always be justified to an REC.

Where it is the investigator's medical opinion that disclosure of the information that would be adequate for consent would be so harmful that it would be unjustifiable, this can only be a decision about individual patients and only in therapeutic research and if the option is approved by the REC. (7.22–7.24)

The Medical Research Council (MRC) was as quick off the mark as the RCP in identifying the need for ethical standards in research on humans to be maintained. As early as 1964 it published its first statement on the subject,[17] explicitly requiring researchers conducting research to obtain consent from their participants. However, the statement goes to some lengths to explain why the formal requirement for consent only holds in the case of non-therapeutic research. It recognised that therapeutic research, conducted in the course of treatment, and to all intents and purposes not different from what the patient might have received anyway, might not warrant a separate consent. This has been the subject of debate ever since, and a subsequent revision and republishing of that statement has widened the requirement to include therapeutic research as well.[18]

The MRC has produced a series of excellent booklets covering different sorts of research and different research populations.[19–22] All of these discuss the issue of consent sensitively and intelligently, fully cognisant of the difficulties there might be in some instances, such as the vexed question about the need to obtain consent for records-based research. If the principle of respect for autonomy were to be upheld, it would be argued that a researcher should always seek the permission of a person before looking at his or her medical records. However, such research typically involves investigating thousands of records, sometimes from right across the country. Seeking consent from patients for this kind of research is at least problematic. The MRC undertakes a highly intelligent discussion of the issues at stake in its guidelines on records-based research.

The Association of the British Pharmaceutical Industry (ABPI) has likewise been prolific in its publications to assist researchers, pharmaceutical companies, hospitals and GP practices in conducting ethical research. Their guidelines cover informed consent under Good Clinical (Research) Practice as follows:[23]

> The investigator must obtain informed consent from trial subjects in accordance with the Declaration of Helsinki before including them in the trial, ideally in writing, otherwise witnessed, indicating the date.

Other ABPI guidelines emphasise the need for consent as well.[24, 25] These guidelines have, however, largely been superseded by the International Conference on Harmonisation Good Clinical Practice Guidelines (ICH GCP),[26] that have statutory force for pharmaceutical companies wishing to conduct medical research on humans. Their status derives from the fact that regulatory authorities in the countries that have signed up to ICH GCP (European Union, US, Japan) will not accept the data from research not conducted according to ICH GCP and hence will not licence a product for marketing in their country. By the same token, if the research is conducted according to ICH GCP then the data holds good for all the countries involved, removing the need to conduct further studies on the same medicine in those countries where the company wishes to obtain a licence for marketing it. ICH GCP includes very strict requirements for consent, detailing the elements that need to be included in the information sheet. This is the extreme end of prescriptivism and leads to information sheets which are long and legalistic. This is what ICH GCP says:

> Both the informed consent discussion and the written informed consent form and any other written information to be provided to subjects should include explanations of the following:
> a) That the trial involves research.
> b) The purpose of the trial.
> c) The trial treatment(s) and the probability for random assignment to each treatment.
> d) The trial procedures to be followed, including all invasive procedures.
> e) The subject's responsibilities.
> f) Those aspects of the trial that are experimental.
> g) The reasonably foreseeable risks or inconveniences to the subject and, when applicable, to an embryo, foetus or nursing infant.
> h) The reasonably expected benefits. Where there is no intended clinical benefit to the subject, the subject should be made aware of this.

i) The alternative procedure(s) or course(s) of treatment that may be available to the subject, and their important potential benefits and risks.

j) The compensation and/or treatment available to the subject for participating in the trial.

k) The anticipated prorated payment, if any, to the subject for participating in the trial.

l) The anticipated expenses, if any, to the subject for participating in the trial.

m) That the subject's participation in the trial is voluntary and that the subject may refuse to participate or withdraw from the trial, at any time, without penalty or loss of benefits to which the subject is otherwise entitled.

n) That the monitor(s), the auditor(s), the IRB/IEC, and the regulatory authority(ies) will be granted direct access to the subject's original medical records for verification of clinical trial procedures and/or data, without violating the confidentiality of the subject, to the exent permitted by the applicable laws and regulations and that, by signing a written informed consent form, the subject or the subject's legally acceptable representative is authorising such access.

o) That records identifying the subject will be kept confidential, and to the extent permitted by the applicable laws and/or regulations, will not be made publicly available. If the results of the trial are published, the subject's identity will remain confidential.

p) That the subject or the subject's legally acceptable representative will be informed in a timely manner if information becomes available that may be relevant to the subject's willingness to continue participation in the trial.

q) The person(s) to contact for further information regarding the trial and the rights of trial subjects, and whom to contact in the event of a trial-related injury.

r) The foreseeable circumstances and/or reasons under which the subject's participation in the trial may be terminated.

s) The expected duration of the subject's participation in the trial.

t) The approximate number of subjects involved in the trial. (4.8.10)

Of course, not everybody, and certainly not every REC, agrees with the requirements for informed consent laid out by ICH GCP, and this has been the cause of a great deal of trouble and controversy. The guidelines were drawn up over a number of years in consultation with the pharmaceutical industries and the regulatory bodies of the countries concerned. In the UK, the bodies involved were the ABPI and the Medicines Control Agency. Although the MCA is a part of the government, it is not located, formally or geographically, within the Department of Health, which has responsibility for RECs. The Department of Health did not know about the formulation of ICH GCP, and felt no need to impart, certainly not to enforce, their requirements on RECs. RECs themselves felt no need to adopt the principles, particularly as they had emerged from the pharmaceutical industry. This was, of course, strictly inaccurate, since it was the regulatory authorities rather than the industry as such that has identified the requirements. However, it was the pharmaceutical companies applying to RECs for ethical approval, rather than the MCA or the Department of Health, who were informing RECs of ICH GCP, and telling them they had to comply or the research would be unacceptable. RECs, unwilling to take advice in any event, were more intransigent than usual about this particular issue.

ICH GCP present the most formulated requirements of all in respect of informed consent. I would argue that they go too far in trying to tell people exactly what they must do to be respectful of the principle of autonomy. Fulfilling their requirements leaves the potential research subject with a highly detailed and legalistic document with little of the sound of care and concern that a doctor might normally expect to make. The consent form, with its required inclusion of a statement by the signatory that he or she will fulfil the requirements of the study, arguably opens the way to not being able to claim compensation should anything go wrong in the study, on the grounds that he or she did not comply in some way with the study requirements.

The uncertain reception and too-detailed requirements of ICH GCP have left much frustration in their wake. Some RECs, in particular MRECs, are coming round to the view that it would be expedient to accept the status of ICH GCP, recognising that if anything they raise standards rather than lower them. But few are happy about the dictatorial approach to informed consent that they demand. In any case, ICH GCP does not apply to research that is not directed towards applying for a marketing licence for a pharmaceutical product.

DIFFICULTIES WITH REGULATING THE CONSENT PROCEDURE

There are two major difficulties with regulating consent. The first is the difference in opinion between research ethics committees as to what constitutes adequate information. The second difficulty is related to whether the requirements of research ethics committees and the guidelines to which they refer can be followed in practice, and even if they are, whether they give rise to the desired effect of properly informed, voluntary research subjects.

Differences between RECs

The difference in opinion between RECs about the consent procedure is felt most keenly by researchers who have to obtain approval from many committees for the same proposal. Until 1997 any multicentre research proposal had to be passed by every local research ethics committee in the centres where the research was to take place. After 1997 new, specially constituted research ethics committees, known as Multicentre Research Ethics Committees (MRECs – as distinct from Local Research Ethics Committees or LRECs) were established to look at trials in five or more centres.[27] However, research in four or fewer centres still has to be passed by more than one LREC; moreover, research which has been passed by an MREC still has to be accepted by the LRECs where the research is to take place, even if the LRECs do not conduct a formal review. One of the aspects of centrally-approved research proposals that LRECs have been most dissatisfied with has been the information sheets and consent forms as found acceptable by the MRECs. This is despite the fact that, like LRECs, the MRECs' most frequent reason for not accepting a study proposal first time is that the information sheets and consent forms are not adequate.[28] The situation is troublesome for researchers since the ethical acceptability of their research is questioned with no clear advice on how to improve it. Many researchers conclude that the concerns of committees are therefore trivial. One serious consequence is that this brings the important principle of patient autonomy into disrespect.

Are the Regulations Practicable?

The second difficulty lies with the practical application of the regulations on consent that research ethics committees impose. Committees scrutinise research proposals; they do not police the research as it is carried out. All they have to work on are the papers which comprise research applications. It is one thing to produce a well-written and informative letter of invitation to a potential research subject and a consent form that clearly identifies his or her rights in that capacity. It is quite another to carry out the consent procedure in circumstances which are often unsuitable for the informed, voluntary decision of a competent person that valid consent requires. Many empirical studies have been conducted which raise questions about the success of the consent procedure. I quote here from one, a qualitative study of parents' understanding of randomisation in the extra-corporeal membrane oxygenation (ECMO) study,[29] a national clinical trial in which neonates with breathing difficulties were randomly allocated to conventional therapy or the novel ECMO. The authors found a considerable level of misunderstanding amongst parents of the randomisation procedure. They cited one couple whom they interviewed:

> They said they could not understand how a decision could be based on only a name, but also had problems when they considered the possibility that the computer had the information about their daughter's case. To them, she clearly needed treatment other than the conventional care she was receiving and with her details to hand it was incomprehensible that she was not given ECMO. They felt the computer had made the wrong decision.

This is one example among many of the evident failure of the consent procedure, whose information sheet had been scrutinised and improved by the numerous research ethics committees to which the research proposal had been submitted. The authors recognised that the time of obtaining consent from the parents was a stressful one and so they may not have been able to take in what they read. However, this observation is true of the majority of situations of seeking consent, and only goes to support the thesis that obtaining consent as demanded by research ethics committees is impracticable, making the regulation of consent in the UK little more than a formality.

SUMMARY AND CONCLUSION

In this chapter I have recounted, as far as it is known, the development of regulation of consent in the UK. Until the late 1960s, paternalism tended to be the prevailing principle of doctors' treatment of their patients, which inevitably extended into the use or justification of patients as research subjects. The growing concern that it was a wrong in and of itself that patients were not being consulted, both within the medical profession and outside it, helped to bring about the establishment of research ethics committees and a plethora of guidelines to help them. These committees are the means by which consent in clinical research is regulated in the UK. Their success is questionable, partly because of the differences of opinion about what constitutes an adequate consent procedure, but more importantly because what research ethics committees ask for, and what patients receive, may well not be the same in all cases, even if the researchers are doing their best to carry out the wishes of the regulators.

My conclusion is not pessimistic, however. In my view it is unavoidable that there will be differences of opinion – and between different committees – about what represents adequate information and appropriate procedures for obtaining consent. There is a general level that may be regarded as reasonable, and as long as practices remain at or around that level, there is no reason to despair. The difficulty in applying the demands of research ethics committees, and latterly of ICH GCP for pharmaceutical company-sponsored research, in practical situations indicates a need for better dialogue between committees and researchers. It also, most importantly of all, demands that researchers retain in themselves an understanding of and a commitment to the need to respect their patients as human beings with rationality to exercise, not simply as means to their research ends, however exciting and ground-breaking those ends may be. Researchers cannot and should not rely upon research ethics committees to be their own ethical guardians, nor should they expect written rules to cover all eventualities and provide an acceptable alternative to their own communication with and care for their patients.

REFERENCES

1. Bradford-Hill A. Medical ethics and controlled trials. Marc Daniels Lecture. *BMJ* 1963; April 20, 1043–5.
2. Editorial. Ethics of human experimentation. *BMJ* 1963; July 6, 5348–9.
3. Editorial. Experiments of human beings. *BMJ* 1955; February 26, 526–7.
4. Hodgson H. Quoted in: Now a voice for the patient. *The Times*. 1963; June 17.
5. Pappworth MP. *Human guinea pigs: experimentation on man*. London: Routledge and Kegan Paul, 1967.
6. Royal College of Physicians. Supervision of the ethics of clinical research investigations in institutions. London: Royal College of Physicians, 1967.
7. Allen PA, Waters WE. Development of an ethical committee and its effect on research design. *Lancet* 1982; May 29, 1233–6.
8. Ministry of Health. Supervision of the ethics of clinical trial investigations. London: HMSO, 1968.
9. Department of Health and Social Security. HSC (1S) 153. Supervision of the ethics of clinical research investigations and fetal research. London: HMSO, 1975.
10. Foster C, Holley S. Ethical review of multi-centre research: a survey of multi-centre researchers in the South Thames Region. *J Roy Coll Physicians* 1998; **32**: 242–5.
11. Foster CM. Manual for research ethics committees. 5th edn. London: King's College, 1997.
12. Nuremberg Code. Taken from Mitscherlich A, Mielke F. *Doctors of infamy: the story of the Nazi medical crimes*. New York: Schuman, 1949; 23–5.
13. World Medical Association. *Declaration of Helsinki*. Latest version: South Africa, 1996.
14. Department of Health. *Local Research Ethics Committees*. HSG(91)5. London: HMSO, 1991.
15. Royal College of Physicians. *Guidelines on the practice of ethics committees in medical research*. London: RCP, 1984, updated 1990 and 1996.
16. Gilbert CM, Fulford KWM, Parker C. Diversity in the practice of district ethics committees. *BMJ* 1989; **299**: 1437–9.
17. Medical Research Council. *Responsibility in investigations on human subjects. Report for the year 1962–3*. (Cmnd 2382), London: HMSO, 1964, pp. 21–5.
18. Medical Research Council. *Responsibility in investigations on human participants and material and on personal information*. London: MRC, 1992.
19. Medical Research Council. *The ethical conduct of research on the mentally incapacitated*. London: MRC, 1991, reprinted 1993.
20. Medical Research Council. *The ethical conduct of research on children*. London: MRC, 1991, reprinted 1993.
21. Medical Research Council. *The ethical conduct of AIDS vaccine trials*. London: MRC, 1991.
22. Medical Research Council. *Responsibility in the use of personal medical information for research*. London: MRC, 1994, reprinted with minor revisions as footnotes, 1995.
23. Association of the British Pharmaceutical Industry. *Good clinical (research) practice*. London: ABPI, 1992.
24. Association of the British Pharmaceutical Industry. *Good clinical trial practice*. London: ABPI, 1995.
25. Association of the British Pharmaceutical Industry. *Guidelines for research ethics committees considering studies conducted in healthy volunteers by pharmaceutical companies*. London: ABPI, 1990.

26. ICH GCP. International conference on *Harmonisation of technical requirements for registration of pharmaceuticals for human use. Guidelines for good clinical practice*, 1997.

27. Department of Health. *Ethical review of multi-centre research*. HSG(97)23. London: HMSO, 1997.

28. Holley S. *MREC procedures*. Talk for Innovex, 20th May, 1998.

29. Snowdon *et al.* Making sense of randomisation: responses of parents of critically ill babies to random allocation of treatment in a clinical trial. *Social Sci Med* 1997; **45**: 1337–55.

A perspective from the USA and Canada

Eric M Meslin

Few topics in bioethics have occupied as much attention in the literature, the legislatures and in living rooms as *informed consent*. A recent annotated bibliography found more than 370 empirical studies alone.[1] In this chapter the history of informed consent in research in the United States and Canada is briefly reviewed, some of the accepted philosophical foundations for implementing consent requirements in research described, and then three challenges to the accepted paradigm that arise from contemporary research are identified, two of which emerged in reports prepared by the US National Bioethics Advisory Commission.

BRIEF HISTORY OF INFORMED CONSENT IN RESEARCH IN THE USA AND CANADA

The received view of the history of informed consent in the human research in the USA and Canada includes several important events and influential documents, some of the latter following directly from the former.[2–4] The ethical transgressions brought to light at the Nuremberg War Crimes Trial had (and still have) a lasting impact on the public's awareness and understanding of human experimentation. The reports of unethical experimentation in the USA including the Tuskegee Syphilis Study, the Willowbrook State School Experiments in which young people were intentionally exposed to hepatitis, and the studies of subcutaneous cancer cell injections at the Jewish Chronic Disease Hospital in New York[5, 6] led to the establishment of the National Commission for the Protection of Human Subjects of Biomedical and Behavioral Research (The National Commission) to review the ethical issues associated with human subjects research, and subsequently to the promulgation of federal regulations for the protection of human subjects by the US Department of Health and Human Services in 1981.[7] These regulations were later adopted by 16 other US federal agencies as the Federal Policy for the Protection of Human Subjects in 1991,[8] and apply to federal agencies that conduct, support, or otherwise regulate human subjects research. The policy is known as the "Common Rule" because these agencies have agreed to be bound by the same set of procedural requirements for the review and conduct of research. As implied by its title, the Common Rule is designed to make uniform the human subjects protection system in all relevant federal departments and agencies.

Recent scholarship by the White House Advisory Committee on Human Radiation Experiments revealed for the first time that informed consent was required as a matter of policy in the USA as early as 1947 when Dr Carroll Wilson, General Manager of the Atomic Energy Commission (AEC), described this requirement in a letter circulated to AEC personnel (ACHRE).[9] Wilson's letter described many of the basic elements of informed consent recognized today. "[P]rior to treatment, each individual patient, being in an understanding state of mind, was clearly informed of the nature of the treatment and its possible effects, and expressed his willingness to receive the treatment."[9 (p. 48)] Although the Wilson letter contains the first mention of "informed consent," and its influence on the evolution of US federal policy was probably minimal, ACHRE's uncovering of this document fills an important gap in history that may warrant further study. In particular, it highlights the necessity of linking ethical rules of conduct with a mechanism for ensuring compliance with and public oversight of those rules. Since the AEC research was "classified", public oversight was impossible.

In Canada, a similar history of cases of unethical research informed the development of research guidelines, especially informed consent. These cases included that of Walter Halushka, a University of Saskatchewan medical student, who suffered cardiac arrest in a study of catheterization procedures (but had not been informed of the extent of the procedure),[10] focusing attention on the different requirements in law (and ethics) regarding disclosure of risks to individuals prior to their enrolment in research.

The *Halushka* decision made clear that the standard of disclosure required in research, as contrasted with medical treatment, is more detailed and specific. In *Weiss v. Solomon*, the family of a research subject who suffered cardiac arrest and died during the course of an ophthalmology study, successfully sued the investigator and institution where the research took place because the consent form failed to disclose the risk of death, judged at less than 1 in 25 000.[11] Canada adopted domestic guidelines published by the Medical Research Council [12, 13] and then considerably revised and expanded them in the policy statement developed by the three major funding bodies in Canada.[14]

PHILOSOPHICAL FOUNDATIONS

Complimenting the factual history of events, guidelines, and regulations is an equally robust history of scholarship, principally in law and ethics, which accounted for what is now regarded as the foundation for the concept and theory of informed consent in research in these two countries. Scholarship in research ethics included extensive argument about the influence of the concepts of personal autonomy and individual liberty in medical experimentation. The National Commission made clear its understanding that informed consent is a particular application of the principle of "respect for persons".[15] Five elements of informed consent have been identified:

- disclosure (of relevant risks and benefits of the procedure);
- competence (on the part of the patient or subject)

to make a decision whether to accept the treatment or to participate in the research;
- comprehension (of the relevant risks and benefits);
- choice (an expressed decision to accept the treatment or participate in the experimentation), and
- voluntariness regarding the choice to accept treatment or to participate in research).[2]

The philosophical foundations supporting Canadian and US requirements for obtaining informed consent in research are, with some important exceptions, quite similar. This should not be surprising given that the world's two largest trading partners interact so regularly in medicine and research. Canada's enactment of the *Charter of Rights and Freedoms* in 1982 has contributed to a jurisprudence more similar to the USA than to the UK. Both countries share a political philosophy based on democratic principles of government, some of which have informed health care decision making.[16] Both countries recognise and emphasise the importance of informed consent in healthcare and research decision-making. The US National Commission's *Belmont Report* explained in simple, yet elegant terms that the ethical justification for obtaining informed consent from potential research subjects is grounded in the principle of respect for persons.[15] Although the *Belmont Report* is now 20 years old, it remains an influential document in US research ethics.[17–20] According to the National Commission, to respect autonomy is to "give weight to autonomous persons' considered opinions and choices, while refraining from obstructing their actions unless they are clearly detrimental to others."[15 (p. 4)]

Similarly, the Canadian Tri-Council Policy adopts the principle of *respect for human dignity*, which it takes to be the "cardinal principle of modern research ethics", one which "aspires to protecting the multiple and interdependent interests of the person – from bodily to psychological integrity."[14 (p. i.5)] In addition, the Tri-Council Policy also adopts the principle of *respect for free and informed consent* which means that "individuals are generally presumed to have the capacity and right to make free and informed decisions."

INFORMED CONSENT REQUIREMENTS REVIEWED BY IRBs

Both the US and Canadian requirements function in much the same way: federally funded researchers (and the institutions in which they work) are required to comply with the respective guidelines or regulations, or risk losing federal funding provided through research grants. For example, in the USA the Federal Policy applies to "all research involving human subjects conducted, or supported or otherwise subject to regulation by any Federal Department or Agency"[8] (sec. 46. 101a) and also includes any research conducted by a research institution, federally funded or otherwise, which has negotiated a contract (called an Assurance) with the federal government's Office for Protection from Research Risks. Similarly, the Tri-Council Policy states that the three councils "adopted this policy as [their] standard of ethical conduct for research involving human subjects. As a condition of funding, [they] require, as a minimum, that researchers and their institutions apply the ethical principles and the articles of this policy."[14] (p.i.2)

The principle of institutional ethical peer review is considered a fundamental component of the US and Canadian systems of protecting human subjects. The authority and responsibility for ensuring that information has been appropriately disclosed to potential research subjects prior to their enrolment in a study funded by the government is given to Institutional Review Boards (IRBs, as they are known in the US), and Research Ethics Boards, in Canada.[21] IRBs have the authority to approve, disapprove, or require modifications to research protocols – including the consent forms and the processes for obtaining consent. However, regulations and guidelines for informed consent must, by their nature, emphasise the *disclosure* requirements necessary to satisfy a standard of legally effective informed consent. For the most part, these guidelines emphasise the procedural aspects of informed consent: whether the consent forms are signed, or whether the consent documents contain sufficient information to protect institutions against liability. Less emphasis is placed on establishing standards for ensuring that potential subjects *understand* what has been disclosed. US federal regulations provide, in considerable detail, the type of information that must be disclosed to research participants prior to obtaining their consent to participate. The US Federal Policy identifies eight "basic elements" of informed consent that must be described in a consent form.[8] (sec. 45 CFR 46.116(a))

1. a statement that the study involves research, an explanation of the purposes of the research and the expected duration of the subject's participation, a description of the procedures to be followed, and identification of any procedures which are experimental;

2. a description of any reasonably foreseeable risks or discomforts to the subject;

3. a description of any benefits to the subject or to others which may reasonably be expected from the research;

4. a disclosure of appropriate alternative procedures or courses of treatment, if any, that might be advantageous to the subject;

5. a statement describing the extent, if any, to which confidentiality of records identifying the subject will be maintained;

6. for research involving more than minimal risk [as defined in 45 CFR 46.102(i)], an explanation as to whether any compensation and an explanation as to whether any medical treatments are available if injury occurs and, if so, what they consist of, or where further information may be obtained;

7. an explanation of whom to contact for answers to pertinent questions about the research and research subjects' rights, and whom to contact in the event of a research-related injury to the subject; and

8. a statement that participation is voluntary, refusal to participate will involve no penalty or loss of benefits to which the subject is otherwise entitled, and the subject may discontinue participation at any time without penalty or loss of benefits to which the subject is otherwise entitled.

For the most part, the Canadian and US guidelines concur on these and both recommend that subjects be given additional information that may affect their continued participation in research depending on the nature of the project itself. The US regulations list six such additional disclosures.[8] (sec. 46.116(b)) Canada's Tri-Council policy lists many of these same items, and others not found in US regulations. For example, the Canadian policy requires that the identity of the researcher be disclosed to the subjects, and that subjects be informed of "the possibility of commercialization of research findings, and the presence of any apparent or actual or potential conflict of interests on the part of researchers, their institutions or sponsors."[14] (sec. 2.4e)

Several recent studies of the IRB system in the US have shown that some committees are considerably overworked and may lack the relevant expertise to review and consider the increasing number of protocols they receive.[9, 22–24] This situation causes two related and worrisome problems: first, with insufficient time to carefully review and make recommendations about protocols, IRBs may spend less time and devote less attention to other important aspects of research ethics review.[18] Secondly, with less time, review committees may spend a disproportionate amount of time on the review of consent forms. *Prima facie* this may not be a bad thing: a detailed discussion of whether potential subjects fully understand the risks and benefits of the study, the nature of the project and/or other substantive matters necessary for making an informed choice are all important judgments made by committees. However, some IRBs have been accused of focusing on minutiae – whether the forms include phone numbers for contacting investigators, and other "boilerplate" disclosures, such as whether the amount of blood removed by venepuncture will be described in mathematical quantities (e.g. millilitres) or more familiar expressions (e.g. tablespoonsful).*

CONTEMPORARY ISSUES: NBAC'S INTEREST IN INFORMED CONSENT

The National Bioethics Advisory Commission (NBAC) was established to advise President Clinton on matters of bioethics policy, and has as its principal focus the protection of the rights and welfare of research subjects, which necessarily includes informed consent.[25] In 1997 NBAC unanimously resolved that "all human subjects should be afforded the twin protections of informed consent and independent review of research." This resolution reflects, in many ways, a central theme in North American research ethics: that the principal procedural mechanisms for protecting the rights and welfare of human subjects involved in biomedical and behavioral research are:

- their own ability to decide whether and to what extent they wish to accept the risks of harm that arise in a study, and
- the ability of a review body – an IRB or REB – to decide whether it is permissible for researchers to approach and invite patients or volunteers to participate in research.

The prevailing model of informed consent in research involving human subjects, and the one reflected in US and Canadian guidelines and regu-

---

*I first heard the term "boilerplate", used by Prof. Benjamin Freedman at a workshop sponsored by the National Council on Bioethics in Human Research, Ottawa, Ontario, Canada, November 1989.

lations, is best understood as one in which a competent, otherwise healthy adult is invited to participate in a clinical trial of a new medication; the consent process follows an expected pattern in which a person (usually a research nurse) provides a consent form to a volunteer, the content of which includes the description of the study, a list of relevant risks and potential benefits, and related details sufficiently detailed to permit a person to make an informed choice regarding participation in a study. The greater the departure from this paradigm, the more this model is subject to challenge. Below, three contemporary challenges to this model are described: research involving individuals who may lack decision-making capacity and are therefore unable to understand fully the information disclosed to them; research involving personal (i.e. medical or genetic) information obtained from biological tissue samples (although in this research the human subject is only indirectly involved in the study); thirdly when research is necessarily undertaken in an emergency situation preventing any manner of realistic consent. The first two of these situations were the subject of reports by NBAC.

Informed Consent when Individuals Lack Decision Making Capacity

Ever since the Nuremberg Code, guidelines and regulations governing the protection of research subjects have attempted to address a particularly nettlesome problem: how and to what extent would it be permissible to conduct research on human beings for diseases that cause these very individuals to lose their ability to participate fully in decisions about the research itself? In the USA, concerns about research on persons with mental disorders housed in state mental health institutions led the early National Commission to focus one of its reports on the subject.[26]

When NBAC first began to address this issue many of the arguments were well known: researchers were enthusiastic about the prospects of treating diseases and conditions that had been resistant to clinical (especially pharmacological) intervention. Moreover, developments in genetic research offered new promise for both identifying the causes of certain conditions such as Alzheimer's and Parkinson's disease.[27] Yet at the same time, concern remained that the conduct of research on persons who cannot themselves voluntarily choose to participate in a clinical trial was seen to compromise a basic tenet of research ethics: the reliance on informed consent. NBAC spent 18 months preparing its report,[19] during which it received considerable public input.[28] While the report focused on those individuals whom, as a result of having certain mental disorder, might lack the capacity to consent, many of the arguments and recommendations also applied to other situations where decisional capacity might be compromised – temporarily, as in the case of someone under anaesthesia, or under the influence of alcohol; intermittently, for example, those persons with bipolar disorder whose capacity "waxes and wanes"; or permanently, as for some people with severe forms of dementia, or following severe head injury.

NBAC made 21 recommendations, principal among them that existing US regulations should be supplemented to include specific protections for persons with mental disorders. The commission further recommended that under certain conditions, individuals could prospectively authorise their future enrolment in research, allowing another to consent on their behalf to the particular protocol.

Research on Tissues and Biological Samples

Among the most challenging of contemporary informed consent problems is the extent to which both prior and prospective informed consent can be obtained from individuals who donate biological materials (e.g. cells, blood, biopsy specimens) for research. When NBAC first began gathering data on this subject in early 1998, the commission conservatively estimated that 282 million specimens from more than 176 million individual cases had been collected and stored in US laboratories, pathology departments and other repositories.[20] Recent estimates are now at 307 million samples, increasing by 20 million samples/year.[29] Millions of these specimens may have been collected as part of clinical and surgical procedures without explicit, prospective, written informed consent to their use in research. Many remain in repositories, long after their progenitors have died.

Currently, the US federal regulations apply only to research involving a "human subject," defined as "a living individual about whom an investigator conducting research obtains: (a) data through intervention or inter-action with the individual, or (b) identifiable private information."[8] Specifically, an intervention includes both physical procedures by which data are gathered (for example, venepuncture) and manipulations of the subject or the subject's environment that are performed for research purposes. NBAC reasoned that, based on this definition, an investigator who obtains a blood or saliva sample is conducting human subject research. The US regulations define "identifiable" to mean that "the identity of the subject is or may readily be ascertained by the investigator or … associated with the information." On the other hand, according to these same regulations, research on samples provided to the investigator with no personal identifiers and without codes linked to personal identifiers would not be subject to regulation (and therefore would not require prior consent or IRB review), because no human subject would be involved. This provision has been the cause of some confusion in the research community. According to the regulations, research on samples that are linked, even through a code, to personal information about the tissue source, constitutes research on human subjects and is subject to the federal regulations.

There are, however, exceptions that are pertinent to research with human biological materials. For example, the regulations state that such an exemption may be applied, for example, to "research involving the collection or study of existing specimens if the information is recorded by the investigator in such a manner that subjects cannot be identified, directly or through identifiers linked to the subjects."[8]

According to US federal regulations, the requirement for informed consent can be waived if certain criteria are met:

- the research involves no more than minimal risk to the subjects;
- the waiver or alteration will not affect adversely the rights and welfare of the subjects;
- the research could not be practicably carried out without the waiver or alteration, and
- whenever appropriate, the subjects will be provided with additional pertinent information following their participation.

Since genetic research on one individual's stored samples may reveal important, even sensitive, information about others, additional attention must be given to disclosure and consent requirements for others. Genetic testing on the deceased, as noted above, can yield information about living relatives. Testing on a number of otherwise unrelated individuals may yield information pertinent to many unrelated people who share important and relevant characteristics, such as ethnicity or the presence of a predisposing medical condition.

Among the problems that arise is how to refocus the process and content of informed consent so as to concentrate on non-physical risks of harm. For example, in most genetic research, the principal risks to which a subject (or group) may be vulnerable are discrimination, labelling, stigmatisation and other threats to an individual's sense of self-worth. In addition, given the absence of universal health care in the USA, employees and patients may be at some financial risk if genetic information arising from this research were used to withhold medical or employment benefits. NBAC argued that it is misleading to suggest that the purpose of informed consent in research on biological samples is to protect a person from physical harm – and yet the disclosure requirements found in federal regulations are oriented towards descriptions and quantification of physical harm.[20]

The central ethical question is whether biological materials that are collected without specific consent to their use in research may be used for that purpose. In NBAC's judgment, where the research uses identified or coded samples from previously collected specimens such uses usually are not justified without the source's consent because the risks to sources and others may be more than minimal. However, the use of unidentified or unlinked samples for research could be justified in some cases if other appropriate protections were in place despite the lack of informed consent.

An additional issue arises when individuals are asked to provide samples for possible use in future studies, even though a research protocol does not yet exist. Two of the NBAC's 21 recommendations focus on these issues in particular (recommendations 8 and 9) and warrant mention here. Recommendation 8 relates to previously collected samples:

> When an investigator is conducting research on coded or identifiable samples obtained prior to implementation of NBAC's recommendations, general releases for research given in conjunction with a clinical or surgical procedure must not be presumed to cover all types of research over an indefinite period of time. IRBs should review existing consent documents to determine whether the subjects anticipated and agreed to participate in the type of research proposed. If the existing documents are inadequate and consent cannot be waived, the investigator must obtain

informed consent from the subjects for the current research or in appropriate circumstances have the identifiers stripped so that samples can be linked.

Recommendation 9 relates to prospectively collected samples:

> To facilitate collection, storage and appropriate use of [HBMs] in the future, consent forms should be developed to provide potential subjects with a sufficient number of options to help them understand clearly the nature of the decision they are about to make.

This latter recommendation lists six options ranging from refusal of future use of materials, to the permitting of coded use of materials for any kind of future study.

While the commission was not unanimous on the number and scope of the options for recommendation 9, taken together these two recommendations reflected an important departure from the standard approach to informed consent: first, that with respect to previously collected samples, research may proceed without consent under certain specific conditions; and secondly, with respect to samples now being collected, individuals may be permitted to prospectively authorise future use in a still-to-be-designed study.

Emergency Research

Research in an emergency setting raises some of the most profound challenges to the concept and practice of informed consent.[30] As discussed above, US federal regulations provide a common set of requirements for informed consent. Separate regulations issued by the Food and Drug Administration (FDA) in 1996 include an exception to the standard consent requirements that allows for the use of a test article without informed consent in emergency situations.[31] These regulations are meant to apply to research carried out under an FDA new drug application or new device exemption. It is generally understood that the drug or device (e.g. a new type of cardiac defibrillator) would be used in the field to save the life of an individual. Under these regulations, IRBs could waive the requirement for signed informed consent, when such prior documentation could not be obtained from the subject or a legally authorised representative, so long as certain conditions were satisfied: prior consultation with representatives of the community in which the research would occur and from which potential subjects would be recruited; secondly, a public disclosure of the purpose of the study, including the potential risks and benefits, and finally, the results of the study must in due course be publicly disclosed. The Canadian Tri-Council Policy also permits emergency research, but requires that a more detailed set of requirements be met.[14] (sec.2.11)

THE FUTURE OF INFORMED CONSENT IN RESEARCH

For the immediate future, informed consent will remain a centrepiece of the system of protecting human subjects in research. Some have argued that this principle is universal, not relative.[32] Given the increase in international collaborative research, considerable progress still needs to be made in ensuring that participants in such studies are fully informed, a point that is treated indirectly in both the US regulations and Canadian guidelines (see, for example, ref. 14, p. 1.12). Neither explicitly describes what constitutes an informed consent in regions or for cultures where signed, written, and witnessed consent is not the norm.

Ongoing use of the regulations and guidelines in these two countries by researchers and review committees has generated considerable academic and policy discussion. The three challenges described above are but a selection from a larger list raised by genetics, public health research, and the delivery of health services, to name but a few. As discussion continues about improving the quality of the informed consent process, it should be self-evident, however, that as a method for *protecting* subjects against potential harms, the informed consent process is only successful if, in the event, potential subjects choose not to participate in a particular study. Informed consent serves its protective role only by providing sufficient information to allow individuals to choose whether to accept the risk of certain known harms, though it can serve other purposes as well. Recently, a number of authors have argued that the emphasis in research ethics should be placed less on the requirements of informed consent, and more on the problem in increasing access to research studies.[33, 34] This change in emphasis – from protection to access – has not yet been fully developed or resolved in practice, but it is likely that as potential subjects (for example those with HIV infection) express greater interest in the design of clinical trials,[35] the role of informed consent may be broadened considerably, and the discussion with a potential participant occurring much earlier in the research activity.

ACKNOWLEDGEMENT

I wish to acknowledge the assistance of Dan Powell in the preparation of this manuscript, and for helpful comments by Harold T. Shapiro on as earlier version.

DISCLAIMER

The views expressed in this chapter are those of the author and do not reflect those of the National Bioethics Advisory Commission or the United States government.

REFERENCES

1. Sugarman J, McCrory DC, Powell D *et al.* Empirical research on informed consent: an annotated bibliography. Hastings Center Report 1999; (January/February) Special Supplement.
2. Faden RR, Beauchamp TL. *A history and theory of informed consent.* New York: Oxford University Press, 1986.
3. Rothman DJ. *Strangers at the bedside: A history of how law and bioethics transformed medical decision making.* New York: Basic Books, 1991.
4. Moreno JD. *Undue risk: secret state experiments on humans.* New York: William H Freeman, 1999.
5. Beecher HK. Ethics and clinical research. *N Eng J Med* 1966; **274**: 1354–60.
6. Katz J. *Experimentation with human beings.* New York: Sage, 1972.
7. Federal Policy for the Protection of Human Subjects. 45 CFR 46 (1981).
8. Federal Policy for the Protection of Human Subjects. *Federal Register* 57; **17**: 28002–28032, revised, June 18, 1991.
9. Advisory Committee on Human Radiation Experiments. *Final Report of the Advisory Committee on human radiation experiments.* New York: Oxford University Press, 1998.
10. *Halushka v. Regents of the University of Saskatchewan,* 52 W. W. R. 608 (Sask. 1965).
11. Freedman B, Glass KC. *Weiss v. Solomon*: a case study institutional responsibility for clinical research. *Law Med Hlth Care* 1990; **18**: 100–109.
12. Canada, Medical Research Council. *Ethics in medical experimentation. Report No. 6.* Ottawa: Medical Research Council, 1978.
13. Canada, Medical Research Council. *Guidelines for*

research involving human subjects. Ottawa: Medical Research Council, 1987.

14. Canada. Tri-Council Policy Statement. *Ethical conduct of research involving humans*. Ottawa: Minister of Supply and Services, 1998.

15. National Commission for the Protection of Human Subjects of Biomedical and Behavioral Research. *The Belmont Report: Ethical principles and guidelines for the protection of human subjects of biomedical and behavioral research*. Washington DC: US Government Printing Office, 1979.

16. Jecker N, Meslin EM. United States and Canadian approaches to justice in health care: a comparative analysis of health care systems and values. *Theor Med* 1994; **15**: 181–200.

17. Beauchamp TL Childress JF. *Principles of biomedical ethics*, 4th edn. New York: Oxford University Press, 1994.

18. Meslin EM, Sutherland HJ, Lavery JV *et al.* Principlism and the ethical appraisal of clinical trials. *Bioethics* 1995; **9**: 399–418.

19. National Bioethics Advisory Commission. *Research involving persons with mental disorders that may affect decisionmaking capacity* (2 vols). Rockville MD: National Bioethics Advisory Commission, December, 1998.

20. National Bioethics Advisory Commission. *Research involving human biological materials: ethical issues and policy guidance* (2 vols). Rockville MD: National Bioethics Advisory Commission, August, 1999.

21. Weijer C, Dickens BM, Meslin EM. Bioethics for clinicians. VII: Research ethics. *Can Med Ass J* 1997; **16**: 1153–7.

22. US General Accounting Office. Scientific Research. *Continued vigilance critical to protecting human subjects*. GAO/HEHS-96-72. March 1996.

23. US Department of Health and Human Services, Office of the Inspector General. *Institutional review boards: a time for reform*. OEI-01-97-00193, 1998.

24. Bell J, Whiton J, Connelly S. *Final report: evaluation of NIH implementation of Section 491 of the Public Health Service Act, mandating a program of protection for*

research subjects. Grant No. NO1-OD-2-2109, June 15, 1998.

25. Executive Order 12975. *Federal Register*. 1995; **60**(193): 52063–52067.

26. National Commission for the Protection of Human Subjects of Biomedical and Behavioral Research. *Research involving those institutionalized as mentally infirm*. Washington DC: US Government Printing Office, 1978.

27. Nuffield Council on Bioethics. *Mental disorders and genetics: the ethical context*. London: The Nuffield Council, 1998.

28. Meslin EM. Engaging the public in policy development: the National Bioethics Advisory Commission report on research involving persons with mental disorders that may affect decisionmaking capacity. *Account Res* 1999; **7**: 227–40.

29. Eiseman E, Haga SB. *Handbook on tissue sources: a national resource of human tissue samples*. RAND Science and Technology Policy Institute, 2000.

30. Abrahamson, Meisel, Safar. Deferred consent: a new approach for resuscitation research on comatose patients. *JAMA* 1986; **255**: 2466–71.

31. 21 CFR 50.

32. Macklin R. *Against relativism: cultural diversity and the search for ethical universals in medicine*. New York: Oxford University Press, 1999.

33. Levine C. Changing views of justice after Belmont: AIDS and the inclusion of 'Vulnerable subjects'. In: Harold Y. Vanbderpool, ed. *The ethics of research involving human subjects: facing the 21st century*. Frederick MD: University Publishing Group, 1996, pp. 105–26.

34. Kahn JK. Mastroianni AC, Sugarman J eds. *Beyond consent: seeking justice in research*. New York: Oxford University Press, 1998.

35. Arras JD. Noncompliance in AIDS research. In: *Ethical issues in modern medicine*. John D. Arras, Bonnie Steinbock, eds Mountain View, CA: Mayfield Publishing Co., 1995, pp. 559–69.

The European Perspective

Richard Nicholson

Progress towards the ethical conduct of medical research on human beings often appears to have occurred in response to various scandals. Public outcry at the abuse of human rights in medical experiments in the Nazi concentration camps, or in the Tuskegee syphilis study, for instance, was met by the writing of the Nuremberg Code and the US National Research Act. Yet a review of the development of research ethics across Europe in the 20th century suggests that such scandals may have made little difference. What does appear to make a difference is the commercial pressure exerted by the pharmaceutical industry to ensure that Good Clinical Practice standards are applied wherever pharmaceutical research is undertaken, to satisfy regulatory agencies. This has been mediated through various transnational guidelines, which individual countries have subsumed as laws or regulations, leading to a marked improvement in the extent to which informed consent, in particular, is sought from research subjects.

EARLY GERMAN SCANDALS

Another perception that needs to be challenged is that informed consent was somehow an American invention after World War II. In fact a legal requirement for the informed consent of the subject of human experimentation was first made in a ministerial directive issued in Berlin in 1900. The need for such a directive arose from the work of Professor Neisser – best remembered nowadays for giving his name to the organisms that cause gonorrhoea and meningitis, *Neisseria gonorrhoea* and *N. meningitidis*. In 1898, when professor of dermatology and venereology at the University of Breslau, and attempting to develop an antisyphilis serum, he injected cell-free serum from syphilitic patients into others – mostly prostitutes – without their full knowledge or consent: some developed syphilis as a result. In 1900 the Royal Disciplinary Court (of Prussia) fined him 300 marks and also levied 1245 marks in legal costs, together representing two-thirds of his annual income.

The Prussian parliament discussed the case and the Minister for Religious, Educational and Medical Affairs obtained detailed reports from doctors such as Professor Rudolf Virchow, and from lawyers. One lawyer stated that research undertaken without consent and not intended to benefit the subject constituted a criminal harm: voluntary consent was a mandatory requirement to make it lawful. At the end of 1900, the Minister issued the following regulation:

Directive to all medical directors of university hospitals, polyclinics, and other hospitals

I.   I advise the medical directors of university hospitals, polyclinics, and all other hospitals that all medical interventions for other than diagnostic, healing, and immunisation purposes, regardless of other legal or moral authorisation, are excluded under all circumstances, if
1. the human subject is a minor or not competent due to other reasons;
2. the human subject has not given his unambiguous consent;
3. the consent is not preceded by a proper explanation of the possible negative consequences of the intervention.

II.   At the same time I determine that
1. interventions of this kind are to be performed only by the medical director himself or with his special authorisation;
2. in all cases of these interventions the fulfilment of the requirements of I (1–3) and II (1), as well as all further circumstances of the case, are documented in the medical record.

III.   The existing instructions about medical interventions for diagnostic, healing and immunisation purposes are not affected by these instructions.

Berlin, 29 December 1900.[1]

Not only was that first regulation of research on human subjects more restrictive than most rules today, but it specifically required consent to be obtained *after relevant information had been given*. What is not clear is how much of an effect it had in practice. By the late 1920s there was frequent criticism in the German press of unethical research undertaken by the medical profession. The extent of the criticism may have been excessive, but it is clear that parts of the medical profession were very uncritical in their relationships with the chemical/pharmaceutical industry, then in a period of great creativity. A spokesman for the National Health Administration listed some of the accusations in 1930: "Naked cynicism; placing the lives of small children on the same level as those of experimental animals; dubious experiments having no therapeutic purpose; science sailing under false colours; crimes against the health of defenceless children."[2]

Press criticism and discussion within the medical profession eventually bore fruit. In February 1931 the German Minister of the Interior issued "guidelines for innovative therapy and scientific experiments on man." Although only guidelines, they were given some force by the introductory statement[3] that the Reich Health Council "has agreed that all physicians in open or closed health care institutions should sign a commitment to these guidelines when entering their employment."

Grodin rightly calls these guidelines "visionary in their depth and scope."[4] They start by acknowledging the need both for "innovative therapy" and "human experimentation" – which today we usually call "therapeutic" and "non-therapeutic" research – and, at the same time, reminding the physician of his "... major responsibility for the life and health of any person ...." on whom he performs research. They go on to stress the importance of keeping to the principles of medical ethics, of prior assessment of risks and benefits, of obtaining consent, of giving extra protection to subjects under 18 years of age, of not exploiting social hardship, of having a senior physician in charge of all research, of training physicians about their special duties when acting as researcher, and of writing up thorough reports of the research. Paragraph 5 reads:

> 5. Innovative therapy may be carried out only after the subject or his legal representative has unambiguously consented to the procedure in the light of relevant information provided in advance. Where consent is refused, innovative therapy may be initiated only if it constitutes an urgent procedure to preserve life or prevent serious damage to health, and prior consent could not be obtained under the circumstances.

Paragraph 12(a) is more succinct: "[Scientific] experimentation shall be prohibited in all cases where consent has not been given."

TREADING WATER

However visionary these guidelines may have been, and even though they remained valid until 1945,[5] they were no match for the Nazi ideology that permitted and encouraged horrendously inhumane "experiments" in the concentration camps, without any semblance of volunteering or of consent. Hence the Nuremberg Code,[6] which is part of the judgment delivered by the tribunal at the doctors' trial in 1947, has an even stronger statement about consent.

Outside Germany there seems, in the first two decades after World War II, to have been no knowledge of the 1900 Prussian Regulations or of the 1931 Ministry of the Interior Guidelines. Even if there were awareness of the existence of the Nuremberg Code among researchers, the long litany of unethical research in Pappworth's *Human guinea pigs* shows that it had little influence on ethical standards in research in the USA or UK. Elsewhere in Europe there has been less evidence of seriously unethical

research, although it is also clear that the Nuremberg Code's assertion that consent is essential was in many countries imperfectly realised, and in some countries totally ignored, until the 1980s.

A fundamental difficulty in providing an accurate picture of the development of informed consent to research in Europe is the lack, until recently, of any empirical studies of the consent process. What laws, regulations or guidelines were in force in any one country at any one time may be ascertained: whether researchers actually complied with them is almost impossible to discover. The only reliable way to find such information would be for research ethics committees to audit the extent to which their requirements for informed consent in individual studies were met. Nowhere in the world is such an audit undertaken in a regular, systematic way even now. So the following comments are necessarily impressionistic.

Although wide publicity about unethical research was generated by Pappworth and Beecher in the 1960s,[7, 8] it seems that the original 1964 Helsinki Declaration had little more influence on the conduct of research in Europe than the Nuremberg Code. Other guidelines in particular countries may have had some influence, but the most important development of the 1960s was probably the setting-up of the first research ethics committees in Europe, initially in response to the US Public Health Service requirement that any clinical research it funded must be reviewed by such a committee. To begin with the quality of such review may not have been very high, but any committee taking its work at all seriously would by then have known the importance of consent.

LEGISLATION AND REGULATION BEGIN

The 1970s was the decade in which laws and regulations for the conduct of clinical research began to be made. There was little uniformity of approach, so that sometimes written consent was mandatory, while elsewhere oral consent was adequate; in some countries no research was permitted on those who could not consent, in others consent could be obtained from relatives, even if they were not legal guardians. Some flavour of the variety is given in the reports of the conferences of CIOMS – the Council for International Organizations of Medical Sciences established by WHO and UNESCO. At the 1978 conference, for instance, William Curran, Professor of Legal Medicine at Harvard, reported on his studies of medical research in Europe, undertaken mainly by interviewing clinical researchers.[9] Among his comments were:

> In most countries of Europe, the concentration of attention is upon the freedom of the patient or subject to consent or not to consent and not upon the "informing" part of the requirement.
>
> ... I saw little evidence in any European country of the use of written, signed consent forms with the possible exception of the Republic of Ireland for projects supported by the Medical Research Council. Some countries, such as Denmark, utilize a written statement of the project which is given to subject-patients on clinical investigation. The patients can read the statement at their leisure and later another person, not the investigator, returns to the bedside to answer any further questions and to obtain the consent or refusal of the patient orally. The precautions taken here are particularly to avoid any feelings of coercion on the part of the patient and to allow time for reflection about participation.

At the same meeting Norman Williams, Head of the Medicines Division of the UK Department of Health and Social Security raised the issue of whether long-stay patients or prisoners could ever give a free consent to participation in research: "Because of such doubts, prisoners are not used as trial subjects in any country in Western or Eastern Europe, although in the USA they are commonly employed as 'healthy volunteers' for the first trials of new pharmaceutical preparations as well as for other investigations."[10]

The Council of Europe's experts concluded that informed consent was always needed when research was not being conducted in the subject's own interest, but had not found the same necessity in therapeutic research:

> Where the trial carried out on patients has a therapeutic element, it is theoretically desirable on ethical grounds to obtain the informed consent of the patient, his family or his legal guardian. However, it is often difficult and delicate to apply this requirement systematically. In any event, even if written informed consent is to be granted by the patient, his family or his legal guardian in full knowledge of the facts, it might be necessary to impose certain restrictions in the patient's own interests. Under certain circumstances, oral consent granted in the presence of a witness and confirmed in writing by the latter might be appropriate.[11]

How human rights in medicine were protected in the German Democratic Republic was discussed at the same meeting (1978) by a representative of its Ministry of Health: it is a delightfully utopian prospect:[12]

> The health protection guaranteed by the Constitution of the GDR enables people to lead a life free of material cares as far as their health is concerned, last but not least because medical care is provided free of charge. This is an important social achievement of socialist society.
>
> ... These social foundations make it possible for medical science to develop freely and for every physician to make full use of his knowledge and skills for the benefit of his patients in keeping with the humanitarian calling of the medical profession. Physicians and patients are not concerned with economic interests or worries that might disrupt the doctor-patient relationship. Thus every citizen of the GDR may have full confidence in his doctor.
>
> ... *The testing of medicaments for use in human medicine.* The testing of medicaments is governed by legal provisions issued on 17 May 1976 .... Consent of the subjects is an indispensable condition. Subjects have the right to withdraw their consent at any time and without stating reasons.

Given, however, what we have learned of East Germany since the fall of the Berlin Wall, one wonders whether consent to participation in research was ever obtained during the communist era. In Scandinavia, on the other hand, the need for consent was recognised, not only in the Danish approach outlined by Curran above, but also in Sweden. A circular on the conduct of drug trials in 1972 stated:

> The doctor is under obligation in good time before the testing to inform the person, if necessary in writing, about the nature and purpose of the experiment as well as the risks connected with the latter, and also to give the person reasonable time for thinking things over before giving his consent.[13]

It was possibly only in Scandinavia, from the early 1970s to the late 1980s, that there was both a recognition of the centrality of informed consent to ethical research and the professional ethos and/or regulations to ensure that it was always obtained. In the UK, for instance, both the legal and ethical importance of informed consent to research were recognised but, in the absence of regulations, the medical professional ethos was not strong enough to prevent some research being done without the subjects' knowledge or consent, thereby causing considerable scandal. In Belgium, as late as 1987, there were notices in the university teaching hospital in Louvain informing patients that by coming to the hospital they had given implied consent to being used as research subjects.[14]

GEOGRAPHICAL VARIATIONS

In the late 1980s there was a measurable difference in approach to informed consent in western Europe between northern and Mediterranean countries. While the benevolent paternalism that had been the norm in Spain in the 1970s had been partly dissipated by a series of legal cases, it was still common in Italy. On entering most Italian hospitals, patients had to sign a form saying that they agreed to any treatments that the doctors might recommend. In Spain, a 1982 ministerial order required clinical researchers to obtain informed consent from any patient before entry into a clinical trial. Yet a survey in 1989 of clinical trials committee members showed that not all of them would do so.[15]

Spanish clinical trials committees in the 1980s were made up of physicians of various specialities, pharmacists and sometimes a statistician, but had no members from outside healthcare. Many members were themselves involved in clinical trials. Researchers were required to inform trial subjects about the purposes, methodology and risks of a trial: if a potential subject agreed to take part, the researcher and a witness, but not the subject, signed the consent form. The 1989 survey found that, while 97% of clinical trial committee members thought that informed consent should always be obtained, only 68% thought it should be in writing, and 58% thought the subject should receive a copy. When asked about the information to be given to potential subjects, less than half the respondents thought it necessary always to supply the following specifics:

- the name of the sponsor of the clinical trial
- the design of the clinical trial
- the experimental procedures involved
- the number of patients to be included
- a statement that subjects would be informed of the clinical trial results.

Other answers, however, showed considerable progress towards fulfilling the requirements of what had recently become known as "Good Clinical Practice".

A survey of researchers who had clinical trials published in the *European Journal of Cancer* between 1990 and 1992 gave some evidence for a North–South divide in approach to informed consent.[16] Eighty-seven clinicians were sent a short questionnaire about how they had usually obtained consent in their reported trials: 60 (69%) responded, of whom 27 came from the South (France, Italy) and 33 from the North (UK, Ireland, Sweden, Denmark, Belgium, Germany, the Netherlands). Six of the Southerners and one Northerner did not inform patients about the trial until after randomisation; 85% of Northerners always told the patient that treatment would be randomly assigned, but only a third of the Southerners did so. Three Southerners did not seek the patients' consent at all; 79% of Northerners gave full information about all treatment options, while 67% of Southerners gave information only on the proposed treatment arm. When trials of supportive care were compared with those of antitumour therapies, the level of consent was found to be much higher in the trials of supportive care.

Research ethics in central and eastern Europe has hardly been mentioned so far, largely because, as understood in the West, it did not exist. For over 40 years those countries shared the common fate of being controlled by the Soviet Union, with all aspects of society permeated by the ideology of Marxism–Leninism. That ideology was the basis of Soviet science, so that a Soviet health minister could write:

> Like all other branches of knowledge, medical science is developing in our country on the basis of dialectical materialism and the Marxist–Leninist conception of the world. The strength of our scientific medicine lies in its close bond with practice and life.[17]

Autonomy, informed consent, patients' rights, and respect for persons were largely absent in a paternalistic system that often gave patients a choice between experimental therapy in a university clinic and little or no treatment, because of financial constraints, in a local hospital. Szawarski concluded:[18]

> Biomedical research was conducted in all socialist countries. In all socialist countries there were proper medical codes and legal rules defining the obligations of doctors regarding human experimentation. It is not yet clear to what extent these rules were observable and enforceable in practice. There is no efficient system of organization to control research on human subjects.

FIRST EUROPEAN GUIDELINES

Before 1990 the Declaration of Helsinki was the only

set of internationally produced research guidelines widely accepted around Europe.[19] Although CIOMS published proposed international guidelines in 1982, they only came to widespread attention when revised in 1993.[20] Simultaneously with the end of the Cold War, however, both major European organisations published guidance on the conduct of medical research.

First came Recommendation R(90)3 of the Council of Europe, recommending member states to adopt legislation incorporating 16 principles. These principles include the need for consent ("No medical research may be carried out without the informed, free, express and specific consent of the person undergoing it"), but then list a variety of exceptions, such as for legally incapacitated subjects, and research in emergencies.[21]

In July 1990, guidelines for Good Clinical Practice prepared by the Committee for Proprietary Medicinal Products of the European Commission were finally approved. Although the guidelines lacked legal force, European drug regulatory authorities expected the pharmaceutical industry to keep to them if the results of their clinical trials were to be considered by the regulators for drug licensing. At 46 pages they were the most thorough European guidance available: within the following guidance on informed consent, for instance, are several elements absent from earlier guidelines:

"1.8. The principles of informed consent in the current revision of the Helsinki Declaration should be implemented in each clinical trial.

1.9. Information should be given in both oral and written form whenever possible. No subject should be obliged to participate in the trial. Subjects, their relatives, guardians or, if necessary, legal representatives must be given ample opportunity to enquire about details of the trial. The information must make clear that refusal to participate or withdrawal from the trial at any stage is without any disadvantages for the subject's subsequent care. Subjects must be allowed sufficient time to decide whether or not they wish to participate.

1.10. The subject must be made aware and consent that personal information may be scrutinised during audit by competent authorities and properly authorised persons, but that personal information will be treated as strictly confidential and not be publicly available.

1.11. The subject must have access to information about the procedures for compensation and treatment should he/she be injured/disabled by participating in the trial.

1.12. If a subject consents to participate after a full and comprehensive explanation of the study (including its aims, expected benefits for the subjects and/or others, reference treatments/placebo, risks and inconveniences – e.g. invasive procedures – and, where appropriate, an explanation of alternative, recognised standard medical therapy), this consent should be appropriately recorded. Consent must be documented either by the subject's dated signature or by the signature of an independent witness who records the subject's assent. In either case the signature confirms that the consent is based on information which has been understood, and that the subject has freely chosen to participate without prejudice to legal and ethical rights while allowing the possibility of withdrawal from the study without having to give any reason unless adverse events have occurred.

1.13. If the subject is incapable of giving personal consent (e.g. unconsciousness or severe mental illness or disability), the inclusion of such patients may be acceptable if the Ethics Committee is, in principle, in agreement and if the investigator is of the opinion that participation will promote the welfare and interest of the subject. The agreement of a legally valid representative that participation will promote the welfare and interest of the subject should also be recorded by a dated signature. If neither signed informed consent nor witnessed signed verbal consent are possible, this fact must be documented with reasons by the investigator.

1.14. Consent must always be given by the signature of the subject in a non-therapeutic study, i.e. when there is no direct clinical benefit to the subject.

1.15. Any information becoming available during the trial which may be of relevance for the trial subjects must be made known to them by the investigator.[22]

NATIONAL LAWS ON RESEARCH IN EUROPE

1990 also saw the start of a period of national law-making across Europe. France had been in a strange position until 1988, in that research on human subjects had no legal standing and was deemed by some legal experts to be unconstitutional. An Act passed in December 1988 – The Protection of Persons Undergoing Biomedical Research – gave authority to carry out research, but its regulations for the lawful conduct of research did not come into force until after it had been amended in January 1990.[23] Part I of the Act had general provisions, part II stated in detail the requirements for valid consent, part III required the setting-up of research ethics committees and outlined their modus operandi, part IV made specific rules on the conduct of non-therapeutic research, while part V laid down penalties for non-compliance. Conducting research without consent, for example, might attract a penalty of 6 months to 3 years' imprisonment and a fine of up to FFr. 200 000.

The French law met with considerable initial resistance from some clinical researchers. As Fagot-Largeault commented,[24] the "French medical profession has had a strong tradition of paternalism and secrecy, including the protection of patients from any 'disturbing' knowledge about their condition." Some specialties, such as paediatric oncology, formed lobbies asking to be exempt from the law, and claiming that it would prevent clinical research. Opposition was short-lived, however, and no diminution has been seen in the amount of research performed.

Ireland, too, found itself in a strange position at the start of 1990. A Clinical Trials Act passed in 1987 had required that informed consent be obtained from all research subjects,[25] but the Act was a disaster because of the burdens it placed on the research ethics committees that it established. Committee members had to guarantee that adequate funds were available to compensate any injured subjects, and rapidly perceived themselves as potential targets of litigation. They called a moratorium on reviewing any research proposals, severely limiting what research was carried out, until an amended Act was passed in 1990.

Spain also legislated in 1990, passing the Drugs and Medicines Act, of which chapter 3 concerned the conduct of clinical trials. This was greatly expanded by Royal Decree 561/1993, so that there are now 47 clauses on clinical trials, subsuming most of the requirements of Good Clinical Practice.[26]

Denmark passed a "Law on a Scientific Ethical Committee System and the Handling of Biomedical Research Projects" in 1992.[27] Its main purpose was to give a legal basis to the research ethics committees in place since 1980. It authorized the Minister of Health to make detailed regulations on obtaining consent to research interventions, and provided for fines or imprisonment for failure to obtain, or adhere to, research ethics committee approval.

The Italian Ministry of Health issued a decree in April, 1992 that gave full legal force to the CPMP Good Clinical Practice guidelines and re-emphasised the need for informed consent; it also resulted in many new research ethics committees being set up.[28]

A law was passed in Portugal in 1993 enacting the requirements of Good Clinical Practice.[29]

FURTHER EUROPEAN GUIDANCE

The two European guidance documents of 1990 were not the last: two more appeared in 1996 and have already led to further national legislation. The first to appear, in May 1996, is known as ICHGCP, the full title being the International Conference on Harmonisation of Technical Requirements for Registration of Pharmaceuticals for Human Use Harmonised Tripartite Guideline for Good Clinical Practice[30] – no wonder the short title is popular! Tripartite in the title reflects the agreement to this guideline of the regulatory authorities in Europe, Japan, and the United States, which require clinical trials for licensing purposes to conform to the guideline.

The informed consent part of the ICHGCP has fifteen sections, one of which alone lists 20 elements that must be on the written information sheet and must also be explained by the researcher to the subject during the obtaining of consent. Many ICHGCP requirements should become part of an European Union directive, being prepared, on the conduct of clinical trials, that would be required to be subsumed into national legislation in EU countries. So far, the European Parliament and the EU Council of Ministers have not agreed on the directive, and the final version will not appear before 2001.

The other guidance produced in 1996 covers more than just research, being the Council of Europe's bioethics convention[31] or, in full: "Convention for the protection of human rights and dignity of the human being with regard to the application of biology and medicine." Only four of its 38 articles are directly concerned with research, although even these are controversial to some, and an additional protocol on biomedical research is supposed to be published in 2000. The controversy concerns a provision that non-therapeutic research may be performed on subjects who are incapable of consenting to it. Such a suggestion is anathema in Germany, explaining why Germany has not signed the convention. Research on children and the mentally incapacitated is only permitted in Germany if there is a real chance of benefit to the subject. Both the laws governing research – the Arzneimittelgesetz of 1976 and the Medizineproduktegesetz of 1994 – and the requirements of the physicians' chambers, ensure that consent to research is obtained (it is too dangerous not to) even though GCP requirements are not yet in the law. Other countries have signed and, in a few cases, ratified the convention, giving it legal force. Finland has only signed the convention but this has resulted in a new Medical Research Act being brought into force in 1999.[32] The new Act follows ICHGCP in requiring written consent – a major change in Finland, where researchers hitherto only obtained oral consent. The National Advisory Board on Healthcare Ethics has had to hold seminars around the country to re-educate researchers.

The Netherlands passed a Medical Research Involving Human Subjects Act that came into force in December 1999.[33] It goes into considerable detail on how consent to research is to be obtained and, interestingly, requires that such consent be obtained from subjects from the age of 12 years upwards.

In Switzerland there is no federal law yet on clinical trials, but several cantonal laws are based on GCP and insist on informed consent to research. There is, however, too much variation between the Cantons, and a federal law is likely to be enacted in the next two to three years. A peculiarly Swiss problem lies in the writing of patient information sheets, since they have to be in at least three languages – German, French, and Italian. One clinical research organisation in Basel was closed down in 1999 for, amongst other deficiencies, bringing Estonian students to Basel as subjects for Phase I studies and providing patient information sheets in English only.

EASTERN EUROPE CATCHES UP

Change is now taking place most rapidly in the former communist countries of central and eastern Europe. The impetus is primarily commercial, since it is much cheaper for multinational pharmaceutical companies to undertake trials than in western Europe. This has put pressure on governments – for whom the investment of research funds is most welcome – to ensure a legal basis for GCP but, although some countries are well advanced towards GCP, others have barely started.

In Russia, a 1993 law on healthcare required ethics committees to be set up to ensure that patients receive adequate information from doctors during routine clinical practice: they are beginning to be effective. In 1997, ICHGCP requirements were adopted in a guidance note from the minister of health. A 1998 law on pharmaceutical products, passed both by the federal and state parliaments, reinforced GCP by requiring, in particular, that written consent be obtained from all patients taking part in pharmaceutical research. Clinical trials are centrally monitored, since they can only be undertaken with permission of the Ministry of Health's pharmacology committee. Clinical trial entry is not permitted for children with no parent, military personnel, prisoners, or pregnant women unless related to pregnancy.

The requirements of pharmaceutical research from the West brought a considerable change in Lithuania's approach to informed consent, which had rarely been obtained in the early 1990s. In 1997 a Ministry of Health decree required it to be obtained. This is likely to be reinforced in 2000 when a law based on the Council of Europe's bioethics convention is expected. The reinforcement is needed, since it appears that research is still sometimes undertaken without consent. There are problems with patient information sheets not being understood, and uncertainty as to whether coercion to enter trials has stopped.

Slovakia had a tradition of greater protection of research subjects than in some parts of the region. Much further progress was expected after the "Velvet Revolution", but at first this was effected only by the setting-up of research ethics committees, and by voluntary adherence by researchers to the principles of GCP. The 1998 Law on Drugs, however, provides for full implementation of GCP in the Slovak Republic.[34]

In the 1980s an annual course on human rights in medicine was held in Dubrovnik, attended not only by Croatian doctors and medical students, but also by bioethicists from both east and west Europe. So it is not perhaps surprising that, since Croatia gained independence, there have been several initiatives dealing with informed consent in research. The Health Protection Law of January 1997 protects patients' rights to refuse both research and treatment.[35] A law on drugs and medical devices in November 1997 mandated the obtaining of informed consent to participate in clinical drug trials. Finally in October 1998 a bye-law introduced the principles of GCP. As elsewhere, the problem lies in how long it takes researchers to take GCP seriously. There is a financial incentive for researchers to take on clinical trials from the West, because the daily struggle to survive is still a fact of Croatian life. Few patients appear really to understand that to which they consent, not least because there is little attempt to write patient information sheets that are easy to understand, and not overoptimistic, making too hopeful assertions about the benefits to patients of taking part.

Some research seems now to be happening in Bosnia, but the patients may not even be informed that it is research. A teacher in Zagreb of postgraduate medical students from Bosnia commented that the idea of informed consent seemed to be entirely new to them.[36]

Surprisingly, the situation of informed consent to research in Poland and Hungary appears closer to that in Bosnia than in Slovakia. In Poland, informed consent is a formality to which lip service only is paid. It is never requested in routine practice, consent forms for surgery usually being blank when signed. There is no law requiring research ethics committees and no satisfactory scrutiny of research proposals. Yet patients are keen to take part in clinical pharmaceutical trials because treatment then becomes free, and since the new drugs usually come from the West "they must be better than anything available locally." This may be an unfair portrait of clinical trials in Poland but, if not, it is surprising because it disregards not only GCP and the Helsinki Declaration but also the Polish Physicians' Code of Medical Ethics, over which there was much lively debate in 1991 and 1992.[37] The code, at paragraph 44, states: "The project of every experiment involving human subjects should be clearly stated in writing and presented to an independent ethics committee for approval." As well as requiring full information to be given, before written consent to research is obtained, the code requires that: "The decision to participate in the experiment on the part of the patients shall not result from their dependence on the physician, nor from any constraint."

The position in Hungary is a little different, appearing to be one of rampant double standards. Research ethics committees have been set up by law, and much reference is made to GCP and the Helsinki Declaration. While there are some good ethics committees with committed members, it is often the leading (in financial terms) researcher at a hospital who chairs the committee and appoints its members. Patients are still very vulnerable to caregivers: it is unheard of for any to refuse to take part in research. In part this is because many patient information sheets are very technical: the most readily understood part is likely to be a statement to the effect: "Congratulations; you are so lucky to be selected for this research." Other worries are that much research is still performed without ethics review, and that many drug trials use placebo controls when there are effective existing treatments.

CONCLUSIONS

During the 1990s there has been a clear trend across Europe to pass laws requiring the informed consent of research subjects to be obtained prior to research interventions being carried out. There are probably three reasons for this:

- the need to protect human rights when medical professions are perceived to be taking too long to grow out of their paternalism;
- to protect commercial interests, since multinational pharmaceutical companies are less likely to invest research funds in countries that do not comply with GCP;
- the desire, fostered by organisations like the Council of Europe, for harmonisation of laws across Europe; such harmonisation now means that most European countries have laws on medical research that mandate the obtaining of informed consent.

It is also clear that scandals about unethical and unconsented research have only local, if any, effect. The scandals of the 1890s and 1920s in Germany did not result in legislation that could prevent the Nazi medical horrors. On the other hand these terrible events did have an effect, but only on Germans, who for many years after World War II were very cautious about what research they undertook.

What is not yet clear is whether all the recent laws are effective at protecting research subjects and ensuring that they give informed consent freely to their involvement. To check this would require more thorough audit of the process of obtaining consent than is yet carried out anywhere: such audit as there is, primarily in clinical drug trials, tracks the paperwork and ensures only that consent forms have been signed. In preparing this chapter, however, the author spoke to doctors and ethicists in many countries across Europe. None of those in countries that have legislated were aware of any serious problems; but the process of GCP is so new to some in eastern Europe that problems with inadequately informed, or inadequately voluntary, consent may continue until all researchers have been more fully educated.

The value of informed consent legislation is perhaps best illustrated by the UK. The UK is now virtually alone in Europe in having neither a law nor legally-enforceable regulations on the conduct of research on humans. There is also a vocal minority in the medical profession still arguing that consent to research is not always needed. As a result the UK is the one country in Europe that has had a regular succession of scandals about unconsented research through the 1980s and 1990s. The latest such scandal, involving neonates in North Staffordshire, led to the setting-up of a government enquiry in 1999.

The lack of legally-enforceable regulations on how research ethics committees (RECs) function in the UK also means that there is a wide variety of responses, some of them distinctly idiosyncratic, to GCP requirements. There are world-renowned medical research centres in the UK whose RECs refuse to work in accordance with GCP – whether the European or ICH variety. A substantial minority of RECs either have no standard operating procedures at all, or ones that are inconsistent in many ways with GCP.[38] The result, according to well-placed sources in the pharmaceutical industry, is that the UK probably loses more than £500 million of investment by multinational companies in clinical trials each year: as harmonised control of clinical trials settles down in the rest of Europe, that figure can only rise.

A basic principle of the Declaration of Helsinki is that "Concern for the interests of the subject must always prevail over the interests of science and society." In most of Europe that concern is, at least in part, being realised by laws that require informed consent to research.

ACKNOWLEDGEMENTS

The author gratefully acknowledges the help of Biserka Belicza, Bela Blasszauer, Eugenijus Gefenas, Soren Holm, Olga Kubar, Salla Lötjönen, Emilio Mordini, Udo Schlaudraff, Zbigniew Szawarski, Bart Wijnberg and Walter Ziegler. Any mistakes are entirely the author's responsibility.

REFERENCES

1. Vollmann J, Winau R. The Prussian regulation of 1900: Early ethical standards for human experimentation in Germany. *IRB: Rev Human Subj Res* 1996; **18**(4): 9–11.

2. Stauder A, Müller F. Die Zülassigkeit ärztlicher Versuche an gesunden und kranken Menschen. *Münch Mediz Woch* 1931; **78**: 104–12.

3. *Reichsgesundheitsblatt*, 11 March 1931; **10**: 174–5. In English translation in *Int Dig Hlth Legisl* 1980; **31**: 408–11.

4. Annas GJ, Grodin MA (eds). *The Nazi doctors and the Nuremberg Code*. Oxford: Oxford University Press, 1992, p. 131.

5. Fischer FW, Breuer H. Influences of ethical guidance committees on medical research – a critical reappraisal. In: Howard-Jones N, Bankowski Z (eds). *Medical experimentation and the protection of human rights*. Geneva: CIOMS, 1979.

6. *Trials of war criminals before the Nuremberg Military Tribunals under Control Council Law 10*. Washington DC, US Govt. Printing Office, 1950; Military Tribunal Case 1, *US v. Karl Brandt* et al. pp. 171–84.

7. Pappworth MH. *Human guinea pigs*. London: Routledge & Kegan Paul, 1967.

8. Beecher HK. Ethics and clinical research. *New Engl J Med* 1966; **274**: 1354–60.

9. Curran WJ. Evolution of formal mechanisms for ethical review of clinical research. In: Howard-Jones N, Bankowski Z (eds). *Medical experimentation and the protection of human rights*. Geneva: CIOMS, 1979.

10. Williams RN. Statutory regulations and ethical conduct. In: Howard-Jones N, Bankowski Z (eds). Medical experimentation and the protection of human rights. Geneva: CIOMS, 1979.

11. Scicluna H. Clinical trials and the Council of Europe. In: Howard-Jones N, Bankowski Z (eds). *Medical experimentation and the protection of human rights*. Geneva: CIOMS, 1979.

12. Rapoport SM. Ethical review practices and protection of human rights in medicine in the German Democratic Republic. In: Howard-Jones N, Bankowski Z (eds). *Medical experimentation and the protection of human rights*. Geneva: CIOMS, 1979.

13. Swedish Board of Health and Welfare. *Circular: 1 November*. Stockholm: SBHW, 1972.

14. Anon. Meeting report: informed consent. *IME Bull* 1988; (37): 4–5.

15. Dal-Ré R. Informed consent in clinical research with drugs in Spain: perspective of clinical trials committee members. *Eur J Clin Pharmacol* 1990; **38**: 319–24.

16. Williams CJ, Zwitter M. Informed consent in European multicentre randomised clinical trials – are patients really informed? *Eur J Cancer* 1994; **30A**: 907–10.

17. Kovrigina Y. In: Medisinskii Rabotnik, 1 November 1957. Quoted in Field MG. *Soviet socialised medicine. An introduction*. New York: Free Press, 1967.

18. Szawarski Z. Research ethics in eastern Europe. *Bull Med Eth* 1992; **82**: 13–18.

19. World Medical Association. *Declaration of Helsinki*.

1964, 1975, 1996 versions reprinted in *Bull Med Eth* 1999; **150**: 13–17.

20. Council for International Organizations of Medical Sciences. *International ethical guidelines for biomedical research involving human subjects*. Geneva: CIOMS, 1993.

21. Council of Europe. *Recommendation R(90)3 of the Committee of Ministers to member States concerning medical research on human beings*. Strasbourg: Council of Europe, 1990.

22. Committee for Proprietary Medicinal Products. *Good Clinical Practice for trials on medicinal products in the European Community*. Brussels: European Commission, 1990.

23. Code of Public Health: Book IIA. *Protection of persons undergoing biomedical research*. Paris: Ministry of Health, 1990. Reprinted in English in *Bull Med Eth* 1991; **66**: 8–11.

24. Fagot-Largeault A. Bioethics in France. In: Lustig BA *et al.* (eds). *Regional developments in bioethics: 1989–1991*. Dordrecht: Kluwer, 1992.

25. Dooley D. Medical ethics in Ireland: a decade of change. *Hastings Center Rep* 1991; **21**(1): 18–21.

26. Vidal-Martinez J. The protection of the person in medical research in the Spanish law. *Eur J Health Law* 1999; **6**: 249–64.

27. *Law on a scientific ethical committee system and the handling of biomedical research projects*. Copenhagen: Ministry of Health, 1992. Reprinted in English in *Bull Med Eth* 1992; **84**: 24–7.

28. Cattorini P, Reichlin M. Bioethics in Italy: 1991–1993. In: Lustig BA (ed.). *Regional developments in bioethics: 1991–1993*. Dordrecht: Kluwer, 1995.

29. Biscaia J, Osswald W. Bioethics in Portugal: 1991–1993. In: Lustig BA (ed.). *Regional developments in bioethics: 1991–1993*. Dordrecht: Kluwer, 1995.

30. *ICH Guideline for Good Clinical Practice*. Paris: International Federation of Pharmaceutical Manufacturers Associations, 1996.

31. *Convention for the protection of human rights and dignity of the human being with regard to the application of biology and medicine*. Strasbourg: Council of Europe, 1996.

32. *Medical Research Act, Statute No. 488/1999*. Helsinki: Ministry of Social Affairs and Health, 1999. Reprinted in English in *Bull Med Eth* 2000; **155**: 8–11.

33. *Medical Research Involving Human Subjects Act*. The Hague: Ministry of Health, Welfare and Sports, 1997. Reprinted in English in *Bull Med Eth* 1999; **152**: 13–18.

34. Glasa J, Bielik J, Porubsky J, Glasova H. Informed consent in health care and in biomedical research in the Slovak Republic. In: *Informed consent in European reality* (conference proceedings). Zagreb: Croatian Academy of Sciences and Arts, 1999.

35. Vrhovac B. Informed consent in Croatia. In: *Informed consent in European reality* (conference proceedings). Zagreb: Croatian Academy of Sciences and Arts, 1999.

36. Belicza B. *Personal communication*.

37. Polish code of medical ethics. *Bull Med Eth* 1992; **82**: 19–25.

38. Griffiths A V. *Impact of the International Conference on Harmonisation Guideline for Good Clinical Practice on research ethics committees in the UK* (MA dissertation). Manchester: Manchester University Faculty of Law, 1999.

15 · Informed consent, medical research and the competent adult

Sheila AM McLean

It has long been accepted that there is a need – social and individual – for medicine to progress. The benefits of medical progress form the basic rationale for the presumption that research is, in general but not inevitably, a good thing, and the fact that laboratory and animal models cannot translate into human results predicts the use of human beings in research. However, the simple logical link between the "good" of progress and the "rightness" of human research does not, in contemporary society, go completely unchallenged. The National Bioethics Advisory Commission (USA) puts the dilemma this way:

> A wide variety of important research studies using human subjects has long played an essential and irreplaceable role in advancing biomedical and behavioral science, thus enhancing our ability to treat illness and better understand human behavior. In recent decades, however, researchers and commentators alike have become increasingly sensitive to the ethical issues associated with such research studies, especially has they concern the rights and welfare of subjects.[1]

This caution is generally taken to stem from the exposure at the Nuremberg trials of the extent to which Nazi Germany's disrespect for human rights was tied up with the callous and careless use by doctors of human subjects – sometimes apparently in pursuit of legitimate scientific knowledge, at other times, apparently, with no real expectation of learning anything of value.[2] Two factors, therefore, predicted the global outcry following the exposure of these appalling abuses of humanity. First, concern was expressed that the subjects had not consented to their involvement in such trials, but secondly, and importantly, was the fact that some "research" was little more than a cruel and hideous exercise of power, unjustified and unjustifiable in terms of real scientific or clinical progress.

The discovery that even clinicians were not immune to the racial and other hatreds that drove the Nazi regime led to the promulgation of the Nuremberg Code which focused on the issue of consent, setting the model for continued debate through the ensuing years. Principle 1 of the Code states unequivocally that "[t]he voluntary consent of the human subject is absolutely essential." In the aftermath of the Nuremberg trials, it has generally been assumed that it is consent that legitimises (or otherwise) the use of human beings in research projects. In considering the sufficiency and efficacy of this consent-based model, it is perhaps worth at the outset explaining what research is taken to be for the purposes of this chapter. In this respect, it is intended to follow the useful distinction succinctly drawn by Mason and McCall Smith, who say:[3 (p. 453)]

> Research and experimentation are commonly used as interchangeable terms – we, however, believe that there is a distinction to be made. Research implies a predetermined protocol with a clearly defined endpoint. Experimentation, by contrast, involves a more speculative, ad hoc, approach to an individual subject. The distinction is significant in that an experiment may be modified to take into account the individual's response; a research programme is more likely to tie the researcher to a particular course of action until such time as its general ineffectiveness is satisfactorily demonstrated.

Not only is this a useful clinical distinction, it is also an interesting legal one. Whereas experimentation may, in the UK, have legal consequences and is arguably subject to legal regulation through the application of the test outlined in the case of *Hunter* v. *Hanley*,[4] as Kennedy and Grubb note, "[r]emarkably, perhaps, there is no specific regime of law regulating research on humans. This is in contrast to the comprehensive legislative framework regulating the conduct of research on non-human animals."[5 (p. 715)] Thus, research, as opposed to experimentation might arguably require greater scrutiny for its ethical import. Not only does it lack a specific legal framework, it is also driven by the imperatives of a satisfactory scientific design, without which its value would be lessened, if not nugatory. On the other hand, of course, the very nature of the design may result in unfortunate consequences, scientifically requiring the continuation of a project even where its outcome might reasonably be predicted before its conclusion, thus putting some subjects at risk – either of the harm occasioned by the new therapy or of not receiving the apparently more effective treatment until the project has concluded its scientific enquiry.

Giesen,[6] for one, has suggested that there may be inherent problems in the dedication of science to particular forms of enquiry. As he said (p. 38):

> It may well be the case, having regard to the statistical model according to which the experiment is constructed, that the test must be continued for a fixed period of time or that a certain number of subjects must be included before a scientifically valid conclusion can be drawn from it. However, if one treatment reveals itself to be more effective in advance of the obtaining of statistically acceptable results, it is submitted that the doctor is obliged to terminate the research and to offer the patient this therapy. The law will not allow doctors to pursue statistical perfection to the detriment of their patients.

However, as has already been suggested, it remains unclear how the law would, in fact, prevent the attainment of "statistical perfection". It may criticise *post hoc*, but it is not certain that it has the capacity to intervene to prevent such an outcome.

Thus, in the absence of clear legal regulation, we have come to depend on a variety of other mechanisms to ensure some clinical and scientific conformity with our aspirational view of research, derived from the Nuremberg Code. However, arguably, our commitment to the ideal of free, voluntary and knowledgeable consent has become less firm as the distance between the demise of the Nazi regime and today's science becomes ever greater. Not even the pioneering work of Beecher[7] and others,[8, 9] highlighting the extent to which non-consensual research was been carried out in the United States even after the Nuremberg Code was promulgated, was sufficient to ensure adherence to the absolute commitments of the Code. Currrent international guidelines can be found in a variety of codes and declarations, but perhaps the most significant of these is the Declaration of Helsinki, promulgated by the World Medical Association in 1964 and last revised in 1996. Garnett suggests (p. 473) that this Declaration "superficially appears to take up the [Nuremberg] Code's torch."[10] However, he nonetheless detects a wavering in its commitments, based perhaps on the "perceived need for more flexible, permissive, and perhaps realistic guidelines for research."

Even while specifying the need for consent (in the case of the competent adult), the Declaration, he suggests (p. 474), "embodies vastly different assumptions about research and experimentation. It promotes a benign rather that a wary, view towards science and research. Written by and for physicians, the Declaration exudes faith in the methods and goals of medical science and accepts the premise that progress requires human subjects."

INFORMED CONSENT

Not least because of this apparent move away from absolutism and towards relativism in the ethics of research, and perhaps most startlingly in recent years in the face of the trials conducted in, for example, New Zealand's Auckland Woman's Hospital,[11] the reliance on consent as a predictor of the ethics and the lawfulness of a proposed research project has been increased. Most notably this is done by using the language of "informed consent" to describe the optimal legitimation for the involvement of humans in research projects. As an aside, it should be noted that, in this chapter, the language of "informed" consent will be eschewed. There are a number of reasons for this. First, the concept is based in American jurisprudence and was, as Robertson[12] points out, specifically designed to expand the liability of doctors. For that reason it may only be tangentially rooted in the rights of subjects and, if this is so, as a conceptual tool it does not satisfy the entirety of the rationale for consent requirements. Second, loose use of the term may encourage emphasis on the outcome rather than the process. In other words, arguably the root of its legitimacy is in the obtaining of an agreement to participate, rather than concentrating – in my view, more appropriately – on the process of discussion (even debate), which should precede a decision, that may, of course, include a decision not to participate. Third, if the last point is accepted, it is little more than tautologous rhetoric. If the critical element in individual decision-making is the extent and quality of the information provided and discussed, then – barring exceptional circumstances – no consent would be real unless it has been "informed".

These exceptional circumstances may occasionally, although not uncontroversially,[13] be found in the routine medical intervention. Full disclosure in clinical practice is not required by law in the United Kingdom[14] or in the United States,[15, 16] although some variations exist. Equally, despite the excitement generated by the Australian case of *Rogers* v. *Whittaker*,[17] that jurisdiction also permits for the non-disclosure of certain information. However, it is generally agreed that an agreement to participate in a clinical trial does require full disclosure, i.e. it requires the disclosure of maximal information – it must be informed in the common sense, rather than legal sense, of the word.

The arguments used to limit the need for full disclosure in the standard medical act – that people wouldn't understand, that they may be distressed by the information, that it is in their "best interests" to receive therapy[18] – are generally regarded as inapplicable where the proposed intervention is research based. This is true whether the research is described as therapeutic or non-therapeutic. Simplistically put, this distinction refers to the difference between research designed to assist the immediate patient group and that which is designed to benefit future patients. A number of cases, such as *Whitlock* v. *Duke University*[19] and *Halushka* v. *University of Saskatchewan*[20] have emphasised the need for, if anything, a higher burden of disclosure where the individual is being invited to participate in research. As was said in the latter case (p. 616–17):

> The duty imposed upon those who engage in medical research ... to those who offer themselves as subjects for experimentation ... is at least as great as, if not greater than, the duty owed by the ordinary physician or surgeon to his patient. There can be no exceptions to the ordinary requirements of disclosure in the case of research as there may well be in ordinary medical practice. The researcher does not have to balance the probable effect of lack of treatment against the risk involved in the treatment itself. The example of risks being properly hidden from a patient can have no application in the field of research. The subject of medical experimentation is entitled to a full and frank disclosure of all the facts, probabilities and options which a reasonable man might be expected to consider before giving his consent.

These sentiments are echoed in the Declaration of Helsinki (Article 9), which requires that each potential subject "must be adequately informed of the aims, methods, anticipated benefits and potential hazards of the study ..."

CONSENT AND RESEARCH

However, none of these aspirations actually addresses the question as to whether or not consent, in these terms, is *possible* in research. The protection ostensibly offered by consent requirements is only significant if they can in fact be met. Arguably, this may mean that the concept requires reanalysis to take account of the peculiarities of research itself. In a hard-hitting critique of the importance of consent in human research, Garnett says: [10 (p. 488)]

> Although informed consent works for noncontroversial, routine experiments that are easily justified and for which consent serves only as a trivial, albeit necessary, condition, it fails us in the hard cases. If we need to perform the experiment in a difficult case, we will. If necessary, we proceed without consent or with only a perfunctory acquiescence, which may reflect desperation, resignation, or simply confusion, but certainly not a robust commitment to human dignity and autonomy. We, in fact, insult human dignity but cloak our affront beneath a fiction or formality, which creates the illusion that we really do value consent, dignity and autonomy.

Here, he exposes but one of the vulnerabilities of the concept of consent in research – namely the extent to which the rhetoric of dependence on consent may obfuscate the reality of the motivations that might underlie an agreement to participate. Thus, the mechanisms built up ostensibly to safeguard the individual may provide a formal system of checks and balances, but do little actually to evaluate the *quality* of the purported consent. Indeed, he even seems to be suggesting that a "need" for a given research project may also drive the enterprise, despite the Declaration of Helsinki's express view (Article 5) that "[c]oncern for the interests of the subject must always prevail over the interests of science and society."

There is, however, a further reason to scrutinise the quality of decisions made about participation in research – namely, that, unlike in the standard medical act (with the exception of idiosyncratic responses), the actual impact on the individual subject will, *ex hypothesi*, be unknown, perhaps even unknowable. For this reason, the Council of Europe's Convention for the Protection of Human Rights and Dignity of the Human Being with Regard to the Application of Biology and Medicine,[21] stipulates that research may only be undertaken if "the risks which may be incurred by [the subject] are not disproportionate to the potential benefits of the research" (Article 16). The Declaration of Helsinki (Article 4) requires that "[b]iomedical research involving human subjects cannot legitimately be carried out unless the importance of the objective is in proportion to the inherent risk to the subject."

The question, however, is how such risk/benefits analyses are to be conducted, and how reliable can they be said to be? If the entire reason for translating animal and laboratory research into the human context is that neither of these can in fact tell us what the effect on human subjects will actually be, then how is such an analysis of risks and benefits to be conducted? It is when hypotheses, however well founded scientifically, are effected on human subjects that the controlled trial, generally randomized (RCT), is needed. As Mason and McCall Smith note (p. 457) "[t]he principle is simple – in order to decide whether a new drug or other treatment is better than an existing one, or is preferable to none at all, the new treatment is given to a group of patients or healthy volunteers and not given to as similar a group as can be obtained."[3]

This apparent simplicity, is, of course, actually rather complex. As Levine points out (p. 174), "… a necessary condition for the ethical justification of … an RCT is that the investigators be able to state an honest null hypothesis – a formal statement of equivalence of the two therapies being compared."[22] However, as he also points out (p. 176):

All too often, before the RCT is begun there are data available to support challenges to the claims of therapeutic equivalence or equipoise required for such justification. Physician-investigators are asked to try to disregard these data – to suspend disbelief – so that they may participate in these studies without violating their patient-centred ethic.

If, therefore, the essential hypothesis may be flawed or challenged, how is the supplementary matter of risk/benefits analysis to be resolved for the protection of the intended research subject? In light of what has gone before, it may be concluded that a genuinely informed agreement (or indeed refusal) to participate in research is difficult, if not impossible, to achieve. Thus, if the concept of consent is derived from the standard medical act and is to be the sole or major criterion for the ethics or legality of research on human subjects, we may be forced to conclude that virtually no significant research could be undertaken, even on the competent adult patient.

DO WE NEED RESEARCH?

For many, if not all, of us, however, this conclusion would be both counterintuitive and overly extreme. Dickens, for example, states (p. 23) that:

A medical professsion which did not seek improved means to conquer disease would be condemned for dereliction of its duty. Members of the public will not accept the current state of the medical arts as finite but feel justified in expecting the development of more effective therapies for illness, and the promotion of improved means of preventive care.[23]

In this extract, Dickens postulates two main reasons for the pursuit of progress, which will inevitably require the use of human subjects. First, he suggests that there would be a professional failure if clinicians did not seek to drive knowledge further and further. Thus, he implies, their professional commitments are not just to do the best they can with existing skills and knowledge but to seek ways of improving them. Secondly, he seems to suggest that the imperative for progress is also driven by public interests or expectations. Doctors, therefore, also have a responsibility to meet these (legitimate?) aspirations. Giesen adds a third issue, saying (p. 22) that "… the development of new drugs and medical procedures which will benefit future patients is in the public interest and that freedom of research and scientific enquiry is, in itself, an important aspect of open societies."[6]

Thus, there are many reasons to argue that research using human subjects is necessary, perhaps even desirable. However, given that there are clear difficulties in providing the quality of consent, which normally legitimates intervention, the final question must relate to how we can reconcile the protection of the individual with the apparently agreed rationales for seeking to progress – to enhance medicine's armoury in the fight against disease and debility.

CONSENT REVISITED

There is, at first sight, a real difficulty in rationalisation here, particularly where the calculation of risks and benefits (however inadequate or uncertain) demonstrates real, as opposed to trivial, possible risks. Indeed, this problem may obtain even where the anticipated risks are relatively trivial. Two questions must, therefore, be addressed. First, does the uncertainty of the clinical trial necessarily invalidate a purported consent, and second, are there limits to what we can consent to? These are intimately linked to each other.

If we accept that the *quality* of information provided to the proposed research subject is necessarily limited, can we then say that a real or valid consent is not feasible? Given the suggestion that a true null hypothesis seldom pertains, it might be thought that consent is adequately provided when such information has been explained (in tandem, of course with the other relevant requirements of a valid consent). However, it might also be said that – if the researcher is aware that evidence already exists that defeats this hypothesis – then any purported consent may have been obtained by fraudulently proceeding to test something the answer to which is at least partially known. To an extent this problem may, of course, be resolved by mechanical changes in research techniques.[22]

However, this still leaves the first question unanswered – namely, if uncertainty truly exists about anticipated risk/benefits, can individuals nonetheless provide an agreement which is both ethically and legally satisfactory? Arguably, if the information required includes, as it seems to, the fact that some things are not known, it is just as much for the individual to accept risks in this as in any other enterprise. We make, and are free to make, contrary or misguided decisions all the time – why should this not include accepting the unknown? As Schuck has said:

> Free individuals, going about their own business with dignity and confidence: that's what the world is all about, we think .... We are uneasily aware that the world isn't quite like that after all ... we make horrible choices all the time. Our actions are often uninformed, self-destructive, neurotically repetitive, floundering and helpless.[24]

In reality, the consent requirement can protect us only so far – thereafter we are in the realms of personal judgement, which arguably should not be overly constrained by ethical or legal considerations. Others, however, might disagree. Any argument that consent to involvement in research, where the level of uncertainty is not disclosed, might be as valid as any other consent would, for example, be challenged by Redmon. In an echo of the judgement in the *Halushka* case, he says (p. 79):

> The physician has some latitude (how much is a matter of great debate) in informing his patient of the risks and other factors in a therapeutic procedure. The researcher has none. One reason is that the physician

is working on *behalf* of his patient and the researcher need not be. Thus, the type of paternalistic behaviour we might allow in the physician is not permissible in the researcher.[25]

Thus, on one thing agreement seems uniform: there is a difference between a valid consent in routine medicine and in research. Whilst doctors may be permitted to withhold certain information in pursuit of a consent to standard intervention, they are not permitted to do so where the intervention is part of a research project. This conclusion is initially intuitively satisfying, yet on reflection perhaps less so. Even disregarding the argument that surrounds whether or not it is justifiable *ever* to withhold information from a patient, the requirement for full disclosure in research may be little more than paying lip-service to autonomy. Arguably, the enhanced disclosure requirement merely demands the disclosure of essentially valueless information – namely, "We don't know". To be sure, such disclosure adds to the information available in terms of extent, but perhaps less so in terms of content.

It is here, however, that we may most acutely perceive a rationale for reflection on whether or not consent in standard therapy and consent in research are essentially equivalent. Consent in the standard medical act is generally taken to be desirable to assist in the expression of autonomy, yet the justification for withholding some information is essentially paternalistic. In research, however, the effect of full disclosure, particularly about unknown hazards, is essentially inviting the autonomous handing over of authority to others. To this extent, the kind of information required may, therefore, differ. If we accept the good of research, then we may need to place less emphasis on the full exercise of autonomy, or at least to recognise that it may be satisfied by transfer of authority to others whose experience and skills reassure us of the safety of so doing. Whether such a transfer of authority is a good thing will depend on the values we ascribe to research – personally and socially – rather than on the atomisation that follows the application of autonomy pure and simple.

The second question concerns the extent to which there are, or should be, limits to what people may agree to. It is well established that consent is no defence to a charge of murder.[26] Nor will consent render the infliction of other serious injuries lawful.[27] In the case of *R. v. Brown*,[28, 29] it was also agreed that, even if a real consent was apparently given, there are public policy issues that prevent the consent from decriminalising certain behaviour. Thus, consent is not an effective justification or protection in all circumstances – it has its limits. However, public policy seems to accept the good of research and is unlikely to have to face the objections raised in the Brown case. Evans and Evans, however, consider that there may be one final problem in the assumption of risks which are more than small. They argue that (p. 66):

> Whilst there are many contexts in which autonomous adults can choose to undertake more-than-minimal risks (sport is an obvious example), clinical research ought perhaps not be among them. The main reason for thinking this is that we should distinguish between the degree of risk someone might privately undergo in an activity of his choice, and the degree of risk it is appropriate for a professional or other public figure to invite a patient to contemplate.[30]

CONCLUSION

It has been said that "… the basic approach to the ethical conduct of research and approval of investigational drugs was born in scandal and reared in protectionism".[31 (p.167)] This brief critique would suggest that this assertion has resonance even today. The creation of international codes and national review structures, such as research ethics committees, arguably has failed to address the crucial questions about what research is actually for. Only when such an analysis is systematically undertaken will the ideological and conceptual bases be clarified, and open for reasoned debate. For the moment, the autonomy model prevails, although it is clear that this model may prove problematic in the area of research. Not only may it raise real issues concerning the quality of consent, but it may also come up against the perceived responsibilities of the state. In emphasising the importance of autonomy, Katz, for example, seems to presume its limitations[9 (p. 3)]:

> When scientists use other human beings as subjects of experimentation, and in so doing jeopardize their rights and welfare, the scientists' freedom of inquiry clashes head on with the right of every individual in our society to personal autonomy. *Therefore, society must retain the right to define and limit the human costs it is willing to bear in order to benefit from advances of knowledge* [emphasis added].

As in *R.* v. *Brown*,[28] therefore, not all apparent exercises of autonomy will be tolerated. To a large extent, however, I would argue that the real focus should not be solely on the apparent exercise of autonomy, but should rather be on the scientific method and justification for research in the first place – either a specific project or research in general. Given that the latter is generally conceded, it may be that the problems surrounding the quality of consent in research may better be circumvented – perhaps obviated – by the extension of the information that must be disclosed beyond the risks/benefits/alternatives model to explanation of the rationale and scientific method, which allegedly mandates the research proceeding at all.

In this way, in problematic cases, less emphasis would need to be placed upon whether research is broadly therapeutic or broadly non-therapeutic, and more would hinge on the extent to which we are permitted to act altruistically. The benefits, and the harms, of research extend more widely than the individuals concerned. Rather they reflect societal values also. Dickens makes the point (p. 24) that "[m]edical experimentation is conducted as a risk which must be weighed against both the prospect of benefit in social terms, and the distribution of benefits in individual terms.[23] Arguably, the application of a more communitarian ethics, rather than an obsession with autonomy, provides the better way forward. Communitarianism can – indeed should – encapsulate autonomy, but it is the autonomy of connectedness rather than the autonomy of selfishness. Thus, while consent remains a critical protector of individuals (and societies), its *protective* limitations must be observed. This is not to minimise the significance of consent, but rather to reinforce it. The need thoroughly to re-evaluate the complexities of consent in research is evident. Any re-evaluation should take account not simply of the fact that information disclosure is a vital component of consent, mandatory in research, but should also confront honestly the limits to, and rationale for, using people in this way. The boundaries of appropriate human research can then be drawn. In the realm of medical research, consent remains the vital cornerstone of an ethically and legally sound intervention, but it should not be taken as its sole justification, without close analysis of its context.

REFERENCES

1. National Bioethics Advisory Commission, *Research involving persons with mental disorders that may affect their decisionmaking capacity.* 1998; **1** (December).

2. *United States* v. *Brandt* (case no 1) 1 Trial of War Criminals 3 (1949).
3. Mason JK, McCall Smith RA. *Law and medical ethics* (5th edn). London: Butterworths, 1999.
4. *Hunter* v. *Harley* 1955 SC 200.
5. Kennedy I, Grubb A. *Principles of medical law*. Oxford: OUP, 1998.
6. Giesen D. Civil liability of physicians for new methods of treatment and experimentation: a comparative examination, *Med Law Rev* 1995; **3** (Spring): 22–52.
7. Beecher HK. Ethics and clinical research. *New Engl J Med* 1966; **274**: 1354–60.
8. Katz J. *The silent world of doctor and patient*. New York: Free Press, 1984.
9. Katz J. The regulation of human experimentation in the United States – a personal odyssey. *IRB: Rev Human Subjects Res* 1987; **9**(1): 1–6.
10. Garnett RW. Why informed consent? Human experimentation and the ethics of autonomy. *Catholic Lawyer* **36**: 455–512.
11. Campbell AV. An unfortunate experiment. *Bioethics* **3**: 59.
12. Robertson G. Informed consent to medical treatment, 97 L.Q.R. 102 (1981).
13. McLean SAM. *A patient's right to know: information disclosure, the doctor and the law*. Aldershot: Dartmouth Publishing, 1989.
14. *Sidaway* v. *Board of Governors of the Bethlem Royal Hospital and the Maudsley Hospital* [1985] 1 All ER 643.
15. *Wooley* v. *Henderson* 418 A 2d 1123 (Md, 1980).
16. *Canterbury* v. *Spence* 464 F 2d 772 (DC, 1972).
17. *Rogers* v. *Whittaker* [1993] 4 Med LR 79.
18. Buchanan A. Medical paternalism. 7 Philosophy and Public Affairs 340 (1978).
19. *Whitlock* v. *Duke University* 637 F Supp 1463 (NC, 1986); affd 829 F 2d 1340 (1987).
20. *Halushka* v. *University of Saskatchewan* (1965) 53 DLR (2d) 436.
21. Oviedo, 4 April 1997. (For a critique of the Convention, see McLean SAM, Elliston S. Bioethics, the Council of Europe and the Draft Convention. *Eur J Hlth Law* 1995; **1**: 1–9.)
22. Levine RJ. "Uncertainty in clinical research". *Law, Medicine Hlth Care* 1988; **16**: 174–182.
23. Dickens BM. Human rights in medical experimentation. *Israel Yearb Human Rights* 1979; **9**: 23–57.
24. Schuck PH. Rethinking informed consent. *Yale Law J* 1994; **103**, 899.
25. Redmon RB. How children can be respected as "ends" yet still be used as subjects in non-therapeutic research. 1986; **12**: 77.
26. *HMA* v. *Rutherford* 1947 J.C. 1.
27. *R.* v. *Donovan* [1934] 2 KB 498 (*A-G's reference (no 6 of 1980)* [1981] QB 715).
28. *R.* v. *Brown* [1993] 2 All ER 75 (HL).
29. *Laskey, Jaggard and Brown* v. *United Kingdom* (1997) 24 EHRR 39.
30. Evans D, Evans M. *A decent proposal: ethical review of clinical research*. Chichester: John Wiley & Sons, 1996.
31. Levine C. Has AIDS changed the ethics of human subjects research? *Law, Medicine Hlth Care* 1988; **12**: 167–173.

16 · Informed consent and clinical research with children

Jonathan Montgomery

Research with children raises a number of issues beyond those relating to adults. These include whether there are some types of research that should be regarded as unethical if children are involved, or whether there are special hurdles to be overcome before such research can be approved. With competent adults, it may be acceptable for ethics committees to approve extremely risky research, provided that they are satisfied that the research subjects are fully aware of the risks involved and can make an informed choice as to whether they are prepared to run them. This may not be the case when children are involved. There may be degrees of risk that we are not prepared to ask children, or their parents, to take. An important distinction needs to be made between therapeutic and non-therapeutic research in this respect. Higher risks may be acceptable in therapeutic studies where it is hoped that the child will benefit.

A second set of problems arises in determining who is in a position to give consent for children to participate in trials. This includes the circumstances when children and young people themselves can give consent, both as a matter of ethics and law. It also raises the question of who can give consent on behalf of a child and whether there are limits to proxy consent. The distinction between therapeutic and non-therapeutic research is again significant because the current legal framework places considerable emphasis on the personal interests of children.

There can be little doubt that these issues are of practical significance. Public confidence in the commitment of researchers to the welfare of child subjects and respect for the rights of parents has been shaken by the initiation of an inquiry into research in North Staffordshire and the revelation that researchers had acquired a "library" of retained organs at Alder Hey. Allegations have been made that research has been carried out without parental consent and even with forged consent forms. The design of studies has been criticised as having exposed children to unnecessary and unacceptable levels of risk. Reassurance that robust legal and professional standards are in place, and adhered to, would go some way to persuading the public that the conduct of vital research does not compromise the interests of children.

This chapter draws on the resources of the law and the guidance from government and professional bodies to disentangle these issues. It must be acknowledged, however, that there remains some uncertainty about the authority of these sources in the absence of clear legal rulings on the subject of research. Consequently, any conclusions drawn about the law are necessarily tentative.

THE LEGITIMATE SCOPE OF RESEARCH INVOLVING CHILDREN

Although the Declaration of Helsinki does not now formally restrict research involving children, merely requiring that proxy consent be obtained (Basic Principle 11), it is usually thought that there should be special limitations on such studies. Two principles have emerged. The first is a presumption against the use of children in research. The second concerns the degree of risk that is permissible in children studies.

The Presumption Against Child Research

Involving children in research raises problems that are not usually present with adults; the vulnerability of subjects, their relative lack of voice, the difficulties of proxy consent, the possibility that any benefits and harms from research might last many years.[1] Consequently, it is generally thought best to avoid these additional complexities unless the research question makes it essential to tackle them. The Department of Health's official guidance indicates that research proposals should only involve children where it is absolutely essential to do so.[2] The Medical Research Council advises that "children should take part only if the relevant knowledge could not be gained by research in adults."[3] The Royal College of Physicians is more precise, precluding non-therapeutic research "unless with the objects of elucidating physiological or pathological conditions peculiar to infancy and childhood or of providing potential benefit to the family, and where it involves no more than minimal risk."[4] This stance creates a presumption against research involving children. Presumptions do not prevent conclusions being drawn, but require clear reasons to be proffered before they can be rebutted. In the absence of a definite reason for involving children in research, studies should not be carried out. The presumption against child research means that the case for involving children must be explicitly made out before trials can be approved.[3]

The presumption can be seen to yield three sub-principles:

- Children should not be asked to be research subjects when the data sought would be available from studies involving adults.
- Research involving children should not be carried out until as much information as possible has been gleaned from adult studies, enabling risks to be assessed as fully as possible.
- Research projects should usually be carried out with older young people who are in a position to consent (or refuse) before younger children are asked to become involved. As the British Paediatric Association advises: "When a choice of age groups is possible, older children should be involved in preference to younger ones, although much valuable research can only be done with younger children and babies."[1]

These sub-principles can be applied in relation to drug trials by requiring a full round of trials into safety and efficacy to be carried out in adults before their usage in children is studied. Protocols for studying the extension of drugs into use with children would need to be justified in terms of the need for further data on child populations. They would need to give an indication of why it is thought that the adult data suggest that this would be worthwhile in terms of efficacy and acceptable in terms of side effects. They

should be carried out in stages where this is possible so that younger children are involved only once results from older consenting children have been analysed.

The Acceptability of Risks

The second principle is that there is a threshold of risk that children can legitimately be asked to undertake in the interests of research. There is broad agreement that this threshold exists, but less consensus on how it should be fixed. A distinction is usually drawn between therapeutic studies, in which there is the possibility or intention of immediate benefit to participants, and non-therapeutic research where any direct benefit to participants is either unlikely or long delayed.[3] Therapeutic studies are seen as raising similar problems to treatment decisions. Innovative treatment that is hoped to assist patients can be acceptable, providing the person with the legal power and responsibility to give or withhold consent is persuaded that the benefits outweigh the risks. The interests of the doctor/researcher are seen as aligned with those of the patient/parent and the matter is generally regulated as a treatment decision rather than a research project. Ethical review is required to ensure reliable data are generated, but not necessarily to authorise an attempt to help the patient by trying something new when more established therapies have failed.

Non-therapeutic studies are regarded with more suspicion. As children cannot always consent for themselves, there is concern that they are asked to run risks that they do not understand. Whilst parents are usually accepted as proxies on behalf of their children, this status is granted in order that they can protect and further the interests of their children, and arguably involving them in research is not for their personal benefit but in the wider public interest. It does not, therefore, follow that because parents can validly consent to treatment that they should also be able to agree to research. Two interlocking arguments come together in this context.

The first draws on the widespread view that children are often vulnerable and that there is a particular obligation on society to protect them from harm. On this view, we should refuse to countenance risky non-therapeutic research because it exploits the vulnerability of children (who lack the voice to object) without offering them any benefit in return. We should look, therefore, for a way to distinguish the degree of risk that is unacceptable from that which may be legitimate if the anticipated broader benefits of research are sufficiently great. This position implies that research placed in the first category should be automatically rejected without balancing the benefits and risks involved in the research because the degree of risk is intolerable, however great the advantage to be secured. This view might be termed a protectionist model because it draws its strength from the claim of children to be protected from the vicissitudes of adult life.

A second approach seeks to normalise the position in which children find themselves to that of those on whom adult rights and responsibilities are conferred. It notes that adults are permitted to run considerable risks if they choose to do so. Further, a blanket ban on risky research would rob children of the opportunities to contribute to scientific and medical advance that adults are granted. It can then be suggested that proxy consent could be used to provide children with parallel opportunities. Those with parental responsibility are trusted to make, on behalf of their children, the sort of judgements that adults make about their willingness to contribute to the public good by assisting in research. Limits to the risks that can be accepted on this basis would then be fixed in the same way that other parental rights are limited and for the same reasons. As we shall see below, under English law, this would require parents to act reasonably in the interests of their children, but would adopt a broad conception of what constitutes those interests.

Both these approaches to identifying the proper scope of research with children can be seen in the literature and legal authorities, and an important historical dimension should be recognised. Over the last few decades, attitudes to this aspect of the involvement of children in research have softened. Priscilla Alderson has traced the gradual extension of the scope of research regarded as legitimate to be carried out with children.[5] In 1963 the Medical Research Council adopted a position that largely ruled out non-therapeutic research on children on the basis that parental consent would be invalid in law if it carried any risk of harm.[6] In 1973 the Royal College of Physicians accepted that non-therapeutic research on children might be acceptable provided that there was no more than "negligible risk or discomfort".[7] In 1980 the British Paediatric Association seemed less sure that there was a threshold of acceptability.[8] However, its 1992 guidance states that "it would be unethical to submit child subjects to more

than minimal risk when the procedure offers no benefit to them, or only a slight or very uncertain one."[1] The Medical Research Council current guidance suggests that a child's participation in non-therapeutic research can only be ethically justified if it involves "no more than negligible risk of harm and is therefore not against his interests."[3]

The dominant contemporary approach of the official guidance offered by the medical profession seems therefore to adopt the search to identify a prohibited level of risk that fits the protectionist model for the limits of research. The Medical Research Council stated that it used:

> the term negligible risk to mean that the risks of harm anticipated in the proposed research are not greater, considering the probability and magnitude of physiological or psychological harm or discomforts than those ordinarily encountered in daily life or during the performance of routine physical or psychological examination or tests.

This approach suggests that it should be possible to assess in the abstract whether any particular procedure should be regarded as carrying no more than negligible risk by examining data on the risks involved. The MRC Committee offered its view that procedures involving only negligible risk would include non-invasive observation and monitoring, developmental assessments and physical examinations, changes in diet, and obtaining blood or urine specimens. No data are offered to support these judgements. A much more detailed analysis was carried out by a working group of the Institute of Medical Ethics on the ethics of clinical research investigations on children, which reviewed and analysed data on adverse effects of various techniques.[9] It showed how difficult it is to make reliable calculations of statistical risks and even harder to ensure that assessments of the significance of risks can hope to achieve general public acceptability. Objective classification of techniques rather than making judgements about individual trials with knowledge of the practice and experience of specific investigators may prove frustratingly elusive. The MRC Committee noted that the requirement of parental consent would provide an additional safeguard.

The minimal risk standard offered by the British Paediatric Association is illustrated rather than defined in the 1992 guidance.[1] It "described procedures such as questioning, observing and measuring children, provided that procedures are carried out in a sensitive way, and that consent has been given. Procedures with minimal risk include collecting a single urine sample (but not by aspiration) or using blood from a sample that has been taken as part of treatment." Crucially, the guidelines rejected the suggestion that only the risks inherent in a procedure were relevant. The sensitivities of the investigation were important in reducing risk to the level of minimal. It was stressed that the level of risk involved should be assessed once steps taken to minimise them were taken into account and that these should include steps to reduce the risks of psychological trauma as well as purely physical difficulties.

The significance and importance of this approach to risk assessment appeared from heated correspondence about the comments made in the BPA Guidelines about the taking of blood samples purely for research purposes. The Guidelines advised that where children feared needles, injections and venepuncture would *for them* carry low rather than minimal risk and should be regarded as unacceptable if they would derive no benefit (emphasis added). Some researchers took this to prohibit the use of venepuncture to collect blood samples and argued that this might discourage important research that could benefit children. To clarify the position, the Guidelines were reissued with a brief commentary from the President of the Association pointing out that the distress of children had to be recognised. If a child was very upset by the procedure, then it should be accepted as genuine dissent to being involved, in the same way as an adult might refuse to be involved in similar research because of an extreme dislike of venepuncture. The fundamental point made by the BPA was that risk assessment had to include consideration of the emotional and psychological effects of subjecting the child to research procedures. It is difficult for research ethics committees to assess these subjective aspects of risk in the abstract. Much will depend on individual children. At least one such committee has tackled the problem by requiring reassurances from researchers that they will not continue in the face of distress from a child at the prospect of a needle being used purely for the purposes of research. Such a condition is required because of the limited protection for children involved in research that the law of consent provides.

CONSENT AND ASSENT FROM CHILDREN

The language of consent covers a range of different issues and circumstances. In law, a valid consent is necessary before any research involving physical contact with a subject is permissible. This narrow function of consent presents a hurdle that must be overcome before research is lawful. The law paints this matter as a clear-cut question, a matter of black and white. There either is consent (in which case the research may be carried out if the other safeguards are respected) or there is not (in which case the research may not proceed). Equally, whether or not a person is legally competent to give a legally valid consent must be answered either affirmatively or negatively. Conceptually there is no grey hinterland between competence and incompetence. It is necessary to determine which category each research subject, patient or parent falls into, and the legal consequences then flow automatically. The test for competence therefore needs to be examined to see which children can consent to research. Consideration also needs to be given to the validity of proxy consent from those with parental responsibility and the overarching role of the court.

There is also a wider dimension to the importance of consent. In the context of treatment, Lord Donaldson has described the "clinical" function, which he explained as the process of securing the patient's trust and cooperation.[10] There is scope for considerable debate about the sufficiency of this understanding to capture to the ethical requirements of the modern commitment to patient autonomy. As a formulation of the ethical function of consent, Lord Donaldson's position is certainly dangerously skewed in the research context, because it assumes that professional and patient/subject share the same objective: promoting the patient's best interests. Securing the patient's cooperation in that project can therefore be presented as an essentially benign process. However, the nature of research is that the pursuit of knowledge competes with concern for the interests of the patients/subjects. The ethical function of consent in the research context is to ensure that any risks involved in the project are freely accepted by the subject. It is not to persuade patients to comply with the therapy prescribed for them by health professionals. This very different function means that legal rules of consent to treatment may not provide a straightforward guide to the principles that govern consent to become involved in research.

"Informed consent" to treatment is a concept essentially alien to English law.[11] While English law has provided a strong guarantee that consent must be given before treatment is lawful, it has accepted that such consent will be valid even if the information given to the patient is minimal. All that is necessary is that there should be information in broad terms about the nature and purpose of the treatment. Side effects, risks and alternatives need not be spelt out in order to make the consent valid (as the law requires in many of the state legal systems in the USA). It is widely assumed that a more rigorous approach would be taken to consent in the research context. If the principal reason for English law's reluctance to require fuller disclosure of information is the assumption that doctors and patients share the same therapeutic objective, then research requires a new legal framework. In research this assumption breaks down because there is the potential for conflict between the interests of the subject and the need to maintain the integrity of the research methodology. Therefore, both law and ethics probably require full and frank disclosure of risks to research subjects before consent can be regarded as valid. This point is general to all medical research on human subjects. The specific problems raised by research involving children concern to whom that disclosure should be made and from whom consent should be gained.

The issues can be seen more clearly if the legal, "clinical" and ethical dimensions of consent are considered separately. The legal issue concerns whether the researchers have done enough to protect themselves against being sued for battery for failing to secure a legally valid consent to their intervention. This requires consent to be given by someone competent in law to give it on the basis of information in broad terms. Under current English law such a consent may be obtainable from more than one person and it is conceivable that it could be obtained from a parent even in the face of opposition from the child subject (see further below). While it now seems clear that this is the position in respect of treatment, there has been no judicial discussion of the implications of the case law for research involving children. It will also be necessary to consider whether there are legal limits to the parental power to consent to research.

The ethical dimension to consent concerns the need to ensure that research subjects (or their representatives) are free to make an informed choice as to whether or not to become involved in research fully cognisant of any risks that they are running. This has a legal aspect, for the rules of negligence require professional practice to be followed in respect of discussion of side effects and risks. Failure to follow established medical ethics might therefore result in a malpractice action. This dimension does not raise difficulties that are peculiar to the context of children and will not be further considered in this chapter.

A version of the "clinical" function of consent may be significant, however. It will be seen that there will be circumstances in which children and young people will not have legal capacity to consent to research procedures. Nevertheless, there is a significant difference between involving "incompetent" but willing children in research and forcing it on those who object to being subjects. The guidelines from the British Paediatric Association use the term "assent" to refer to acquiescence from children to cooperate in research projects. This term does not have legal significance, but it is valuable as a tool to distinguish collaborative research with those who cannot consent from coercive imposition upon them. Professional guidance supports the view that coercion is unacceptable, although the law is less clear.

Children's Capacity to Consent

There is no statutory provision that governs consent to research procedures. From the age of 16, young people are presumed to be competent to consent to treatment as if they were adults, but this does not cover research.[12] In the absence of statutory guidance the matter is governed by the test for competence set out in the *Gillick* case.[13] In this case, the House of Lords had to determine when young people could consent to care on their own behalf and when parental consent alone would suffice. It was held that young people could give valid consent to health care provided that they had "sufficient understanding and intelligence to enable [them] to understand fully what is proposed." Although the test was formulated in the context of family planning, it is now used as a test of general application. Thus, children who satisfy this test for competence can give a valid legal consent to being involved in research. This would remove the legal need to seek parental consent, although the guidance usually suggests that parental assent should still be obtained.[2, 3, 4]

To be *Gillick competent* the child must have the ability to appreciate the nature of the procedures (what would be involved, including the fact that they might not receive active treatment in a placebo-controlled trial), and their purpose (that they are for research and something of the reason for carrying out the study). In the research context, some understanding of the risks involved would also be necessary, although no legal case has yet arisen in which this has had to be established. This test is to be applied to each project individually rather than to assess the general level of maturity of the child. Thus, the same child may have sufficient understanding of one study but not another, or even of only some stages in a single study. This also means that developmental concepts such as mental age have no relevance to the assessment of *Gillick competence*. The understanding, relevant knowledge, and experience of each child must be individually assessed. Researchers would be wise to have a record of this assessment to forestall criticism should things go wrong.

Children who are not *Gillick competent* could not be involved in research without parental consent. Very few justifications are recognised by the courts for giving care to children without parental consent. In *Gillick*, Lords Scarman and Templeman suggested that this would be permissible only as a temporary measure. They cited as examples cases where it is immediately necessary and a parent cannot be found, where the parents have abandoned the child, or where the child has been abused by the parents.[13] Lord Templeman observed that, in general, it would be wrong for doctors to usurp the responsibility of parents to take decisions about their children's care. The only other category in which care without consent is permissible is life-saving treatment. Here, it is widely accepted that treatment can be given without parental consent, although it is still advisable that a court is asked to resolve disputes if it is practicable to do so.[11] The restrictiveness of these limitations on treatment of children without consent indicates that the law is unlikely to countenance research on children unless a valid consent has been obtained. They are intended to secure children's best interests pending full consideration by parents or the courts, rather than to evade the need for consent entirely.

Even where the legal test for competence is not satisfied, it is good practice to take active steps to seek the child's assent. The Royal College of Physicians and the Medical Research Council suggest that the "willing cooperation" of the child should be sought.[3, 4] The British Paediatric Association advises that positive agreement of school-age children should be sought and that steps should always be taken to ensure that the child does not object.[1] This helps ensure that coercion is avoided. The situation where children do not wish to be involved with research to which their parents agree is explicitly covered in professional guidelines, although the legal position remains somewhat obscure. Article 12 of the UN Convention on the Rights of the Child 1989 provides that any child capable of expressing their views (i.e. whether or not those views have been competently formed) has the right to do so and to have them given due weight according to their age and maturity. This right of participation is not directly enforceable in British courts. However, it is clearly supported by professional guidelines about the involvement of children and good practice indicates that children should be encouraged to play as full a part as possible in healthcare decisions from an early age.[14]

The Reluctant Child

The view expressed by the Department of Health in 1990 was that consent from parents could never justify overriding a refusal from a competent child.[2] This was probably based on legal advice that may no longer be so clear as it seemed at that point. Since the guidelines were issued, the Court of Appeal has held in a number of cases that parental consent to treatment remains valid even when the child or young person concerned is able to consent.[10] In principle it would seem that the parental power to consent is legally valid to override a child's refusal. However, Lord Donaldson expressly relied upon the strength of medical ethics to protect children from the inappropriate use of parental powers to consent. He said that it would be this that would protect young women from having terminations of pregnancy forced upon them by their parents.

There is no clear indication that the parental power to override a child's refusal would exist in relation to research. The general position in relation to parental responsibility is that, where parents have powers, they may exercise them independently, unless a court order restricts their right to do so. In some areas, the courts have limited the unilateral exercise of powers in cases of disputes between parents. This has been done in relation to the removal of the child from the jurisdiction so as to alter their place of habitual residence and change of surname. Most importantly, however, it has been held that a father could not validly consent to the non-therapeutic circumcision of a made child in the face of opposition from the mother.[15] In these cases it is now necessary to bring disputes before the court. It is possible that a similar limit might be placed upon the exercise of consent to research in the face of opposition from the child. However, these examples are exceptional and until a case comes before the courts it is impossible to be sure how it would be decided. It is also possible that the courts would adopt the view that forcing a child to become a research subject should be analysed as a purported use of the parental power to administer reasonable chastisement. Given that the coercion was not used in response to any misbehaviour by the child and not in the child's interests at all, it could be strongly argued that it would be an abuse of parental power. In the light of this uncertainty, it is probable that professional ethics is a more important guide than speculation about the likely response of the courts.

Professional guidelines show a strong consensus that it would not be permissible to carry out research involving children against the opposition of the subjects. The Helsinki Declaration requires the consent of the minor in addition to that of the parent or guardian (Basic Principle 11). The Royal College of Physicians advises that where a child obviously objects that rejection must be respected.[4] Its guidelines refer to cases where "assent or agreement" is withheld, suggesting that a refusal need not be "competent" in the legal sense to be respected. The concurring views of the British Paediatric Association and the Medical Research Council have already been noted. Thus, even if the legal position is unclear, ethical considerations preclude including reluctant children in research studies. This covers both those who are competent to give a valid consent and decline to do so and also those whose resistance is not regarded as based on an informed understanding.

PROXY CONSENT AND ITS LIMITS

Where a legally valid consent has not been forthcoming from the child involved in the research it will be necessary to approach someone with parental responsibility for the necessary consent as a proxy on behalf of the child. The rules on who has parental responsibility are complex, and details are to be found in the Children Act 1989 and the Human Fertilisation and Embryology Act 1990. The mother will always have such responsibility for her children. In cases of assisted reproduction where the genetic and gestational mother are different, it will be the woman who gives birth who is classified as the mother for these purposes. Genetic fathers will not

automatically have parental responsibility. They will acquire it if they are married to the mother, if they register a formal parental responsibility agreement with the High Court in London, or if they obtain a parental responsibility order from a court. A non-parent or local authority will also have parental responsibility if a residence or care order has been made in their favour.

While the rules set out in the previous paragraph are technical they are reasonably clear. The same cannot be said of the law on parental consent to the involvement of their children in medical research. In 1963 the Medical Research Council considered that the law precluded proxy consent for most non-therapeutic research. It suggested that it would be acceptable to seek parental permission for research procedures that were intended to benefit a child. However, research that provided no particular benefit to the subject and which might carry some risk of harm was thought to be beyond the scope of parental consent.[6] This view was compatible with the sparse relevant legal authorities, but there was no directly applicable legal ruling. Legal commentators have suggested that the position may in fact be less strict.[9,16,17] The dominant view now seems to be that non-therapeutic research is acceptable provided that the risk involved to the child is minimal, and parents can consent to such studies on behalf of their children on the basis that it would not be against their child's interests to do so.[1] Given the continued absence of any clear legal ruling on this point it is important to appreciate the reasoning that supports this position, and its reliance on drawing analogies with other areas. Only then can the strength of the argument be assessed.

The *Gillick* decision established that parents were given powers and rights in order to protect the interests of their children rather than to protect a conception of parental rights or family privacy that demanded that society did not interfere.[18] If the parental power to consent to medical intervention has to be exercised in the interests of their children, it is easy to justify their involvement in therapeutic studies. There it is hoped that the child will benefit directly, and it would be quite reasonable for parents to accept a degree of risk in order to secure the possibility of that benefit. However, in non-therapeutic studies there is no obvious benefit to be gained and it can be suggested that children are being put at risk for no possible gain and that this cannot be in their best interests. If parental consent can only be given in the *best interests* of their children, this presents a considerable difficulty. It would imply that a decision that was later found to have been less than optimum would have been void and invalid.

However, the courts have accepted a slightly more relaxed understanding of the law. First, they do not usually hold that there is only one acceptable view to be taken of the interests of the child. They recognise that determining what is best for children is a complex exercise. In relation to challenges to judicial judgements on this point the appeal courts leave to trial judges a margin of interpretation and interfere only if they are found to be "plainly wrong." It is likely that they would take a similar line to disputes about the legitimacy of decisions about children's treatment, holding that, so long as parents act within the boundaries of reasonableness, then their decisions should not be regarded as invalid. This would not prevent the courts taking their own view of the merits of a case if a dispute arose, but they would supersede rather than invalidate the original decision.

Secondly, the courts have taken a broad view of the conception of a child's interests. In paternity disputes it has been held that knowing the truth is generally to be regarded as a benefit, even if the practical implications of discovering that a man is not the child's father might be negative. It could therefore be accepted that research into a condition that might affect the child is similarly within a broad conception of benefit. In cases of family break-up, the value of mutual support between siblings within familes has been recognised. This might support the involvement of children in research that might produce benefits for their families, even if they themselves might not receive direct advantages. Such reasoning has been used to justify a mentally incapacitated adult donating bone marrow to her sister. The court accepted that it was in the woman's interests to preserve her links with her mother, which would be damaged if the sister did not receive the bone marrow.[19] Formal and informal eductional advantages are also considered relevant in child care disputes. It might be argued that participating in the search for knowledge is an educational enterprise and that children may benefit from feeling that they are contributing to medical advances. However, this seems unlikely to persuade the courts unless the risks involved are extremely small and the child plays an active role in the research rather than being a passive subject.

There has been one area in which the courts have concluded that the parental power to consent to medical intervention cannot validly be exercised. This is non-therapeutic sterilisation. Such procedures on children can only be authorised by a court.[20] If they regarded experimentation as generally unacceptable, then you would expect it to be treated in the same way. Whilst there have been few cases in which it was necessary to give a ruling, judges have indicated the categories of case that they think might be treated in this way without identifying research. They include refusal of life-saving treatment, abortion, and donation of non-regenerative tissue for transplantation. These are all irreversible decisions that significantly narrow the scope for future choices. If it is this that provides the common factor, it could be argued that medical research does not belong in the same category.

It is most likely that the courts would approach the problem by asking themselves whether the parents could reasonably argue that it was safe to involve their children in the research. This would not be plausible if there were any significant risks involved. However, if the risks were negligible then it could be said that consenting to their involvement did not compromise their interests because it was not actually against them.[21] This approach has been adopted by most advisers and has led to the way in which the concepts of minimal or negligible risk have become significant in the professional guidelines. It would be possible to seek a court ruling under the Children Act 1989 as to whether it was in the best interests of a particular child to be involved in a project. This might clarify the legality of involving children in research, but it is more likely that the courts would be reluctant to lay down general rules and would confine their ruling to the specific circumstances.

CONCLUSION

As in most research, the notion of informed consent plays a vital part in studies that involve children. However, consideration must be given to the stake of both the children themselves and their parents in the agreement to participate. Good practice indicates that unless both the child and their parent agree, then it would be improper to recruit the child to a project. It may be that only one consent, from either a competent child or a parent, is required for legal purposes. However, assent from both is recommended by professional guidance. It would be advisable for researchers to ensure that there is a record of the assessment of the child's views, and that all investigators understand the importance of respecting the reluctance of children to cooperate. It is hard to see how coercive research can ever be justified. Paediatric research needs to maintain the confidence of the public and particularly parents, and careful adherence to the principles for involving them and their children that have been explored in this chapter would go a long way to reassure them.

Researchers will maintain public confidence only if they are trusted to protect the vital interests of the children in their care. The limitations on the risks to which children should be subjected in the name of research provide a source of reassurance. In therapeutic research, the possible benefits to the child should be weighed against the risks to them and there is no clear guidance on what is regarded as acceptable. Each case should be considered on its individual merits. Where non-therapeutic research is concerned, the risks involved should be carefully assessed in order to ensure that no more than minimal risk is involved before children and parents are invited the consent. Professional guidance indicates that studies involving more than minimal risk should not be undertaken (although the definition of the risk threshold varies slightly between documents). Such risks should be understood to include their subjective emotional and psychological aspects. Care should also be taken to ensure that risks are minimised. These principles aim to secure for children as a group the benefits of rigorous research without compromising the interests of any individual child.

These principles present challenges both to research ethics committees and research teams. Assessments of risk, scrutiny of proposals for securing legally valid consent and for gaining cooperation from children are essential parts of the approval process for protocols. The special difficulties encountered in considering projects involving children may require paediatric medical or nursing input to committees.[1] Even where the projects themselves appear sound, however, researchers retain considerable responsibilities in implementing them. Obtaining consent, particularly to unfamiliar procedures, requires both time and skill.[14] Standardised consent forms, however child-friendly, cannot replace the need to build up relationships with children in order to win their confidence. The effort required to do these tasks effectively cannot justify ignoring the ethical and legal principles that require them. Ignoring those principles is likely to undermine public confidence, and without public confidence cooperation with research will dwindle. Commitment to the proper conduct of research is

thus also commitment to the future of care for children. Without evidence, improvements to such care will be difficult to obtain, but without public confidence the evidence will rapidly become unavailable.

REFERENCES

1. British Paediatric Association. *Guidelines for the ethical conduct of medical research involving children*. London: BPA, 1992. Reprinted. *Arch Dis Child* 2000; **82**: 177–82.
2. Department of Health. *Local research ethics committees*. London: DoH, 1990.
3. Medical Research Council. *Issues in research with children*. London: MRC, 1991.
4. Royal College of Physicians. *Guidelines on the practice of ethics committees in medical research involving human subjects*. 3rd edn. London: RCP, 1996.
5. Alderson P. 'Did children change, or did the guidelines?' *Bull Med Eth* 1999; **150**: 38–44.
6. Medical Research Council. Responsibility in investigations on human subjects. In: *Report of the Medical Research Council*, 1962–63. Cmnd. 2382 pp. 21–25.
7. Royal College of Physicians. *Supervision of the ethics of clinical research investigations and fetal research*. London: RCP, 1973.
8. British Paediatric Association. *Guidelines to aid ethical committees considering research involving children*. *Arch Dis Child* 1980; **55**: 75–7.
9. Nicholson R ed. *Medical research with children: ethics law and practice*. Oxford: Oxford University Press, 1986; pp. 76–124.
10. *Re W* [1992] 4 All ER 627.
11. Montgomery J. *Health care law*. Oxford: Oxford University Press, 1997.
12. Family Law Reform Act 1969, s. 8.
13. *Gillick* v. *W Norfolk AHA* [1985] 3 All ER 402.
14. Alderson P, Montgomery J. *Health care choices: making decisions with children*. London: Institute for Public Policy Research, 1996.
15. *Re J (child's religious upbringing and circumcision)* [2000] 1 FCR 307.
16. Dworkin G. Legality of consent to non-therapeutic medical research in infants and young children. *Arch Dis Child* 1978; **51**: 443–6.
17. Dworkin G. Law and medical experimentation: of embryos, children and others with limited legal capacity. *Monash University Law Rev* 1987; **13**: 189–208.
18. Montgomery J. Children as property?' *Modern Law Rev* 1988; **51**: 323–42.
19. *Re Y* [1996] 2 FLR 787.
20. *Re B* [1987] 2 All ER 206.
21. *S* v. *McC; W* v. *W* [1972] AC 24.

17 • Informed consent and clinical research in psychiatry

Phil Fennell

In passing judgment on the atrocities committed by Nazi doctors on concentration camp inmates, the Allied Military Tribunals laid down the 10 principles known as the Nuremberg Code, to regulate medical experimentation on human subjects. The first and fundamental principle is this:

> ... The voluntary consent of the human subject is absolutely essential.
>
> This means that the person involved should have the legal capacity to give consent; should be so situated as to be able to exercise the free power of choice, without the intervention of any element of force, fraud, deceit, duress, overreaching, or other ulterior form of constraint or coercion; and should have sufficient knowledge and comprehension of the element and subject matter involved to enable him to make an understanding and enlightened decision.
>
> This latter element requires that before the acceptance of an affirmative by the experimental subject there should be made known to him the nature, duration, and purpose of the experiment; the method and means by which it is to be conducted; all inconveniences and hazards reasonably to be expected; and the effects on his health and person which may possibly come from his participation in the experiment.

The Nuremberg Code has since been supplemented by the Declaration of Helsinki (1964), and as we shall see it is now seen as acceptable in certain circumstances for patients who lack capacity to participate in clinical research. Nevertheless, the first Nuremberg principle immediately points up the ethical problems for research in psychiatry. Many psychiatric patients do not have the legal capacity to consent. Many are detained, and are therefore not well-situated to exercise the power of free choice. This essay examines the role of informed consent in clinical psychiatric research, the possibilities to carry out such research without consent, and the impact of the Human Rights Act 1998 on the activities of local research ethics committees (LRECs).

CLINICAL RESEARCH IN PSYCHIATRY

Clinical research is medical research combined with professional care. Research is generally categorised as therapeutic or non-therapeutic. The difference lies in the primary aim of the research and the directness of benefit to the patient. Therapeutic research involves trying out new methods of treating illness with a view to more effective treatment or reduction of adverse side effects, where the primary aim is to benefit the patient. For research to be therapeutic, there must be some prospect of direct and significant benefit to the patient. Non-therapeutic research is intended primarily to further medical knowledge for the benefit of future patients, with no direct or identifiable benefit to the patient.

Clinical research may include therapeutic and non-therapeutic components:

> Research is defined as clinical if one or more of the components is designed to be diagnostic, prophylactic or therapeutic for the individual subject of the research. Invariably, in clinical research there are also components designed not to be diagnostic, prophylactic, or therapeutic for the individual subject; examples include the administration of placebos and the performance of laboratory tests in addition to those required to serve the purpose of medical care. Hence the term 'clinical research' is used, rather than therapeutic.[1]

Clinical research in psychiatry may involve trials of drug or other treatments. It may involve research into the causes of mental disorder, or its epidemiology. It may involve randomised controlled trials. Clinical research in psychiatry is complicated by five main factors:

- The stigma associated with mental disorder, even in societies esteeming themselves enlightened, which places a premium on confidentiality.
- Mental disorder may impair or destroy completely

a person's capacity to consent to treatment or research.

- Mentally disordered patients may be detained under mental health legislation, which means that they can be given drug or ECT treatment for their mental disorder without their consent, subject to a statutory system of second opinions. Detention under the Act does not automatically entail incapacity to consent to or to refuse treatment Detained status means that clinicians and Local Research Ethics Committees must anxiously scrutinise the genuineness of consent. In *Freeman* v. *Home Office*,[2] the Court of Appeal held that the fact that the prison doctor had a say in a patient's eligibility for release on licence was not coercion, even though refusal would have made release less likely. The judge at first instance offered valuable guidance on the right approach where the doctor could influence the prospects of release from detention:

> The right approach in my judgment, is to say that where, in a prison setting, a doctor has the power to influence a prisoner's situation and prospects a court must be alive to the fact that what may appear, on the face of it to be a real consent, is not in fact so. I have borne that in mind throughout the case.[3]

The same caution must apply to detained patients where the prospects of discharge will be greatly influenced by the opinion of the patient's responsible medical officer (RMO), the psychiatrist in charge of the patient's treatment. Whilst the psychiatrist may not put pressure on the patient, there will be a natural tendency for the patient not to want to displease the RMO.

- Psychiatric treatments can have unpleasant and harmful side effects (such as the risk of tardive dyskinesia with certain neuroleptic drugs) and this gives rise to complex issues in terms of entitlement to treatment information where the benefits are uncertain.

- Extra care must be taken to ensure the genuineness of consent with therapeutic research where the benefits of a treatment are uncertain and the potential risks great. Additional safeguards are necessary where research is non-therapeutic. As the Law Society and the BMA put it in their guide *Assessment of Mental Capacity*, "a greater evidence of understanding is required if individuals are being asked to consent to their participation in

something which brings them no likelihood of direct benefit."[4]

HUMAN RIGHTS AND LOCAL RESEARCH ETHICS COMMITTEES

The Human Rights Act 1998 comes into force in October 2000; it requires all public authorities to act compatibly with the European Convention on Human Rights (ECHR), and public authority is defined in functional terms as "any person or authority certain of whose functions are of a public nature." In 1991 the Department of Health issued Guidelines on Local Research Ethics Committees (LRECs), which state that; "No NHS body should agree to any research involving NHS patients without the approval of the relevant LREC. No research should proceed without the approval of the relevant NHS body."[5] As Kennedy and Grubb observe, although the authority wielded by LRECs is informal and extra legal, "that authority should not be minimised."[6] Research funders usually stipulate LREC approval. Researchers within the NHS will be denied access to patients without such approval. Once an LREC constitutes itself and considers a research proposal that affects the rights of patients, it takes on important legal duties. LRECs authorising access to be granted to patients for clinical research will surely be regarded as exercising public functions, and therefore the committees will be obliged to act compatibly with Convention Rights, most particularly the right not to be subjected to inhuman or degrading treatment (Article 3) and the right of privacy (Article 8).

The ECHR was drawn up in the immediate aftermath of the Nazi horrors and it is important to remember that the rights that it guarantees are to be seen as a floor, not a ceiling. The Human Rights Act obliges UK Courts, wherever possible, to interpret UK legislation compatibly with Convention Rights. Article 3 of the Convention protects against torture or inhuman or degrading treatment. In principle, medical treatment is capable of breaching Article 3, but treatment will be considered inhuman only if it reaches a certain level of gravity causing physical or mental suffering, and will only be degrading if the person undergoes humiliation or debasement attaining a minimum level of severity. Moreover, a measure deemed to be a therapeutic necessity by a responsible body of medical opinion will not breach Article 3. Nevertheless, the European Commission on Human Rights has stated that "medical treatment of an experimental nature without the patient's consent can, under certain circumstances, be considered as being contrary to Article 3,"[7] without specifying what those circumstances might be.

Article 8 of the European Convention protects the right of privacy and family life. Privacy has been held to include medical confidentiality.[8] It has also been held that "a compulsory medical intervention, even if it is of minor importance," must be considered an interference with the right of privacy under Article 8. However, these rights can be limited in accordance with the law where necessary in a democratic society in the interests of (*inter alia*) prevention of disorder or crime, for the protection of health or morals, or for the protection of the rights and freedoms of others.[8, 9] Considerable breadth is afforded by the European Court of Human Rights to these exceptions.

In addition to the Convention, there are other international instruments, which, although of a non-binding nature, carry great weight. The core concerns of all of them are human dignity and the requirement of informed consent as the key safeguard of the sanctity of the person. Both notions are fundamental to the World Medical Association's Declaration of Helsinki (1964), which lays down authoritative guidance on therapeutic and non-therapeutic research, as well as to International Ethical Guidelines for Biomedical Research involving Human Subjects issued in 1993 by the Council for International Organisations for Medical Sciences and the World Health Organisation. The Council of Europe Committee of Experts on Bioethics saw the "essential foundation of human dignity" as being that "all human beings are equal and that everyone has a value unto himself as a subject. The human being may never be regarded as a means or an object."[10] This is reflected in Article 7 of the International Covenant on Civil and Political Rights, which not only prohibits torture and inhuman or degrading treatment, but also particularly stipulates that "no one shall be subjected without his free consent to medical or scientific experimentation." Principle 3 of the Council of Europe Recommendation R (90) 3 provides that no medical research may be carried out without the informed, free, express, and specific consent of the person undergoing it.

Articles 16–18 of the Council of Europe Convention on Human Rights and Biomedicine* deal with research.[11 (p. 210)] It is important to note that the Biomedicine Convention, unlike the European Convention on Human Rights (ECHR), has not been signed or ratified by the United Kingdom. Even if signed and ratified, the Biomedicine Convention does not confer a right on individuals to make an application to the European Court of Human Rights. Article 29 of the Biomedicine Convention confines the Court's role to that of giving advisory opinions. However, acts that are a violation of the Biomedicine Convention may be considered in proceedings under the ECHR, if they also constitute an alleged violation of one of the rights conferred by the ECHR. So, for example, in a country which has signed and ratified the Convention, a failure to obtain informed consent contrary to Article 5 of the Biomedicine Convention could be brought before the ECHR as a violation of the right of privacy under Article 8 of the ECHR.[12]

In relation to research, Article 16 provides that, before clinical research can be undertaken, there must be no alternative of comparable effectiveness to research on humans, and the risks run by the patient must not be disproportionate to the potential benefits of the research. The project must have been approved by the competent body, after independent examination of its scientific merit, including assessment of the importance of the research and multidisciplinary review of its ethical acceptability. The research subject must have been informed of his or her rights, and the free and informed consent necessary for medical treatment under Article 5 of the Biomedicine Convention must have been given expressly, specifically and must be documented. The subject must be free to withdraw consent at any time.

Research on people unable to consent is authorised under Article 17 if, in addition to the Article 16 requirements, two further conditions are met. These are that the results of the research must have the potential to produce real and direct benefit to the subject's health, and that research of comparable effectiveness cannot be carried out on individuals capable of giving consent. Proxy consent in written form is necessary from the patient's representative,

---

*The Convention for the Protection of Human Rights and Dignity of the Human Being with regard to the Application of Biology and Medicine: Convention on Human Rights and Biomedicine Adopted by the Committee of Ministers, Council of Europe, on November 19 1996, submitted for signature and signed by 21 Member States in Oviedo on 4 April 1997. Six Member States have already ratified the Convention. They are Denmark, Greece, San Marino, Slovakia, Slovenia and Spain.

or a person or body provided for by law, and this can be withdrawn in the subject's best interests at any time. The article also lays emphasis on encouraging the individual to take part as far as possible in the decision to participate.

The Convention authorises participation of incapable adults in non-therapeutic research in exceptional circumstances. These are where the research has the aim of contributing through significant improvement in the scientific understanding of the individual's condition, disease or disorder, to the ultimate attainment of results capable of conferring benefit to the person concerned or to other persons in the same age category or afflicted with the same disease. The research must entail only minimal risk and minimal burden for the individual.

The European Commission Guidelines on good Clinical Practice for Trials of Medicinal Products in the European Community restrict research on subjects incapable of giving personal consent to that which promotes the welfare and interest of the subject.

Five key principles animate the approach of international human rights instruments to clinical research. They are:

- the dignity of human beings and their right to be treated as subjects, not objects;
- the requirement of informed consent, based on knowledge that the treatment is experimental, as the key protection for the sanctity of the person;
- a relationship of proportionality between the potential therapeutic benefit of the experimental treatment and the extent of the risk to the subject;
- effective supervision of research into vulnerable groups such as detained or mentally incapacitated patients;
- a presumption against the involvement of incapacitated or detained patients in non-therapeutic research.

At the root of all these principles is one fundamental right. The right to know that one is involved in a research project, and whether the research has a therapeutic or non-therapeutic intent.

With clinical research the doctor's duty, as with other treatment, is to act in the patients best interests and to do no harm. This has three main consequences for the conduct of trials, described in these terms by Kennedy and Grubb:[6] (p. 1043)

First, if the trial consists in testing a new treatment, the doctor must have reasonable grounds for believing that the treatment may be efficacious. For example that the necessary research on animals and other studies have been carried out.

Secondly, patients not receiving any new treatment which is the subject of the trial (i.e. those in the control group) must receive the best available established treatment.

Thirdly, the trial must contain an appropriate mechanism ('a stopping rule') whereby it may be discontinued if (a) a new treatment proves less beneficial than established treatment; or (b) a new treatment proves more beneficial that existing therapies; or (c) therapy A shows a marked benefit over therapies B or C.

These principles and rules apply to all research carried out with consent. The complicating factors with psychiatric research stem mainly from the fact that many psychiatric patients are detained, and of those who are not detained, significant numbers lack the necessary mental capacity to consent. At 31 March 1999 there were 13 000 patients detained in hospital, and between 1 April 1998 and 31 March 1999 27 100 patients were admitted compulsorily under the Mental Health Act.[13] Over 90% of psychiatric patients are informal. 'Informal' does not mean the same as voluntary admission. It simply means admission without using the powers of detention under the Act. It does not necessarily mean that the patient is capable of consenting to hospital admission and has consented. Informal admission is not only for the capable volunteer. It may also be used for the incapable, non-resisting patient. A significant proportion of informal patients lack capacity to consent to admission or treatment, but have not been detained because they are not resisting being in hospital.[14]

The concluding sections of this essay consider the position of informal and detained psychiatric patients in relation to therapeutic and non-therapeutic research.

INFORMAL PATIENTS: CAPACITY AND INCAPACITY

The *Mental Health Act Code of Practice* does not refer to "informed consent", preferring "valid consent", and emphasising the personal responsibility of a doctor to determine whether each patient whom he or she proposes to treat has capacity to give a valid consent. Assessment of capacity is a matter for "clinical judgment, guided by current professional practice and subject to legal requirements."[15] The Code stresses that mentally disordered people are not necessarily incapable, and that capacity is to be assessed in relation to the patient in question, at the particular time, with relation to the treatment proposed. Similarly, the fact that a person has been detained under the Mental Health Act does not render them automatically incapable of consenting to or refusing treatment.[15] The explanation of the treatment given by the doctor should be appropriate to the level of the patient's assessed ability.[16] (para 15.12)

A person's capacity to consent to research is assessed in the same way as their capacity to consent to treatment. Additional safeguards, however, come into play when the research is non-therapeutic. Greater evidence of understanding is required if individuals are being asked to consent to their participation in something that brings them no likelihood of direct benefit. Even if there is a prospect of therapeutic benefit, the greater the risk attendant on the research the higher the threshold of capacity required to consent to take part.[17]

Consent to clinical research is effectively consent to treatment, but with added requirement, such as that the patient be made aware of the fact that he or she is participating in research. Kennedy and Grubb argue that failure to disclose the intention to conduct research would amount to fraud sufficient to vitiate any consent which might be forthcoming.[6] (p. 1045) The person must also be told that they may refuse to take part in the research project with no adverse consequences in terms of their subsequent treatment. The person must also be informed if the nature of the research is such that he may be a member of a control group. If so the researchers would normally be expected to tell the patient that they will review the emerging data at intervals, and if the treatment is proving to be the most effective, he or she will be offered that treatment. The patient must also be informed if the research is part of a randomised controlled trial, and what that means.

Mental capacity

In order for consent to be valid, the subject must have the necessary mental capacity, as is evident from the following passage from Lord Donaldson's judgment in *Re T*:

An adult patient who ... suffers from no mental incapacity has an absolute right to choose whether to consent to medical treatment, to refuse it or to choose one rather than another of the treatments being offered ... This right of choice is not limited to decisions which others might regard as sensible. It exists, notwithstanding that the reasons for making the choice are rational, irrational, unknown, or even non-existent.[17 (p. 102)]

Treatment includes diagnostic procedures.[18]

Capacity is the gatekeeper concept to decision-making autonomy. Capable adults have the right to have their decisions respected. Patients who lack capacity have the right to be treated in what their doctor considers to be in their best interests. In *Re F (mental patient: sterilisation)*, the House of Lords held that doctors have a power and, in certain circumstances, a duty to give patients who lack mental capacity treatment, which is necessary in their best interests.[19] The decision whether the treatment is in the patient's best interests is to be determined in accordance with a responsible body of medical opinion which is logically supportable. A person lacks capacity if some impairment or disturbance of mental functioning renders the person unable to make a decision whether to consent to or refuse treatment.

There is a presumption of capacity, and it is for the clinician alleging incapacity to satisfy him or herself that some impairment or disturbance of mental functioning has rendered the person unable to make a decision whether to consent to or refuse treatment. As the Mental Health Act Code of Practice puts it:[15]

An individual is presumed to have the capacity to make a treatment decision unless he or she:
- Is unable to take in and retain the information material to the decision, especially as to the likely consequences of having or not having the treatment – this includes information about the likely benefits and risks; or
- Is unable to believe the information – this means that he or she is prevented from believing it by some delusion, compulsion, or phobia (such as a belief that a blood transfusion is poison because it is red); or
- Is unable to weigh the information in the balance as part of a process of making the decision.

In order to be capable of giving informed consent to clinical research, patients must be able to take in and retain the information that the treatment is given as part of a research project. Where the treatment is experimental, the patient has a right to know this. In *R v. Mental Health Act Commission ex parte X*, Stuart Smith stated that "no doubt consent has to be 'informed consent' in that [the patient] knows the nature and likely effects of the treatment" (p. 86). In the particular case, where an anticancer drug (goserelin) was being put to novel use as a sexual suppressant, the judge held that it was important that the patient should know this. However, he went on to reject the proposition that "a patient must understand the precise physiological process involved before he can be said to be capable of understanding the nature and likely effects of the treatment or can consent to it" (p. 87). The Mental Health Act Commission Third Biennial Report says that the "knowledge communicated by the therapist may vary in detail from 'broad terms' to great detail, depending on the patient's ability and the complexity of the treatment being offered, with the final criteria ... being that the patient is capable of understanding the nature, purpose and likely effects of the treatment."[21]

A person who is competent can consent to research provided they are given the necessary information. The fact that a patient is suffering from mental disorder does not mean that they will necessarily lack capacity. However, where mentally disordered patients are giving consent to involvement in clinical research, and where the benefits are uncertain and the known risks significant, those running the research project will need to ensure that the patient is capable, and to have documented their assessment in the notes.

INCAPACITATED PATIENTS

Where a person lacks capacity to decide for themselves, no other person has the authority to give consent on their behalf. However, involvement in a research project may be justified if it is approved by the LREC and is expected to produce a direct and significant benefit to the incapacitated person. The principle in Re F which authorises treatment in the patient's best interests means that therapeutic research may be carried out on incompetent patients. Article 17 of the Biomedicine Convention authorises research on people unable to consent provided that the results of the research have the potential to produce "real and direct benefit to the subject's health", and that research of comparable effectiveness cannot be carried out on individuals capable of giving consent. However, Article 17 requires proxy consent in written form from the patient's representative or a person or body provided for by law, which can be withdrawn in the subject's best inter-

ests at any time. No such arrangements for proxy consent exist under English law. Nor, it seems, will they in the near future. The 1999 White Paper *Making Decisions*[22] has indicated the Government's intention not to take forward the Law Commission's recommendations for regulating research on incapacitated people in their 1995 Report *Mental incapacity*.[23]

In 1995 the Law Society and BMA publication *Assessment of mental capacity* concluded (p. 82) that: "Although the involvement of persons lacking capacity in non-therapeutic research is increasingly regarded as ethical, it is doubtful that carrying out such research is lawful."[4] This was based on the Law Commission's view that:

> If ... the participant lacks capacity to consent to his or her participation, and the procedure cannot be justified under the doctrine of necessity, then any person who touches or restrains that participant is committing an unlawful battery. The simple fact is that the researcher is making no claim to be acting in the best interests of the individual person and does not therefore come within the rules in Re F.[23 (para 6.29)]

The Biomedicine Convention authorises participation of incapable adults in non-therapeutic research in exceptional circumstances. These are where the research has the aim of contributing through significant improvement in the scientific understanding of the individual's condition, disease, or disorder, to the ultimate attainment of results capable of conferring benefit to the person concerned or to other persons in the same age category or afflicted with the same disease. The research must entail only minimal risk and minimal burden for the individual. The Law Commission's proposals would have been in line with the Biomedicine Convention because they would have provided that research, which was unlikely to benefit the participant, or whose benefit is likely to be long delayed, should be lawful if (a) the research is into an incapacitating condition with which the person is or may be affected, and (b) the approval of a new statutory committee were obtained. Although the Law Commission's recommendations will not be implemented in England, a Bill on Incapacity has been presented to the Scottish Parliament which provides for a central research ethics authority for research on people who lack mental capacity. The Scottish arrangements would comply with the Biomedicine Convention, should the United Kingdom sign and ratify it. Regardless of the Biomedicine Convention, under existing principles of English law the lawfulness of non-therapeutic research on incapable patients is extremely doubtful. The Scots have recognised that if research on incapable people is to be legally and ethically acceptable, this will only be achieved by providing extra safeguards to ensure that the ethical issues have been fully considered.

RESEARCH WITH DETAINED PATIENTS

A key question in relation to detained persons is whether their status as detainees precludes them from giving valid consent. In *Re C (mental patient) (medical treatment)*,[24] it was held that a detained patient suffering from schizophrenia had the capacity to refuse amputation of his gangrenous foot. This was an important reminder that the mere fact that someone is suffering from mental disorder or is detained under mental health legislation does not necessarily mean that they are incapable of making a treatment decision. In their Sixth Biennial Report (1993–1995),[25] the Mental Health Act Commission drew attention to the ethical implications of research being carried out on detained patients. A person may be detained under mental health legislation and yet still retain the capacity to consent to or refuse treatment at common law. In January 1997 the Commission published a position paper on "research involving detained patients."[26]

Whilst asserting that the Maudsley Hospital's "elevation of involvement in research to a right goes too far", the position paper proceeds from the principle that the "freedom" to take part in research is not taken away by the Act. Therefore it "was to be assumed that a detained patient is not prevented from taking part in research" provided the following three conditions are met[26]:

- he/she has the capacity to consent and does consent;
- such involvement does not conflict with any provision of the 1983 Act, or any prohibition or restriction imposed by law;
- such involvement is not otherwise inconsistent with the patient's status as a detained patient.

Crucial to the legal and ethical acceptability of research carried out with the consent of a detained patient, as with all patients, is the right to know that one is involved in a research project, and whether the research has a therapeutic or non-therapeutic intent.

Moreover, Kennedy and Grubb's three principles (outlined above) apply. The doctor must have reasonable ground for believing that the treatment may be efficacious, the control group must receive the best available established treatment, and there must be "a stopping rule" applying equally to research carried out on detained patients.[6 (p. 1043)]

The Mental Health Act Code of Practice emphasises that although Part IV can be used to authorise treatment without consent, the psychiatrist in charge of the patient's treatment (RMO) must always seek the patient's valid consent before giving treatment.[15 (para 16.11)] If the patient is capable of consenting and has consented to ECT or medicine, the RMO certifies this on Statutory Form 38.[27] Unlike the consent forms used in general medicine, the statutory consent form does not require the patient's signature, only that of the RMO. The RMO must certify that two criteria are met: that the patient is capable, and that he or she consents to the treatment. Consent may be withdrawn at any time.

The statutory test of capacity under Part IV is that the patient is capable of understanding the nature, purpose and likely effects of the treatment. In *R v. Mental Health Act Commission ex parte X (orse W)*,[20] Stuart Smith LJ noted (*obiter*) that, "the words are 'capable of understanding', and not 'understands.'" Thus the question is capacity and not actual understanding."[20 (p. 85), 28] Despite this, the advice from the Mental Health Act Commission to second opinion doctors is that, in assessing validity of consent, they should look not just at capacity to understand in the abstract, but at actual understanding of the treatment proposal.

There has also been some debate as to whether the amount of information required to be given under section 58 is greater than the common law duty to give the amount of information that a responsible body of medical opinion would give. In *ex parte X (orse W)*, Stuart Smith LJ stated that "no doubt consent has to be 'informed consent' in that [the patient] knows the nature and likely effects of the treatment."[20 (p. 86)] In the particular case, where an anticancer drug was being put to novel use as a sexual suppressant, the judge held that it was important that the patient should know this. However, he went on to reject the proposition that "a patient must understand the precise physiological process involved before he can be said to be capable of understanding the nature and likely effects of the treatment or can consent to it."[20 (p. 87)] The Third Biennial Report says that the "knowledge communicated by the therapist may vary in detail from 'broad terms' to great detail, depending on the patient's ability and the complexity of the treatment being offered, with the final criteria [*sic*] ... being that the patient is capable of understanding the nature, purpose and likely effects" of the treatment.[21]

The Mental Health Act *Code of Practice* does not refer to "informed consent", preferring "valid consent". The Code emphasises the personal responsibility of a doctor to determine whether each patient whom he or she proposes to treat has capacity to give a valid consent, and that assessment of capacity is a matter for "clinical judgment, guided by current professional practice and subject to legal requirements."[15] It goes on to stress that mentally disordered people are not necessarily incapable. Therefore capacity is to be assessed in relation to the patient in question, at the particular time, with relation to the treatment proposed. The explanation of the treatment given by the doctor should be appropriate to the level of the patient's assessed ability.[15 (para 15.12)]

Part IV of the Mental Health Act 1983 provides that certain treatments may be given only with the patient's consent. Research involving these treatments cannot therefore be carried out without consent. Part IV also allows treatment for mental disorder to be given without consent, so therapeutic research involving detained patients may be lawful, even without the consent of the participant, provided the safeguards required by the 1983 Act are observed. The Mental Health Act Commission's position paper stipulates five conditions which should be observed in relation to research on detained patients:

1. Research involving detained patients must be clearly identified and described as research, separate from routine or established forms of treatment.
2. Such research should be clearly identified and described to show whether it is considered to be therapeutic or non-therapeutic.
3. If a patient has capacity to consent to participation in research, and does in fact give actual and informed consent, then participation should not be prevented unless:
   • involvement conflicts with any provision of the 1983 Act; or
   • involvement is inconsistent with treatment being received as a detained patient.
4. If a detained patient does not have the capacity to consent to participation in research, his or her

involvement can only be justified if the research forms a part of that patient's treatment under the Mental Health Act.
5. Local research ethics committees should establish agreed protocols designed specifically for research that may involve detained patients.

Before examining the issues that are to be covered by these LREC protocols, it is important to consider the situations where psychiatric research requires consent, and where it may lawfully be carried out without consent.

Research Requiring Consent

Therapeutic research

Clinical research is treatment, and the 1983 Act allows for detained patients to be given certain treatments for their mental disorder without consent. This would appear to indicate that therapeutic research may be carried out without consent. However, there are some treatments for mental disorder for which consent is necessary. No psychiatric patient, detained or not, may participate in research involving psychosurgery or the surgical implantation of hormones to reduce male sex drive, unless they are capable of understanding its nature purpose, and likely effects, and have consented to it. Their consent must be certified as genuine by a panel of three people appointed by the Mental Health Act Commission. Moreover, the medical member of that panel must certify that the treatment ought to be given, having regard to the likelihood that the treatment will alleviate or prevent deterioration in the patient's condition (section 57). In the unlikely event of research involving these treatments, the patient's consent is therefore necessary, together with compliance with the statutory second opinion procedures, together with LREC approval.

Non-therapeutic research

The other type of research requiring consent, even from a detained patient, is non-therapeutic research which does not involve any element of treatment. Here, as with non-psychiatric patients, participation must depend on capacity, informed consent, and LREC approval.

Therapeutic Research Without Consent

Part IV of the Mental Health Act authorises treatment without consent. Medicine or ECT for mental disorder may be given without consent subject to a second opinion under section 58. Treatments for mental disorder other than medicines or ECT may be given without consent under section 63 if it is at the direction of the psychiatrist in charge of the patient's treatment. Emergency treatment may be given without consent or a second opinion, if it is immediately necessary to save the patient's life or to meet one of the emergencies defined in section 62.

ECT and medicines for mental disorder

Section 58 of the 1983 Act provides that no detained patient may be treated with medicine or electroconvulsive therapy (ECT) unless either (a) they are capable of consenting *and* consent to it; *or* (b) an independent second opinion psychiatrist appointed by the Mental Health Act Commission has certified that the treatment ought to be given. This means that detained patients, who are unable to consent or are refusing treatment, may be given drugs or ECT subject to a favourable second opinion. The second opinion doctor must consult a nurse, and another person, not a doctor, who has been professionally concerned with the patient's care. The decision as to whether the patient is to have the treatment without consent is based on the likelihood that the treatment will "alleviate or prevent deterioration in the patent's condition." The approach to be applied in authorising treatment is outlined in the circular DDL 84(4) which states that second opinion doctors should not ask themselves, "Is this a treatment I would recommend?" but rather "Is this a treatment which other responsible doctors would recommend?" This is a version of the so-called *Bolam test*. "Has the treating doctor prescribed a treatment which accords with a responsible body (not necessarily the majority) of medical opinion, skilled in the specialty?" This should now be modified in the light of *Bolitho*, which requires that the responsible body of medical opinion must "be supported by logic." Nevertheless, the overriding legal criterion to which the second opinion doctor must have regard is "the likelihood that the treatment will alleviate or prevent deterioration in the patient's condition." This is important in the case of experimental treatments. It is submitted that if there cannot reasonably be said to be any likelihood of alleviation or prevention of deterioration, the treatment may not lawfully be authorised.

A detained patient who cannot or will not consent

to ECT must have a second opinion immediately, unless there is an emergency covered by section 62 of the 1983 Act. The procedure is somewhat different for medicines. Although attempts should always be made to obtain consent, a detained patient may be required to accept medicines for mental disorder for up to three months before becoming entitled to a second opinion. If medicine is to be given thereafter, either the patient's consent is required or a statutory second opinion must be obtained. Nonconsensual research cannot therefore extend beyond three months unless a favourable second opinion is obtained, and in addition the LREC has approved the involvement of detained patients without consent.

Other treatments

Treatments for mental disorder not involving psychosurgery, surgical hormone implants to reduce male sex drive, ECT or medicines may be given without consent under section 63 of the 1983 Act. The Mental Health Act Commission position paper states that the consent of a patient to therapeutic research involving these "other treatments" is not necessary provided two conditions are met:

- the research falls within the definition of medical treatment given to him or her for the mental disorder from which he or she is suffering; and
- the treatment is given by or under the direction of the Responsible Medical Officer.[26, 47]

Section 145 of the Mental Health Act broadly defines medical treatment for mental disorder as including "nursing, care habilitation and rehabilitation under medical supervision." It has been held to include not only treatment for the core disorder, but treatment of "the symptoms and sequelae" of mental disorder. The intention of section 63 was to authorise routine, not controversial or untested treatments, and so the Commission's bald statement that "consent is not necessary" gives insufficient weight to the need for caution in authorising experimental treatment without consent.

Emergency treatment

Section 62 is intended to allow treatment that would normally require a statutory second opinion to be given to cope with an emergency. At the same time it seeks to protect patients against hazardous or irreversible treatment unless that treatment is immediately necessary to save their own lives. Emergency treatment that is hazardous or irreversible may only be given without consent or a second opinion where it is immediately necessary to save the patient's life. A treatment that is hazardous (but not one that is irreversible) may be given if it is to prevent a serious deterioration in the patient's condition. Emergency treatments immediately necessary to alleviate serious suffering by the patient may be given as long as they are neither hazardous nor irreversible. Finally treatments that are neither irreversible or hazardous may be given if immediately necessary and if they represent the minimum interference necessary to prevent the patient behaving violently or being a danger to himself or others.

The *Mental Health Act Code of Practice* (para 16.40a) stresses that the treatment must be given by or under the direction of the RMO and must be necessary to achieve one of the objects specified in the section. It is insufficient for it simply to be "necessary" or "beneficial".[15] The Mental Health Act Section 62(3) deems treatment irreversible if it has unfavourable irreversible physical or psychological consequences, and hazardous if it entails "significant physical hazard". The *Code of Practice* (para 16.40b) states that the RMO is responsible for deciding whether a treatment is irreversible or hazardous "having regard to generally accepted medical opinion."[15] Where a treatment is immediately necessary to prevent serious suffering on the part of the patient or to prevent him or acting violently or endangering self or others, it must be neither irreversible nor hazardous. It is difficult to envisage circumstances in which experimental emergency treatments could be given as part of research, given that for the most part they must be neither hazardous nor irreversible.

CONCLUSION: LREC PROTOCOLS FOR RESEARCH INVOLVING DETAINED PATIENTS AND CONVENTION RIGHTS

The Mental Health Act Commission position paper recommends that LRECs develop protocols concerning research on detained patients. These should address seven points:

- the need for the involvement of detained patients in research at all, or in the particular study;
- the need for the approval of the patient's RMO for the research;
- whether or not written consent from the patient should be obtained;

- the desirability of consultation with the patient's nearest relative, subject always to the consent of the patient;
- the desirability of consultation with the patient's ASW and other members of the multidisciplinary team;
- the need for clear explanation (both oral and written) to the detained patient of the nature of the research and whether or not any information personal to the patient, will be used (and if so how, and for what purpose);
- the need for the protection of patients' confidentiality.

On the assumption that LRECs will be public authorities for the purposes of the Human Rights Act 1998, these points need to be considered in relation to Convention Rights, so that protocols may be adopted which are "Convention compliant". The main issues which need to be borne in mind are that, where the right of bodily integrity is concerned, LRECs need to ensure that they are aware of the potential impact of Articles 3 and 8 described above, and the potential for the Biomedicine Convention to be used as an aid to construction of those Articles. Above all, they should take full account of what has been described as "the situation of vulnerability and powerlessness of detained psychiatric patients"[52] in assessing the need for valid consent and the need for detained patient participation in the research.

REFERENCES

1. Council for International Organisations for Medical Sciences and the World Health Organisation. *International ethical guidelines for biomedical research involving human subjects.* 1993, p. 11.
2. *Freeman* v. *Home Office* [1984] QB 524.
3. *Freeman* v. *Home Office* [1984] 2 WLR 130.
4. BMA and Law Society. *Assessment of mental capacity.* London: BMA, 1995, p 81.
5. Department of Health. *Guidelines on Local Research Ethics Committees (LRECs).* 1991, (HSG(91)5), para. 1.4.
6. Kennedy I, Grubb A. *Medical law: text with materials* (2nd edn). 1994.
7. *X* v. *Denmark* 9974/82 Decision of 2 March 1983 DR 32, p 82.
8. *Z* v. *Finland* (1997) 45 BMLR 107.
9. *MS* v. *Sweden* (1997) 45 BMLR 133.
10. Council of Europe. *Medical and biological progress and the European Convention on Human Rights.* 1994, p. 26.

11. Nys H. Physician involvement and patient's death. *Med Law Rev* 1999; **7**: 208–246.

12. Explanatory Report No. 165.

13. Department of Health. *In-patients formally detained in hospitals under the Mental Health Act 1983 and other legislation, England: 1988–9 and 1994–5 to 1998–9.* DoH Statistical Bulletin 1999/25. London: DoH.

14. Fennell P. Doctor knows best: therapeutic detention under common law, the Mental Health Act, and the European Convention. *Med Law Rev* 1998; **6**: 322–53.

15. Department of Health and Welsh Office. *Mental Health Act 1983 Code of Practice*. London: HMSO, 1990. (As revised by amendments laid before Parliament on 19 May 1993), para. 15.9.

16. *Re C (adult) (mental patient: medical treatment)* (1993) 15 BMLR 77.

17. *Re T (adult) (medical treatment)* [1993] Fam 95.

18. *Re H (mental patient) (sterilisation)* [1993] 1 FLR 329.

19. *Re F (adult) (mental patient: sterilisation)* [1990] 2 A.C. 1.

20. *R v. Mental Health Act Commission ex parte X (orse W)* (1988) 9 BMLR 77.

21. Mental Health Act Commission. *Third Biennial Report 1987–1989*. London: HMSO, p. 25.

22. *Making decisions* 1999 Cm 4465, para. 12. London: The Stationery Office, 1999.

23. Law Commission. Mental incapacity. London: Law Commission, p. 231.

24. *Re C (mental patient) (medical treatment)* [1994] 1 All ER 819.

25. Mental Health Act Commission. *Sixth Biennial Report 1993–1995*. London: HMSO, para. 5.17.

26. Mental Health Act Commission. Research involving detained patients. *Bull Med Ethics* 1997, July 8–11.

27. Mental Health (Hospital, Guardianship and Consent to Treatment) Regulations 1983 SI 1983 No 893, reg 16(2)(b) and Schedule 1.

28. Fennell P. Sexual suppressants and the Mental Health Act 1983. *Criminal Law Rev* 1988; 660.

29. *Herczegfalvy v. Austria (1992)* 18 BMLR 48.

18 · Informed consent and surgical research

Alan G Johnson

We may be sure that future ages will be very critical in their judgement of us, a present race of surgeons, and demand to know what use we made of our unparalleled opportunities, and whether we went astray amidst all the light that was given us.

BMJ 1899; **ii**: 337

The above quotation refers to the dawn of antiseptic surgery, but the challenge is equally relevant 100 years later. There is an ethical imperative for both surgeons and patients to undertake research to develop and evaluate new procedures. As we enjoy the fruits of past research, so it is our duty to improve treatments for present and future patients. This is part of a surgeon's duty of care and, with the increasing emphasis on evidence-based medicine, it is important to know which surgical operations are most effective and which give the best value for money. It is equally important to know which are not effective and should be abandoned. There is a significant list of operations such as blood-letting, nephropexy for floating kidneys and gastric freezing for bleeding ulcers, which enjoyed great popularity in the past but have since been abandoned. At the present time in the UK there are 60 different types of artificial hip joint being inserted at widely varying cost. We do not know if millions of pounds are being wasted each year on expensive prostheses or if cheaper alternatives are equally effective. To take another example, it is important to know whether large and radical operations for cancer, which carry an increased operative mortality and morbidity are, indeed, more likely to give a cure than a smaller, safer procedure. Experience with breast cancer has concluded that they are not. Why are we so unsure about the effectiveness of common operations?

The first and simple reason is that, until recently, surgical operations, unlike drugs, could be introduced into practice without any compulsory evaluation of safety and efficacy. The second reason is more controversial. The Editor of the *Lancet*[1] reviewed nine general surgical journals (see Box) and considered that, "Cynics might even claim that the personal attributes that go to make a successful surgeon differ from those needed for collaborative multi-centre research." This was not warmly welcomed by surgeons, as the correspondence columns of the *Lancet* testified! However, it may have more than a grain of truth. The second box gives the result of a survey in which 61% of a simple of surgeons said that they would not put patients into randomised controlled trials (RCTs) and gave their reasons. However, the common practical reason is that the hassle, bureaucracy, and organisational problems that have to be overcome, together with the great pressure on hospital beds and operating sessions, mitigate against any prolongation of the operation or hospital stay. Solomon *et al.*[2] concluded that, for various reasons, "Only 39% of surgical procedures could be subject to RCTs." Having said that, a considerable amount of surgical research has been done in all specialties over the last 25–30 years.

Survey of nine general surgical journals from January 1996[1]	
• Total articles	215
• Original work	175
• Case series	80(46%)
• Randomised controlled trials	12(7%)

Principle reasons given by surgeons for not performing randomised controlled trials (61% of sample)[2]	
• Uncommon condition	24.2%
• No community equipoise	10%
• Methodology issues	1.2%
• Patient preference	23.1%
• Surgical preference	2.3%
• Other reasons	0.4%

HOW DOES RESEARCH IN SURGICAL DISCIPLINES DIFFER FROM THAT IN OTHER BRANCHES OF MEDICINE?

It is the nature of the "assault", the potential for harm and the irreversibility of many procedures, that distinguishes surgical operations from other types of medical care. Patients must exercise an extraordinary degree of trust to allow a surgeon to cut them open with a knife and remove various important organs. Surgical operations are distinct events in the management of disease, which are easy to identify and subject to consent. Most medical treatments can be stopped half way, be changed or reversed; but once an organ has been removed, it cannot be put back. In addition, the patient is usually anaesthetised and unconscious during the procedure, which means that any unexpected findings cannot be discussed with the patient before the surgeon continues. Surgeons, then, need to know the patient's wishes on options that they may have to decide about in the middle of the procedure. This includes decisions whether to proceed, for example, to a large operation on the result of a frozen section biopsy, and how much risk to take in an attempt to remove a tumour. Fortunately, good imaging beforehand means that unexpected decisions during operations are becoming less common.

"Informed" (valid) consent implies that enough information is given to the patient to take a rational decision whether to choose a certain operation. The patient can never be fully informed, as all the facts are not known. This puts a considerable burden on surgeons to anticipate likely developments and obtain the patient's opinions beforehand, and to interpret with integrity the wording on the Consent Form: "Any other procedure that may be found *necessary* during the operation." If a completely unexpected disease is found in any other organ than that which is being operated on, unless waiting will put the patient at significant risk, any extension of the operation should be deferred to a second procedure, after discussion and consent. An exception might be if a patient has a particular risk from an anaesthetic, when a second would be more than doubling this risk. It is because patients are to be rendered unconscious that written, rather than verbal or implied consent is required.

There is, therefore a strong moral and legal obligation for consent for surgical operations so as to preserve the patient's autonomy during such an intrusive treatment. Without consent in ordinary rela-

tionships, cutting someone with a knife would be the criminal offence of "assault and battery". Formal consent protects the surgeon as well as the patient. There is always discussion and debate about the amount of information that should be given before consent is obtained. In the USA, patients are given details of every possible risk, however small, whereas, in the UK, only major or significant risks are given and there is no legal obligation to disclose every possible complication. Since 1957, the law has been judged by the Bolam principles: these resulted from a judgement which stated that the amount of information given to a patient should be what a reasonable body of doctors would give in similar circumstances. However, this principle is increasingly being questioned and, as the Lord Chancellor has pointed out,[3] may gradually shift towards what "a reasonable body of patients would be expect to be told in order to make an informed decision."

There is, in theory, a fundamental difference in the nature of consent for treatment on the one hand and research on the other. During treatment, the patient is ill and has come to the surgeon requesting help – indeed, requesting treatment that the patient is unable to give to himself. Alastair Campbell has pointed out that consent normally implies agreeing with reluctance, "acquiescence to or acceptance of something done or planned by another."[4] This, he points out, may be appropriate for consent to research, but not for treatment. He argues that it should be called "Informed request" for treatment by the patient.[5] This is a helpful distinction, although it may have no legal validity. The surgeon gives patients advice and options for different treatments with their possible results, and the patients, when they have as much information as they wish, request the surgeon to undertake a certain procedure. For research, on the other hand, it may be future patients who benefit, and the patient is consenting to an invitation to take part in such an investigation, i.e. research "planned by another". The more the research could be jointly planned by patient and surgeon together, the less this concept of acquiescence is relevant. However, there is an important grey area where treatment blends into research and research into treatment. Operations are evolving all the time, and it is often difficult to define when a major modification of the existing procedure becomes a new operation, or when an experimental procedure becomes routine practice.

The Belmont Report in the USA noted that the standards of consent for research had to be higher than standards of consent in medical practice.[6] Why should duty of disclosure be greater for research than for treatment? If the research is unconnected with treatment, when there is an extra study added on, then refusal would make no difference to the patient's management. If, on the other hand, two treatments are being compared, then refusal to join the trial does not mean that the patient receives no treatment at all. Indeed, the ethics of such a trial is that the patient's treatment will proceed irrespective of whether or not he agrees to go into the study. However, if the explanation for the research leads to the patient refusing an operation, it could have serious consequences, and if the consent has been requested in such a way as to make refusal more likely, it has important implications. The responsibility of not worrying a patient inappropriately is as relevant as giving the important facts. Katz[7] has suggested that different degrees of disclosure are required for different types of treatment according to the urgency and seriousness of the disease (see Box). Ethical theory has to be anchored in the real world where time is often the limiting factor. If patients do not want to know all the facts about their treatment, that is their decision. There is no obligation to force information about operative risks on them, even if the surgeon might like the relatives to know the risks to protect him from future accusations should something go wrong.

Variable consent according to situation

- Acute life threatening (essential facts only: as no alternative treatment)
- Elective procedures (formal discussion respecting patients wishes)
- Fatal outcome likely (slow and sensitive)
- Very minor "procedures", no formal consent (verbal sufficient)
- Cosmetic and non-essential (very full disclosure)

Does the same principle hold for research? If a subject of a research study says, "I trust you – I'm happy to take part, don't confuse me with the facts," should the surgeon go ahead with the project, as he might do if he were discussing a treatment? We will return to this matter later.

PATTERNS OF SURGICAL RESEARCH

The principles of research with patients who happen

to be in a surgical ward are the same as those in the other medical situations considered elsewhere in this book. Here we are dealing with research that only a surgeon or anaesthetist can do. There are five situations in which research most commonly occurs in direct relationship to surgery (see Box).

Different types of clinical surgical research

- Controlled trials or other assessments of surgical treatments
- Studies in the immediate postoperative period
- Implanting recording apparatus at surgery
- Intraoperative studies – *new anaesthetic and physiological measurements*
- Removing tissue for research
  - *the organ being removed*
  - *other tissues*

Assessment and Controlled Trials of New Operations

Surgical techniques have developed rapidly over the last 30–40 years, but most of them have been introduced into clinical practice without proper appraisal of safety and cost-effectiveness. Indeed, the terms of reference of hospital ethical committees in Britain and many other countries have encouraged this: because they are *research* ethics committees, which only consider formal research protocols. Therefore a surgeon can introduce a new operation without any proper controlled evaluation and make no reference to the ethics committee; whereas, if he wants to do a proper randomised controlled trial, he has to get permission from the ethics committee to do so! Nothing has illustrated this better than the introduction of laparoscopic surgery over the last 10 years, which Professor Cuschieri has described as "The biggest unaudited free-for-all in the history of surgery."[8] Belatedly the Academy of the Medical Royal Colleges has set up an organisation known as SERNIP (Safety and Efficacy Register of New Interventional Procedures),[9] which classifies procedures into four categories (see Box). However, referral to this body is still voluntary. Unfortunately, control will be by lawyers unless something more comprehensive is developed. The Medical Devices Agency checks the soundness of a piece of apparatus, such as an artificial joint, but not its effectiveness in use. The new organisation in Britain – The National Institute of Clinical Excellence (NICE) – does assess the effectiveness of new procedures, but can only cover a few at a time. The pressures that led to the free-for-all of a new type of operation have been well summarised (see Box) by Dr Hiram Polk in the USA.[10] The key question is not whether it is ethical to do randomised trials of a new technique, but whether it is ethical to introduce them *outside* randomised trials?

SERNIP classification of new procedures[9]

- Safety and efficacy established; procedure may be used
- Sufficiently close to a procedure of established safety and efficacy to give no reasonable grounds for questioning safety and efficacy; procedure may be used subject to continuing audit
- Safety and efficacy not yet established; procedure requires a fully controlled evaluation and may be used only as part of systematic research, comprising either:
  - an observational study in which all interventions and their outcomes are systematically recorded
  - a randomised controlled trial and advise the Standing Group on Health Technology accordingly
- Safety and/or efficacy shown to be unsatisfactory; procedure should not be used

---

Danger signs for new laparoscopic procedures[10]

- The attractiveness of methods to patients who were informed by the news media of possible benefits without complications
- The attractiveness of the methods of surgeons who saw "bread and butter operations" threatened by non-surgical treatment
- The strong influence of instrument manufacturers for whom rapid dissemination of technology was good business
- The absence of safeguards inherent in the traditional surgical education and the numerous short training courses that were promoted

---

Prospective Randomised Controlled Trials (RCTs)

Prospective randomised controlled trials are famil-

iar methods when a new drug is being compared, either with an existing drug or a placebo (inactive compound). Usually the two drugs are concealed in the same outside capsule or tablet so as to prevent bias, because then neither doctor nor patient knows which is which. It is well known, for example, that certain coloured tablets have more non-specific effect than other colours. When surgical trials are being designed, "blinding" those involved has even greater importance because of the huge placebo (non-specific) effect that surrounds such a dramatic and invasive procedure.[11] (Some estimate that placebo accounts for about 35% of the total effect of the operation). The simplest trial is to compare two operations that are done through the same incision so that the outside looks the same: the Box lists the different methods of blinding. When incisions are different they can be concealed from patients and assessors by applying the same dressings over the wounds.[12]

Methods of "blinding" in surgical trials

- Same incision/approach
  - different procedures inside, e.g. different operations for peptic ulcer[13]
  - sham procedure, e.g. internal mammary ligation[14]
- Different incision – similar dressings, e.g. laparoscopic vs minicholecystectomy[11]
- Same procedure – different effects due to other agents, e.g. sensitisers for photodynamic therapy for Barrett's oesophagus[18]
- Blinding assessors, e.g. non-surgical vs surgical treatment (lithotripsy vs surgery for gallstones)[19] – *essential for adequate assessment of symptoms*

As with drugs trials, placebo (sham) operations have been used in surgical research. An early example from the 1950s was to test whether tying an artery behind the ribs would improve patients with angina by diverting blood to the heart, as some surgeons had claimed. Patients were randomised to a skin incision alone or skin incision plus ligation of the artery.[14] Patients were assessed postoperatively by a doctor who was unaware which operation had been done and he found no difference! The operation was therefore abandoned. Recently a new operation was introduced for Parkinson's disease in which fetal tissue was transplanted into the brain of patients with the disease.[15] Because of doubt about its efficacy, the

National Institutes of Health (NIH) in the USA sponsored a double-blind trial. For patients in the placebo (sham) operation group this meant two anesthetics, a scalp incision, and burr holes nearly through the skull as well as treatment with cyclosporin, a drug given to inhibit rejection of the cells. Patients were told the details of the trial and consented voluntarily, but they were also told that, if they happened to be in the placebo group and the transplant was proved to be successful, they could have it themselves. Drug treatment for the Parkinson's disease was continued in both groups. However, there was a vigorous debate in the medical press about whether or not the trial was ethical.[16, 17] With appropriate safeguards and informed voluntary consent, placebo surgery can be ethical, and the ethics of consent will depend on the degree of risk and what the patients are told to preserve their autonomy.

Another example of a placebo intervention is the laser treatment of Barrett's oesophagus – a premalignant change in its lining.[18] This particular kind of treatment is known as photodynamic therapy (PDT), when a laser light interacts with a sensitising "dye" that is taken up only by the abnormal cells. If the green laser light is shone on cells that do not contain the sensitiser, they are not damaged. The sensitiser is taken by mouth disguised in orange juice so that neither patient nor surgeon knows what is in the drink. Half the patients randomly take the sensitiser, and half do not; both groups have an endoscope passed down their oesophagus and have the light treatment, and in only one group are the premalignant cells damaged. The effect of the treatment is studied some weeks later by two endoscopists who do not know whether or not the sensitiser was given. This blinding is ethical because the risk of the endoscopy is only very slight, and it is carried out with the full knowledge and consent of the patients, who have consented to be randomised for PDT. As in the previous example, the promise that, if the treatment did turn out to be effective, it would be given to the placebo group also makes it ethical, because the patients are not being deprived of possible benefit, only having it delayed. In any case, patients may feel more of a sense of partnership with their surgical researcher if both are blinded in the way they normally are in drug trials.

Intraoperative Studies

A patient under general anaesthetic provides a unique opportunity for research in both human pathophysiology and anaesthetic techniques. Studies of new and different anaesthetic agents come in the same category as trials of new drugs or new surgical techniques and needs special consent. Monitoring physiological response to the operation is part of treatment and is covered by consent to the anaesthetic, unless some apparatus is introduced that carries extra risk, i.e. using a jugular venous catheter to sample blood from the brain or a Swan–Ganz catheter to measure pulmonary arterial pressure in the heart. This is used routinely in some operations but will be an extra procedure in others. However, undertaking another study that is not part of the intended operation, e.g. seeing the response of the gallbladder to hormonal stimulus in patients having a hernia repair, is similar to the second example in the previous section and requires distinct and detailed explanation and consent. If the patient declines, it should in no way affect the operation or the surgeon's attitude to the patient.

Sometimes, surgeons are requested by colleagues to use the opportunity of an open abdomen to implant recording devices for later research, once the patient has recovered from the operation. One example is the use of miniature electrodes on the wall of the intestine to measure intestinal motility (the wires coming out alongside a drain that would normally be inserted during the operation and removed later). Again, two slightly different scenarios can be imagined, one where the operation is on the intestine, so the information obtained directly relates to the procedure, and secondly when the operation is on a different organ. Although both require direct permission from the patient, the type and timing of consent may differ, the first being more closely linked to the consent for treatment.

PATTERNS AND TIMING OF CONSENT FOR SURGICAL RESEARCH

In any clinical research, patients must not be regarded as "guinea pigs" but as partners in the research enterprise – willing partners and indispensable partners without whom the research cannot be done. The ethics of biomedical research involving human subjects have been guided by the Declaration of Helsinki since the 18th World Medical Assembly in Finland in June 1964. It has been amended four times since and is, at present, being updated again. The Declaration makes a distinction between research that is part of treatment and research that is not. When the research involves comparing two operations for the same disease, this is clearly "therapeutic research", but when a non-therapeutic procedure is being done as part of a therapeutic operation, the distinction can easily be blurred. For example, if a patient is joining a randomised controlled trial of two operations, e.g. laparoscopic versus open cholecystectomy, the consent for the trial is a consent for treatment. Of course surgeons must make it clear that patients will be treated if they do not wish to join the trial, but by joining the trial they waive their right to choose one or other treatment. Therefore once the trial has been explained (including the fact that the surgeons do not know which is best, otherwise they would not be doing the trial in the first place), patients are asked to consent to a "trial cholecystectomy" on their treatment consent form.

In the trial that we conducted, which included 200 patients,[12] only two refused to be randomised, one insisting on the first operation, and the other on the second! This typed consent is termed *prerandomisation consent*. The alternative – to randomise first and then obtain consent – can imply that one or other operation has been chosen for the patient, rather than decided by random. The *randomised consent design* has been described by Zelen[20]: those randomised to the standard operation are consented for it as usual. Those randomised for the new operation are asked if they would consent to have it instead of the standard procedure. Those who agree and those who refuse can both combine for analysis on an "intention-to-treat" basis. However, in addition, those who refuse the new operation are combined with the "standard" group for analysis and, if only a few refuse, then the new operation can be assessed properly. If half refuse, then the analysis is more difficult. Alternatively, there are statistical designs, e.g. Bradley–Brewin,[21] that incorporate the patient's choice (*patient preference trials*). In this method patients are divided into four groups, two where the assignment is randomised to one or other operation and two where the patients themselves have chosen one or other operation, having refused to be randomised. If the chosen group are evenly distributed and the patient characteristics are similar, then the data can later be combined, even though other sources of bias may creep in.

When the research is not part of the treatment, e.g. physiological studies during anaesthesia, the consent for treatment can and must be separated from the consent for research. The separation is best achieved by someone other than the operating surgeon obtaining the research consent. Consent in the immediate postoperative period also needs consent separately from the operation, because the studies are not part of the operation. However, it could be argued that consent should wait until afterwards so as not to confuse it with consent for surgery. In the immediate postoperative period the patient is receiving analgesics, many of which also have a sedative effect, and may not be feeling very well: this is not the ideal situation for obtaining free and voluntary consent! It is best then to obtain consent before operation but also make it clear that there will still be a further check or "let-out clause" after operation in case the patient has a change of mind. This of course is not possible with intraoperative research.

Research on organs or tissue that are removed as part of the operation has been the subject of a study by the Nuffield Bioethics Group. This recommends that separate consent for the removal and use of tissue for research should be obtained if the link with the patient is not broken and it is anticipated that the patient may be recontacted at some future date as a result of the research. Patients should also be informed of, and agree to, any intent on the part of researchers to make commercial use of the tissue or to grow "immortalised" cell lines from it. Conversely, if the link between the patient and tissue is broken and the patient has expressed no interest in retaining it, then it can be used without consent. Because of the broken link, the patient can no longer have any control over, or personal interest in, the tissue, other than clinical benefit that might accrue for anyone with similar health needs. Removal of tissue that is not part of the procedure must have separate consent.

The *timing* of consent for research as part of treatment is more controversial. On the one hand, it is important to separate the research element to make it clear that the surgeon's argreement to treat the patient will not alter if he or she declines to join the research study. On the other hand, it could be alarming to add the research element on at the last minute, just before the patient is about to have an operation. It is sometimes important to know before the hospital admission whether or not the patient is to be involved with the project. Therefore the research aspect should usually be mentioned in principle at the initial consultation when the request to treatment is agreed. This allows sufficient time for patients to reflect on the decision: but there should also be an arrangement for withdrawing the consent later if they wish. Timing of consent in relation to randomisation has been discussed above.

The Use of Written Material

Information leaflets are being used more and more in addition to verbal explanations about operations. It is difficult to write these in an appropriate level of detail to suit a wide range of patients. In a carefully planned study where a combination of verbal information and specific or general leaflets were used in patients having wisdom teeth extracted,[22] patient satisfaction (if that is the right criterion) did not relate to the use of leaflets. Other studies have shown greater satisfaction and better postoperative progress if leaflets are used.[23] Research ethics committees usually request to see the exact wording of the explanation leaflet to the patient. Again, having this written down and put in an objective, rather than an emotional way, is important for not prejudicing the patient's decision. However, a study in the USA[24] found that 156 institutions had 549 different consent forms for radiological treatment and research. The clinical forms were shorter but harder to interpret. Many of them needed 15 years of education to understand and some at least college level education! Patients must be given time to read and think about written explanations, not have them pushed into their hands and after a few seconds asked to "sign here". Many surgeons have a research nurse or person independent of the care team to talk to patients after they have had verbal and written explanations, to check that they understand and to answer any questions.

PROBLEMS OF OBTAINING CONSENT FOR SURGICAL RESEARCH

Surgeons' Problems

Only a small proportion of patients are entered into surgical trials. The reasons are various, but include all the extra work and trouble that a trial brings. However, there are situations where a surgeon is so sure that one operation is superior to another (even though he may be wrong) that he does not think it right to randomise and will not agree to take part. Is he acting ethically or should his autonomy be overruled? We have already noted the reasons that surgeons gave in a survey for not putting patients into randomised trials (see Box at p. 193). There are many logistic problems with pressure on operating time and the extra time needed to discuss trials with the patient, but the main reason is lack of equipoise: surgeons do not think (for whatever reason) that the operations could be equally effective or safe or they are not prepared to admit to the patient that they do not know which is best. A surgeon finds this particularly difficult if he or she has invented the new operation!

The surgeon's second problem is how much information to give a patient. This applies to consent for treatment as well as for research. All communications with patients should aim to give information that produces the right understanding. Words can have very different meanings for different people depending on past experience or what has been gleaned from the media. The surgeon is rightly concerned that the patient's consent is based on a real, balanced understanding of the issues and not an emotional overreaction to catch-phrases. Unnecessary or inappropriate anxiety may make a patient refuse a life-saving treatment or refuse to join an important research study. Alternatively, an overoptimistic explanation for research may cause patients to take risks because they have a rose-coloured view of the possible benefits. Written material theoretically overcomes the subjective optimism or pressures of a conversation, but has to be pitched at an average level of understanding and knowledge.

Is there any evidence that giving every detail of possible complications leads to inappropriate anxiety that could lead to a decision that could harm the patient? In order to test this hypothesis, 96 male hernia patients were randomised to receive simple or full information, and the anxiety levels, measured by Speilberger Scores, were assessed before and after.[25] There was no difference between the groups, but this finding cannot be extrapolated to much more serious operations where the risks are considerably greater.

Recall of "informed" consent in 100 patients interviewed 2–5 days after operation[26]

- All aware they had had an operation
- 27 unaware which organ was operated on
- 44 unaware exact nature of operation
- Age (>60) positively correlated

A number of studies have assessed the recall by patients of information that they were given before they consented to operation. The results are not very encouraging[26] (see Box). Does that matter if they remember and understand at the time of signing or agreeing to an operation? A patient needs sufficient information to make the decision valid, but the surgeon can only give information based on means or averages, and many people do not appreciate that it is impossible to give an accurate probability of risks for any individual patient.

Surgeons increasingly worry about the problem of litigation and are always thinking of ways of covering themselves against this risk. In clinical practice, this means a fully documented discussion of the main benefits and risk of the procedure. In research, surgeons are far more protected because Ethics Committees have screened the design and the information that will be given to the patient. Sometimes, legal constraints may override ethical principles (see below) where a patient, for example, does not want to know, and yet the surgeon insists on giving details for his own protection in case, at some future date, the patient changes his mind or his attitude. This brings patients' autonomy into conflict with surgeons' autonomy. Patients need the important facts, but they also have a perfect right not to know facts that they would rather not discuss. The surgeon's dilemma is whether to force facts, like operative death rates, on frightened patients so that relatives are also aware of the dangers and do not blame the surgeon should the patient fail to survive. On the other hand, surgeons have no right to talk to relatives of a fully competent patient without his or her consent. Increasingly, patients and relatives are being told about risk, which only serves to frighten them but to protect the surgeon. When comparing two operations in a trial, surgeons may be required by Ethics Committees to give more detailed information that would be required for standard treatment. If the patient does not want to know, should the information be forced on them just because the treament is part of a trial? Not only are the results of the new operation largely unknown, but information about operations that have been around for many years is often incomplete. Unfortunately, patients often receive "hyped-up" details about a new procedure through the media. Speculative information or spurious data are not part of the consent process. The most important thing for the patient to know is that the surgeon generally does not know!

Should the Learning Curve be Included in a Randomised Controlled Trial?

It is sometimes argued that the trial of a new operation should wait until the learning curve is over and the surgeon has done a certain number; yet the risks are greatest during this period. The patient must know that a procedure is new and untried even if it is not part of a trial, but it is better to start the prospective evaluation early on and use statistical adjustments to allow for the learning process. The learning curve cannot be ignored.

Patients' Problems with Consent for Randomisation

Patients find it unnerving to discover that their surgeon does not know which is the best operation for them. The proposal that one of two operations will be chosen at random by a computer smacks of science fiction. Even more worrying is the suggestion that the surgeon may be "blinded" to which of the two operations he is going to perform until he walks into the operating theatre! However, the concept that the person assessing the results of the operations later will not know which has been done is more acceptable. Time has to be spent explaining to patients why randomisation is necessary and how it is justified when we do not know which operation is best. The blanket principle of "doing no harm" cannot apply to surgery because all operations have a potential for harm. Patients vary in the degree of risk that they are prepared to take. Some of them are prepared to take significant risks, either from altruism or because they hope that they may benefit. What degree of risk is justified, and should the patient be left to decide what risk they are willing to take in the hope of receiving some benefit? Or should they be protected from their own ability to take risks?

Certainly, Ethics Committees see themselves as guardians of the patients against risks suggested by doctors, but should they be protecting patients from themselves? According to the USA federal regulations on research involving human subjects, "Minimal risk means that the probability and magnitude of harm or discomfort anticipated in the research are not greater in and of themselves than those ordinarily encountered in daily life or during the performance of a routine physical or psychological examinations or tests."[27] Another standard that has been suggested is that "sham" surgery should carry no greater risk than that involved in going to the dentist. However, these are referring to patients with mild or no disease. When the treatment of a serious or disabling disease is considered, the degree of justified risk is different. The risk should be related to the *degree of possible benefit*. The more serious the disease the more potential for benefit there is, and the greater the risk patients are prepared to take. Here there is a responsibility of the researchers to ensure that the patients' expectations are not unreal. In this sense they may need to be "protected from themselves".

There is, quite rightly increasing pressure from groups advising on new procedures to suggest that they should only be available to patients within a prospective randomised trial because of the risk of using something new without proper evaluation. This means that the patient can only obtain certain treatments by agreeing to take part in a trial. Is this blackmail, overriding patients' autonomy? The history of the risks of untried operations makes this ethically justified, although it is difficult for some patients to appreciate that they are being protected from unnecessary risk because of the constraints and controls of the research design.

When a serious condition is being treated by two methods, and death or severe disability are possible outcomes, the statistical design can help protect patients. Instead of planning that a fixed number of patients must be entered into each group before any analysis is done (power calculation), a *sequential design* or *group sequential design* can be used, which allows continuous analysis or analysis of small groups as the trial proceeds. This means that differences between the two treatments can be picked up at the earliest opportunity, providing the end points of the trial have been predefined. Ideally, no more patients than absolutely necessary should be exposed to the risk of one treatment or miss the benefit of the other treatment. When patients are deciding whether to join a trial, the philosophy behind the statistical design should be explained as part of the consent process.

CONCLUSION

Surgical research is important, and the orderly evaluation of new procedures is more important than ever. In order for the practice of surgery to flourish, there must be a high degree of trust between surgeons and patients, but that trust must be honoured in all aspects of research by honesty, openness, and respect. When the patient becomes a partner in the research enterprise, and there is careful research design, then scientific progress for the benefit of future patients can coexist peacefully with patient autonomy. Patients should be allowed to take risks in the research enterprise, provided they are given the facts (as far as they are known) and that the risk is commensurate with the potential benefit and the prognosis of the condition. Autonomy is not necessarily honoured by forcing information on an unwilling patient, but by giving patients the freedom to ask for the information they require. The degree of disclosure of information varies in clinical practice according to the seriousness and the urgency of the treatment and availability of alternatives. The same applies in therapeutic clinical research. However, when the research is either of little or no benefit to the patient, the surgeon has a greater duty of disclosure than when it is concerned with treatment.

Patients can be safeguarded by careful research design and statistical planning and all sorts of long legally binding documents can be drawn up: but unless there is mutual trust and partnership between the surgeon and patient, with a large measure of common sense, surgical research will become more and more contentious and future patients will be the losers.

REFERENCES

1. Horton R. Surgical research or comic opera: questions but few answers. *Lancet* 1996; **347**: 984.
2. Solomon MJ, McLeod RS. Should we be performing more randomised controlled trials evaluating surgical operations? *Surgery* 1995; **118**: 459–67.
3. The Lord Chancellor. The Long Fox Memorial Lecture, Bristol Medico-Chirurgical Society, 1998.
4. Hanks P, ed. *Collins dictionary of the English language*. London and Glasgow: Collins, 1982.
5. Campbell AV. Personal communication.
6. National Commission for the Protection of Human Subjects of Biomedical and Behavioural Research. *The Belmont report: Ethical principles for the protection of human subjects of research*. OPRR Reports. Washington, DC. US Government Printing Office, 1979.
7. Katz J. Reflections on informed consent: 40 years after its birth. *J Am Coll Surg* 1998; **186**: 466–74.
8. Cuschieri A. Whither minimal access surgery? Tribulations and expectations. *Am J Surg* 1995; **169**: 9–19.
9. SERNIP – Academy of Medical Royal Colleges, 1 Wimpole Street, London W1M 8AE, UK.

10. Polk H. Quoted by Bernard HR, Hartman TW. Complications after laparoscopic cholecystectomy. *Am J Surg* 1993; **165**: 533–5.

11. Beecher HK. Surgery as a placebo. *JAMA* 1961; **176**: 1102–7.

12. Majeed AW, Troy G, Nicholl JP *et al.* Randomised, prospective, single blind comparison of laparoscopic vs. small-incision cholecystectomy. *Lancet* 1993; **165**: 9–14.

13. Goligher JC, Feather DB, Hall R *et al.* Several standard elective operations for duodenal ulcer: ten to sixteen year clinical results. *Ann Surg* 1979; **189**: 18–24.

14. Cobb LA. Evaluation of internal-mammary-artery ligation by double-blind technic. *New Engl J Med* 1958; **258**: 113–15.

15. Hauser RA, Freeman TB, Snow BJ *et al.* Long-term evaluation of bi-lateral fetal nigral transplantation in Parkinson's disease. *Arch Neurol* 1999; **56**: 179–87.

16. Freeman TB *et al.* Use of placebo surgery in controlled trials of a cellular-based therapy for Parkinson's disease. *New Engl J Med* 1999; **341**: 988–92.

17. Macklin R. The ethical problems with sham surgery in clinical research. *New Engl J Med* 1999; **341**: 992–5.

18. Ackroyd R, Davis MF, Brown NJ, Stephenson J, Stoddard CJ, Reed MWR. Photodynamic therapy for Barrett's oesophagus: A prospective randomised placebo controlled trial. *Endoscopy* 1997; **29**: E17.

19. Nichol JP *et al.* Randomised controlled trial of cost-effectiveness of lithotripsy and open cholecystectomy as treatments for gall bladder stones. *Lancet* 1992; **340**: 801–7.

20. Zelen M. Randomised consent designs for clinical trials: An update. *Stat in Med* 1990; **9**: 645–56.

21. Brewin CR, Bradley C. Patient preferences and randomised clinical trials. *BMJ* 1989; **299**: 313–15.

22. O'Neill P, Humphries GM, Field EA The use of an information leaflet for patients undergoing wisdom tooth removal. *Br J Oral Maxillofacial Surg* 1996; **34**: 331–4.

23. Edwards MH. Satisfying patients' needs for surgical information. *Br J Surg* 1990; **77**: 463–5.

24. Hopper KD, Ten Have TR, Hartzel J. Informed consent forms for clinical and research imaging procedures: how much do patients understand? *Am J Roentgenol* 1995; **164**: 493–6.

25. Kerrigan DD, Thevasagayam RS, Woods TO *et al.* Who's afraid of informed consent? *BMJ* 1993; **306**: 298–300.

26. Byrne DJ, Napier A, Cuschieri A. How informed is signed consent? *BMJ* 1988; **296**: 839–40.

27. 45 CFR 46 (1991).

19 • Informed consent and genetic research

Ruth Chadwick

Does genetic research raise any special issues with regard to informed consent? While there are different views about the importance that should be accorded to informed consent in research, and about the extent to which exceptions to it are permissible, there are also differences of opinion as to whether genetics itselfs gives rise to any specific questions. This has sometimes been discussed under the aspect of whether genetic information should be regarded as special or as just another form of medical information. Article 13 of the UNESCO Declaration of Human Rights and the Genome[1] states that "the responsibilities inherent in the activities of researchers ... should be the subject of particular attention in the framework of research on the genome." What is the basis of this view?

In what follows I shall not be addressing the theoretical basis of informed consent *per se*, in terms of ethical theory. Nor shall I be discussing problems specific to certain vulnerable groups. I take as my starting point the argument of Len Doyal[2] that those who volunteer to participate in research are liable to face risks over and above those normally encountered in the course of medical treatment and therefore they must have the information required to protect themselves, both about those risks and about the goals, methods and possible benefits. I shall address the possible aspects in which informed consent is particularly problematic in genetics and shall divide the areas of possible difference into two categories. The first consists of problems associated with the "informed" aspect of informed consent in genetic research. This category can be subdivided into (a) factors affecting what counts as 'informed' in genetic research and (b) particular features of the information in genetic research, related to the risks and benefits involved. The second category encompasses issues associated with the "consent" aspect of informed consent in genetic research. This includes

facts about the particular nature of consent in genetic research and issues about commercialisation and exploitation. I shall conclude with some reflections on whether there are grounds for regarding informed consent in genetic research differently from its role in other contexts. First, however, it is necessary to ask what is meant by genetic research.

WHAT COUNTS AS GENETIC RESEARCH?

The term "genetic research" is very broad, starting with basic research on the human genome; research into the genetic mechanisms involved in disease; research into the genetic basis of behavioural traits; genetic population research; and trials on gene therapy. The particular kind of genetic research at issue may itself have implications for informed consent. Genetic research on samples collected from particular populations, for example, may pose specific problems for informed consent relating to group consent. Again, there might be differences in potential harms arising out of research or in the type of information at stake. In order to focus particularly on the ways in which informed consent differs from informed consent in other clinical research, I am going to consider the incorporation of a genetic element into clinical trials. What then becomes the focus of analysis is, first, genetic research on the genetic basis of susceptibility to side effects from particular treatments for a condition. Afterwards, the discussion will be broadened to include a wider interpretation of genetic research.

I propose to proceed by examining various scenarios, concerning the collection of samples for genetic research. I do not include here the issues relating to genetic research on samples previously obtained for another purpose, where informed consent was not obtained specifically for genetic research.

Scenario One

Pharmaceutical company Hi-tech is conducting a randomised controlled trial to test the safety and efficacy of a new drug, Extrastrong, for condition Longsuffering. As part of the protocol Hi-tech proposes to collect DNA samples from the population of research subjects receiving Extrastrong (all of whom suffer from Longsuffering) to establish whether there is any relationship between genetic make-up and their response to Extrastrong in terms of either recovery or side effects. The subjects will be asked to give separate consent to taking part in the trial of the drug, on the one hand, and to the genetic aspects of the trial, on the other.

In Scenario One the genetic research is being done on subjects with regard to their specific condition and its treatment. One of the most problematic areas from an ethical point of view, however, concerns the collection of samples for genetic research, which may be on a wide range of genes and conditions. This research need not be carried out on samples collected in the context of a clinical trial but, for present purposes, it will be helpful to complicate the picture by introducing this extra feature. Hence Scenario Two.

Scenario Two

Hi-tech proposes to keep some samples from the trial in Scenario One in order to do research on other genetic markers and the possible links between these markers and conditions other than Longsuffering. In this case those who agree to participate will have their samples stored after the end of the clinical trial in a DNA bank for research on an unspecified range of conditions. The subjects who participate in the aspect of the trial involved in Scenario One will be asked to give a separate consent to the use of their research samples in Scenario Two.

Is there any reason to think there might be specific problems as regards consent to the DNA aspects in Scenarios One and Two, when compared with the drug trial aspect? Looking at the case studies should enable us to identify the potential differences in informed consent in different phases of the trial. This identification will also have relevance for the issue of informed consent in other types of genetic

research. The fact that Scenario Two, in particular, involves the setting up of a DNA bank, is significant because Doyal has presented the case of stored tissue from anonymous donors as one of three exceptions to the requirement for informed consent. However, he goes on to state: "This third exception does not apply to research into the genetic causes of or predispositions to disease where research materials have not been strictly anonymised and where there is any possibility of further patient contact. Here informed consent should always be obtained."[2]

Having outlined these possible scenarios I shall now proceed to examine the aspects in which informed consent might be different in genetic research, beginning with the "informed" part.

BEING "INFORMED" IN GENETIC RESEARCH

What Counts as "Informed" in Genetic Research?

The suggestion that informed consent is particularly problematic in genetic research might be made for a variety of reasons: the degree of public awareness of genetics; the sensitivity of the "information"; and doubts about whether it is *possible* to be informed in this field.

Public awareness and understanding of genetics

Over the past few years there have been calls for raising public awareness of the issues raised by developments in genetics,[3] particularly as applied to medicine. More recently, however, the issue of genetically manipulated food has come to the forefront of public opinion.

There are different aspects to the debate about public understanding. The first relates to worries that genetics is not only poorly understood but that it is also difficult to understand. Despite the claim of the gene's role as a cultural icon,[4] the explanation of what a gene is, is no simple matter, quite apart from differential gene expression. Thus individuals may have a very imprecise idea of what they are consenting to regarding genetic information. Such impressions can be fuelled by representations of genetics in the media and in popular culture, which have produced a vision of choice as compromised between extremes. On the one hand, genetics is depicted as offering cures for genetic diseases: on the other, fears are expressed of scientists "playing God" with all the frightening associations of that phrase.[5] One possible construal of the situation is that people are being sold a narrative of progress in connection with the Human Genome Project, portrayed as the answer to disease (via the promises of gene therapy and designer drugs). On the other hand there is concern that individuals have lost trust in science and therefore in the genetic "information" that they are given, although there is evidence to suggest a difference in attitudes towards medicine and food.

In the light of this situation one view, based on what is described as the "deficit model", is that more information is required to make good the deficit in information, and that public acceptance of new technologies will be facilitated by greater understanding. The deficit model has been increasingly challenged, however, both by querying the notion of a homogeneous unaware "public" and by pointing to the importance of lay interpretations in this area that may reflect mistrust of science for very good historial reasons.[6, 7]

An important distinction must be drawn between the information required for a better understanding of genetics *per se* and the information necessary for individuals to appreciate the implications of genetic information for themselves. In contexts of clinical genetics, the nature of differences of perceptions of risks has long been recognised – individuals may have very different attitudes towards a given lifetime risk of developing breast cancer, for example. It is not only a question of individual attitudes to risk, however, of how "risk-averse" they are, there are also issues about making clear the difference between being genetically *determined* and genetically *predisposed* to develop a condition.

The nature of the information

The second concern about genetic information is that it is particularly sensitive. The considerations that support the (not uncontroversial) view that genetic information is different from other medical information have included the facts that we share genetic information with relatives and that it is not specific to time. This gives such information a predictive aspect, for both individual patients and their relatives, which in turn make the dangers arising out of disclosure particularly acute, because of the possibility of adverse effects on the future course of someone's life. Some have argued for a right not to

know such information.[8] Whilst all these features may be true to a greater or lesser degree of other medical information, these features seem to give rise to different possible interpretations and implications, which may make more likely the unintentional inflicting of harm by researchers.

Another worrying feature of genetic information is the potential way in which it is perceived as intricately bound up with our identities as persons. It has been suggested that DNA is the modern secular equivalent of the soul, or at any rate the guarantor in some sense of who we are.[4] However well grounded this view may or may not be, in this respect the information takes on a new significance, which may affect the nature of informed consent. This is because people are not just taking decisions about allowing the use of some piece of medical information that is incidental to their identity; they are making choices about what may appear to them to be in a deep sense part of themselves. The sensitivity of genetic information thus resides not only in the harms that may ensue from its use, but also from a perception of its association with what is most intimate and personal. This suggests the need at least for special care in informing research participants about what will become of their samples.

It is possible for anyone to be informed?

The third concern about the possibility of being "informed" in this area relates to the idea that it is simply not possible to be genuinely informed of all the risks and benefits in genetic research. The idea behind this concern is that no one can be adequately informed, because it is not possible to foresee the range of uses to which genetic information about someone might be put. It is necessary here to address specifically an important difference between Scenario One, which concerns "narrow" consent related to a specific condition and Scenario Two, which involves "broad" consent on an unspecified range of conditions. It might be argued that it is only broad consent to which this worry relates. On the other hand, even in the case of narrow consent to genetic research on a specific condition, the legal and ethical regulation of this area is still developing, so that individuals are making choices about their samples in an uncertain situation. It is nevertheless possible to inform research participants of the *type* of research, its risks and benefits, and implications for them. It is at this point we need to turn to a specification of the nature of the risks and benefits.

The Nature of the Risks and Benefits

It might be helpful to begin by examining a list of concerns typically expressed about genetic research before placing in that context the particular risks and benefits that might arise from the Longsuffering study. The list of concerns found in the HUGO Statement on the principled conduct of genetic research provides a fairly typical list of the kind of potential harms arising from genetic research:[9]

- fear that genome research could lead to discrimination against and stigmatisation of individuals and populations and be misused to promote racism;
- loss of access to discoveries for research purposes, especially through patenting and commercialisation;
- reduction of human beings to their DNA sequences and attribution of social and other human problems to genetic causes;
- lack of respect for the values, traditions and integrity of populations, families and individuals;
- inadequate engagement of the scientific community with the public in the planning and conduct of genetic research.

Whilst some of these may be several stages removed from a given individual asked to consent to provide a sample for genetic research, it is arguably because of these wider implications that the issue of informed consent is thought to be particularly problematic in the genetic context. Discrimination, in particular, is a live issue relevant to the consent process. It is to a large extent because of the potential for stigmatisation and discrimination, e.g. from insurers and employers, that the informed consent issues involved in genetic research have been so concerned with privacy and confidentiality. The question of racism is also an important one in so far as individuals, who have not consented to participate in a particular research project, may be affected by it, because, for example, a research project may result in information showing that there are predispositions to particular conditions or treatments that are specific to certain minority ethnic groups. This information may be disadvantageous (as well as having potential advantages to people seeking information facilitating their own health-related decisions) not to individuals participating in the trial but to members of the group generally.

In addition to these wider factors, however, there are potential harms for individuals arising, not out of possible actions of third parties, but from their own responses. These are of three kinds: misunderstanding, psychological consequences such as anxiety, and challenges to people's self-concept. On the other hand, as noted above, genetic information also has the potential to benefit individuals by enabling them to make choices about their future, including preventive health interventions. Given the different types of harms and benefits, a crucial factor in the informing process will relate to access to information by third parties and access to information by the research participants themselves, including the possibility of feedback on the results of research on their samples.

Having looked at the range of types of interests that might be affected, let us focus on the Longsuffering trial. The subjects affected by Longsuffering are primarily participating in a trial of a new drug, Extrastrong. For this they will have been informed of the mechanics of a randomised controlled clinical trial and of the possible risks and benefits of taking the trial drug. In addition, however, they are to be asked if they are willing to provide a blood sample that will enable researchers to undertake research into what, if any, is the genetic basis for their response to Extrastrong, if they are taking it.

It is clear, first, that the nature of any possible benefit is very different from what might be involved in the drug trial. In the trial, any given individual might be receiving a placebo, but on the other hand might stand to benefit from a more effective (and immediate) treatment for Longsuffering. In the genetic study, there is no chance that any individual will gain immediate benefit from more effective treatment. Here, the purpose of the research is to find out why some people respond and others do not. The overall aim is to provide more effective treatments in the long term, so that people who do not respond will not be prescribed Extrastrong and vice versa. It is conceivable that trial subjects will be among those who benefit in the long term, but there is no prospect of immediate benefit for any of them. So that is one clear difference: no possibility of immediate benefit, although participation in genetic studies involves the use of blood to test for drug resistance or susceptibility to different types of currently untreatable illness.

What of the risks? Whereas in the drug trial the risk arises out of the possible effects of the drug, in the genetic part of the trial the taking of the blood sample poses a small hazard. Here, it is not the clinical intervention itself that is the focus of concern.

Rather, the risks of giving blood for genetic analysis accrue from the information gained itself, in ways indicated above.

In Scenario One, what people are being asked to consent to is to have their DNA analysed to see if there is any relationship between their DNA and their response to Extrastrong. There is of course potential for misunderstanding of this in so far as it might be thought that participating in this branch of the research would make them more likely to be protected against the side effects of Extrastrong. The problems of mistakenly thinking that individuals might gain therapeutic benefit from participating in a trial, however, are not specific to this context. The truth is that it will not help them but could help other people with their condition in future with regard to appropriate prescribing for that condition.

In Scenario Two, samples are being kept back so that further genetic research may be done in future, with reference to an unspecified range of diseases or conditions. There is a specific issue here about the interpretation of the information. If subjects who agree to participate are informed that research will be done that may link their DNA profile to susceptibility to certain other diseases, there is, of course, potential for misinterpreting this to mean that the research will show that they are inevitably going to develop those diseases. Even if some information is discovered showing them to have a genetic *predisposition* to developing a certain condition other than Longsuffering, however, the question arises of the extent to which feedback is possible in the different scenarios and gives rise to the potential harm arising from distressing information. If the subjects do not have access to the information, they will be protected from the adverse psychological consequences arising from either misunderstanding or correctly understanding the information.

An important difference becomes clear at this point between Scenario One and Scenario Two. For the research in Scenario One to be possible it will be necessary to be able to link the sample with an identified subject, as the point is to track the subject's response to the drug against the genetic basis for this response. In Scenario Two, however, the genetic research is not linked to the specific condition or drug involved in the clinical trial. Scenario Two involves the longer term storage of samples from which identifying references to individual subjects can be removed.

The anonymising of samples, while devised for the protection of subjects against the potential risks of genetic information, may be perceived by some as a disadvantage. This could occur if some discovery arose out of research on an individual's sample that could be of benefit to them. Under conditions of anonymisation, however, there is no possibility of recontacting.

There are different issues involved here and these should be disentangled when informed consent is being discussed. Doyal[2] has suggested that genetic research, where there is the possibility of recontacting, requires informed consent, although research on stored anonymised tissue may be an exception. Where there is no possibility of recontacting, however, subjects need to be informed of this very fact, including the lack of potential benefit to the subjects themselves. It is clear, however, that the issue of identifiability is separate from that of recontacting. Even if the subjects who have given the samples are identifiable, as they must be in Scenario One, it does not follow that they will or should be recontacted. Whether recontacting is permissible or desirable is an ethical issue in its own right. There is a view that if the information is of clinical relevance (as opposed to research results of uncertain value) to identifiable subjects, those subjects have a right to it,[10] but from the perspective of informed consent the essential requirement is that the information must include the procedures relating to the subject's potential access to information: what they will and will not be told.

It becomes clear then, that in the genetic context elements that have to be covered in the informing process include the measures to protect the security of the samples and the identity of the sample sources: who will have access to them and the research results; are they to be coded or will it be possible to break the code; will they be anonymised? The differences with respect to these issues in Scenarios One and Two will need to be explained. The techniques for ensuring anonymity, however, are themselves a possible source of misunderstanding. The degree to which anonymisation can be assured is one area of concern. The explanation of the difference between coded, non-identified, and anonymised is ripe for misunderstanding.

In the context of explaining the risks and benefits, another aspect on which subjects need to be informed concerns the possibility of withdrawing from the study. Individuals may conclude at a later date, perhaps following publicity about harms arising from genetic research, that the risks and benefits are such that they no longer wish to participate.

If subject Jones has contributed a sample in both Scenario One and Scenario Two, what does "withdraw" amount to? If the sample cannot be identified as hers, how can she withdraw? Does this entail physical destruction of the sample? What about the information? Just as different individuals interpret risk differently, they are likely to have differing understandings of concepts such as "anonymise", "destroy".

Having looked at the respects in which the informing process might be particularly problematic in genetic research, I now turn to the issues specific to consent.

CONSENT

The Nature of Consent in Genetic Research

Although the "informed" and the "consent" parts of informed consent are here discussed separately with regard to genetic research, they are of course intimately linked. Incomplete or inadequate information is one way in which consent can be undermined. There are other potential problems, however, that are more closely associated with the "consent" side of the process of obtaining agreement to participate. Uncertainties about voluntariness and coercion are examples. The potential problems to be guarded against (where there is no question of incompetence) are typically specified as duress and undue influence. Once again, however, we must remind ourselves of how genetic research in particular might be relevant to these potential worries. Individuals may, of course, participate in trials because they want to please the doctor – there is a view that even to ask people to participate in research may be coercive to some degree. It might be argued that if subjects have already agreed to participate in a drug trial, they are more likely to agree to participate in the DNA aspects. However, even if there is a chance of this occurring, mention has already been made of concern over the context in which choices are made, with reference to extreme, competing, images of genetics. There are also the historical factors of abuse of genetics. Against the possible "please the doctor" factor, there is a competing pull from fear of what is involved, in terms of exposure to potential harm, in surrendering genetic information about oneself.

Perhaps the most significant way in which the consent might be argued to raise different issues in the case of genetics relates to the subject who is asked to consent. In the case of a drug trial, subjects volunteer to undergo physical risks to their own health. In the context of genetic research, however, an individual's consent may have implications for others, such as their blood relatives. As has already been mentioned, that consent to participate in research by some individuals may indirectly have consequences for groups beyond blood relatives, by demonstrating a genetic predisposition prevalent in a particular minority ethnic group. Indeed, the requirements of protecting communities as opposed to individuals are increasingly an issue,[11] and this is particularly relevant in genetic research.

Commercialisation and Exploitation

Another issue relating to consent is the question of commercial interests in genetic research. It is by now a commonplace that major commercial interests exist in genetic research, interests that shape its pattern and direction. Individuals participating in such research are liable to be asked specifically to sign away any rights that they may have arising out of the commercial exploitation of their samples. Is this problematic for informed consent?

Let us consider Scenario Three.

Scenario Three

Subjects Smith and Jones, who suffer from the condition Longsuffering, agree to participate in the trial of the new treatment Extrastrong. They also agree to participate in the genetic research linking their response with genetic predispositions, and agree to their sample being put in a DNA bank for further as yet unspecified genetic research. Unfortunately Extrastrong does not help Smith and Jones. During the genetic research on their samples, however, it is found that they have a particular genetic characteristic that leads to the development of a highly effective treatment for the condition Ultracommon. The pharmaceutical company markets Miracle-Cure for Ultracommon and makes a substantial profit. Smith and Jones are not entitled to any share in these profits because they signed a consent form acknowledging that they had no right to any commercial benefits arising out of the research.

Arguably this is more of an issue of fairness than of informed consent *per se*. The possibility of financial considerations undermining the possibility of genuine consent is more typically construed as a problem when subjects are being offered inducements, not when they are signing away access to them. It is one thing to say that someone cannot give genuine consent if there are financial considerations involved; it is another to say what is a fair distribution of benefits. If we confine ourselves strictly to the issue of consent, the question turns on first, whether the informed consent process made sufficiently clear the position with regard to the possibilities of commercial exploitation (it will be important that the participants are aware of relevant commercial interests in addition to any humanitarian benefits of research); and secondly, whether the context was one of voluntariness.

This is a real issue, especially with regard to populations or population groups where group consent might be involved. The issue of whether some kind of benefit is owed to research subjects is increasingly discussed. At the time of writing, the Human Genome Organisation (HUGO) is preparing a statement on benefit sharing. In the present context however, Smith and Jones as individuals will have consented to give up any commercial rights and in any case in Scenario Two they cannot be contacted for any sharing of benefits.

DOES GENETIC RESEARCH MERIT A DIFFERENT STANDARD OF INFORMED CONSENT?

There may be concern that informed consent requirements in the context of genetic research are being watered down in the face of strong commercial interests. There are, however, already suggestions that there are types of research to which there may be exceptions to, or different standards of, informed consent. The question seems to turn on what the rationale is for this. There seem to be three main lines of considerations. The first relates to the potential for harm to the subject; the second relates to the likelihood of the harm occurring. In genetic research the potential for harm appears to be significant not only to individual subjects but also to groups of which they form a part. The nature of the harm tends to be associated with the use of and access to information. That is why there is so much emphasis on the confidentiality and privacy issues in genetic research, and why Len Doyal insists on fully informed consent where there is any possibility of recontacting.

There is a third consideration, however, and that relates to the practicability of the research. In the case of long-term research on samples in DNA banks, it would be impracticable to contact all the sample sources for each and every piece of research, and this could itself constitute a source of harm. This point suggests a trade-off. Some degree of informed consent is traded against the benefits of genetic research, via extra protection in the form of anonymisation.[12]

CONCLUSION

We have seen that there are indeed significant respects in which genetic research raises particular problems for informed consent. The nature of the informing process is complicated by the sensitivity of the particular subject matter and the social context in which it is delivered. The risks arise out of the information itself, which leads to the issue of privacy protection becoming central; and there is no possibility of benefit to the sample source in the scenarios we have been considering. Consent of an individual may have implications for others and the debate takes place in the context of vast commercial interests.

It is also clear that the number of options for potential research subjects includes a number of variables. The US National Bioethics Advisory Commission lists six different permutations, according to whether subjects wish to permit identified or only unidentified use of their samples; whether they wish to participate in one particular study only or in any research; and whether they wish to permit further contact or not.[13] Some empirical research has been undertaken on potential participants' concerns and willingness to take part in such research, but more is needed with different population groups.[14]

In the current situation the essential questions are: what are the interests that need to be protected, and by what mechanisms can they be safeguarded? Specifically, can informed consent can adequately protect the interests of research participants? On the one hand calls for raising public awareness constitute an attempt to address the perceived deficit in information and understanding about genetics, an attempt to change the context in which choices are made. On the other hand there is a view that where long-term storage of samples is concerned, anonymisation constitutes a protection that reduces the need for informed consent. In the light of the pressures arising from the feasibility of certain types of research and the potential harms to groups, too much cannot be expected of individual informed consent, a doctrine that was not designed to deal with scenarios of this type and scale. In so far as informed consent does have a role in protecting interests in genetic research, it has been argued here that what is both different and important for the informed consent process is the type of research; the particular nature of the risks and benefits; the possibility of access to one's own results and protection from access by others; and the commercial interests involved. This is a necessary starting point. Genetic technology is leading us to revisit and rethink traditions of medical ethics, however. More work is needed on what would count as sufficient protection of relevant interests.

REFERENCES

1. UNESCO. *Universal declaration on the human genome and human rights*. 1997.
2. Doyal L. Journals should not publish research to which patients have not given fully informed consent – with three exceptions *BMJ* 1997; **314**: 1107–11.
3. Nuffield Council on Bioethics. *Genetic screening: ethical issues*. London: Nuffield Council on Bioethics, 1993.
4. Nelkin D, Lindee MS. *The DNA mystique: the gene as cultural icon*. New York: W. H. Freeman, 1995.
5. Chadwick R. Playing God. *Cogito* 1989; **3**.
6. Kerr A, Cunningham-Burley S, Amos A. The new genetics and health: mobilizing lay expertise. *Publ Underst Sci* 1998; **7**: 41–60.
7. Kerr A, Cunningham-Burley S, Amos A. Drawing the line: an analysis of lay people's discussions about the new genetics. *Publ Underst Sci* 1998; **7**: 113–33.
8. Chadwick R, Levitt MA, Shickle D (eds) *The right to know and the right not to know*. Aldershot: Avebury, 1997.
9. Human Genome Organisation (HUGO) Ethics Committee. Statement on the principled conduct of genetic research. *Genome Dig* 1996; **3**: 2–3.
10. Medical Research Council. Human tissue and biological samples for use in research: report of the Medical Research Council Working Group to develop operational and ethical guidelines. London: MRC, 1999.
11. Weijer C. Protecting communities in research: philosophical and pragmatic challenges. *Cambridge Qu Healthcare Ethics* 1999; **8**: 501–13.
12. HUGO Ethics Committee. Statement on DNA sampling: control and access. *Genome Dig* 1999; **6**: 8–9.
13. National Bioethics Advisory Commission. Research involving human biological materials: ethical issues and policy guidance. Rockville, Maryland: NBAC, 1999.
14. Merz JF, Sankar P. DNA banking: an empirical study of a proposed consent form. In: Weir RF (ed.), *Stored tissue samples: ethical, legal and public policy implications*. University of Iowa Press, 1998.

20 · Informed consent and HIV: public health versus private lives

Rebecca Bennett

Estimates from the Joint United Nations Programme on HIV/AIDS (UNAIDS) and the World Health Organization (WHO) suggested that 32.4 million adults and 1.2 million children will be living with HIV by the end of 1999. In 1999 alone around 5.6 million people became infected with HIV and around 2.6 million people died from HIV/AIDS; 95% of all those infected with HIV live in the developing world.[1] With so many affected by HIV and this number continuing to rise, research into the disease and work on the development of possible treatments and vaccines is of vital importance. However, whilst information gathering is important, this must be balaced against the individual's rights to autonomy and privacy. Thus, when considering policy on HIV research, we are faced by the familiar tension between the interests of public health and interests of individuals.

This chapter argues that, rather than patient autonomy being a reason for demoting the importance of the interests of individuals, public health interests are best served if patient autonomy is upheld in the area of HIV research. The requirement of informed consent in HIV medical research not only removes any confusion as to the nature and the purpose of such studies but also allows a valuable opportunity to provide information about HIV to individuals in a non-coercive atmosphere, a recognised contributing factor to prevention. Whilst research studies may suffer in terms of levels of participation, this risk is outweighed by the benefits upholding patient autonomy and increasing knowledge of HIV and AIDS.

AUTONOMY, INFORMED CONSENT, AND PUBLIC POLICY

The last two decades have not only witnessed a dramatic increase of individuals effected by HIV, but also the gradual evolution of a doctrine of patient autonomy. Respect for patient autonomy is fully endorsed in the writings of most ethicists and at least partially now recognised and enforced by the law and observed in medical practice. Patient autonomy is increasingly and rightly perceived as a manifestation of the individual's rights of self-determination and privacy, universally regarded as a pillar of civil liberty. It is acknowledged that the state should refrain from intervention in private lives save where the individual's health state or lifestyle endangers others. Health, more and more, is a matter of private choice, as is the decision as to whether or not to undergo medical treatment.

Whilst it is held to be important that individuals are able to exercise their own choices with regard to their health and lifestyle, it is also assumed that nation states are responsible for the protection of citizens against threats to their lives, including threats in the shape of illness or disease. Thus, when considering social policy in the area of public health, we are faced with a "balancing act" between respecting individual autonomy on the one hand and the state's responsibility to protect others on the other.

The development of social policy relating to HIV/AIDS illustrates this tension between individual autonomy and public health responsibilities. The threat posed to the community by HIV/AIDS has forced a reconsideration of any concept of absolute autonomy. It is held as important that individual autonomy and privacy should be protected, especially when we are dealing with a disease that may not only have disastrous health consequences but may also lead to stigmatisation and discrimination. It is, however, also imperative that greater knowledge of HIV is developed, including the undertaking of surveys to discover the distribution and transmission routes, and clinical trials to discover the effects of the disease and the effectiveness of possible treatments. The urgent need to develop effective preventative and therapeutic measures appears at times to conflict with the principle of patient autonomy and, in particular, the issue of informed consent.

Informed consent is generally seen as essential in the testing and treatment of HIV. In the 1980s non-consensual testing of individuals and even so-called "high risk groups"[2] was not uncommon, but it is now usually assumed that such policies are not only morally offensive but also ineffective in terms of disease prevention. Non-consensual testing of individuals and groups occurred in the 1980s, particularly in Eastern European Countries including Bulgaria, Hungary, Romania and Poland. It has been argued,[3] for instance, that while the testing process is an important part of any AIDS prevention strategy, it may be that it is the information given in pre- and post-test counselling that is important not necessarily the test itself. If testing is undertaken in a non-consensual or coercive situation, then it is less likely that information and counselling given will be easily accepted. It is for this reason that it is normally assumed that an HIV test should not only be undertaken on a voluntary rather than coercive basis, but that it should also be accompanied by adequate pre- and post-test counselling.

Legislation, such as the British Public Health (Control of Disease) Act 1984 or the German Federal Law on Contagious Diseases (1964), does set public health precedents regarding the non-consensual treatment of individuals infected with communicable diseases. However, such legislation was originally designed to cope with communicable diseases such as cholera, typhus, and tuberculosis, which differ in significant ways from HIV/AIDS. Diseases such as cholera, typhus, and tuberculosis are both more highly contagious than HIV and communicable in circumstances that allow little scope for an individual to protect himself from contracting that disease. Moreover, treatment for such diseases is generally available and effective, and patients contracting the disease are unlikely to be subject to social ostracism once the treatment takes effect. The Public Health (Infectious Diseases) Regulations 1988 extend to HIV provisions of the UK. Public Health Act 1984 providing for the compulsory detention and treatment of people with AIDS. However, owing to the differences that arguably set HIV apart from other communicable diseases, there is a great reluctance to invoke its powers to compel testing and treatment in the case of HIV and AIDS. In fact there

has only been one reported occasion where this power of coercive treatment has been used in the UK. Generally, policy regarding HIV testing and treatment has strongly emphasised the need for informed consent. For instance, the UK General Medical Council (GMC) argues that explicit informed consent must always be given for named HIV testing.[4]

This tendency to treat those with HIV/AIDS differently from individuals with other communicable diseases has been described as "HIV/AIDS exceptionalism".[5] Instead of the traditional approach to communicable disease control, policy relating to HIV and AIDS emphasises medical confidentiality and informed consent. Happily in the therapeutic and preventative aspects of HIV, the interests of the individual appear to coincide with the wider public health interests of the community. There is little to be gained by non-consensual testing and treatment: informed consent for testing may actually be an important factor in prevention. However, there are strong arguments to suggest that insistence on informed consent is not always conducive to efficient research programmes in the area of HIV and AIDS. A number of these claims focus on the practices of anonymous HIV testing as part of serosurveillance programmes, HIV testing in blinded clinical studies, and consent issues with regard to vaccine and treatment trials in developing countries.

ANONYMOUS SEROSURVEILLANCE TESTING FOR HIV

It is estimated that around half those infected with HIV in England and Wales remain undiagnosed.[6] Without any mandatory screening programmes it is likely that there will always be a considerable proportion of those infected with HIV who remain undiagnosed. Voluntary testing, by its very nature does not provide an accurate picture of HIV infection. In order to be able to gain detailed and accurate understanding of HIV and its transmission routes, effective epidemiological surveillance systems need to be put into place. Many countries have implemented anonymous or unlinked testing to give a picture of HIV infection while protecting the autonomy and privacy of the individual.

Anonymous HIV serosurveys, such as those developed in the United Kingdom, normally entail the testing of blood already taken for other purposes and inevitably involve the testing of specific groups in society. For instance, in the United Kingdom such testing involves the testing of patients attending antenatal care, general practices, genitourinary medicine (GUM) clinic services, and hospitals. Patients attending participating centres are notified by leaflets and notices that their blood may be tested anonymously.

Those who advocate the use of anonymous screening programmes for HIV argue that informed consent is not necessary for this kind of HIV test. They maintain that this type of screening involves no adverse consequences for the patient. The testing procedure is non-invasive as it tests "left-over" blood taken for other clinical reasons. Since any information gained by the test is coded and cannot be traced back to the individual, no one, including the patient, will ever be aware of any named individual's HIV status as a result of the screening. To require informed consent for participation in these HIV serosurveys would require time and money being spent on informing patients and may result in an increase in the numbers of patients refusing to participating in the survey.

Those opposed to this type of research argue that involuntary screening of this kind constitutes an unjustifiable violation of patient autonomy. Two apparently very different arguments have been used. First, it is argued that it is the lack of explicit informed consent that constitutes a violation of patient autonomy. Just as individuals are normally assumed to have a right to refuse any medical treatment, they should be made aware of any additional tests being made and have the opportunity to refuse permission for these tests. A second kind of argument against the present system of anonymised testing argues that those tested have the right to know the result of the test, especially if the test is positive, in order to make fully autonomous choices about their future. It is claimed that, if information exists that could influence an individual's future choices then that information must be disclosed in order for the individual to make fully informed choices about the future. We will consider these two criticisms of anonymous screening in turn.

Does a lack of explicit informed consent present an unjustifiable infringement on patient autonomy?

Whilst The World Medical Association Declaration of Helsinki strongly emphasises the prerequisite of

informed consent for any human research, it does contain a clause that states that there may be circumstances in which informed consent is not required.[7] Len Doyal echoes this, arguing that whilst in general informed consent must be gained before individuals may participate in any medical research, anonymised testing of tissue or other stored clinical material (for example, blood) is an ethically justifiable exception to this rule. If every effort is made to assure anonymity of these samples, then it seems that there is little chance of adverse consequences for individuals and the research data should be of great value to many.

However, although there are compelling reasons to accept the lack of informed consent for these kinds of anonymised testing programmes, it is not clear that requiring informed consent would be a less preferable option. We will return to this later.

Do patients have a right to know the results of anonymous testing? Do healthcare professionals have a duty to tell them?

It has been argued that anonymous screening is unethical, as it not only compromises individual autonomy by "denying" individuals information about their health state but also compromises the healthcare professional's duty of care towards the patient. For example, focusing on the anonymous testing of pregnant women, Paquita de Zulueta argues that "the ethics of anonymised testing urgently needs reappraisal."[8] She explains:

> This situation is analogous to non-therapeutic research, and should meet the same rigorous criteria for informed consent. The *procedure* is not important. The blood is being taken anyway for other tests (which she has presumably consented to), and only if there is some left over is it tested anonymously for HIV. It is the anonymisation of the *result* which is crucial. Since the woman is being asked voluntarily to relinquish the opportunity to learn the result, she needs to know the advantages and disadvantages of doing so. Put it another way, she needs to know the benefits and burdens of receiving the result.

Zulueta argues that anonymisation deprives pregnant women of the opportunity to benefit. If a woman is aware that she is HIV positive, she will be able to seek treatment. She may take measures to protect others from infection and can make more informed choices about her future. Information about one's HIV status may be even more poignant for pregnant women. If a pregnant woman is aware of her HIV positive status, she may be able to take measures to reduce the chance of passing on the infection to her future child.

Results from an American–French trial that involved the use of zidovudine during pregnancy, labour, and in the neonatal period, indicated a two-thirds reduction (from 25.5 to 8.3%) in the risk of infection for the infant.[9] Evidence also exists that breastfeeding approximately doubles the risk of HIV transmission,[10] and that delivery by caesarean section may reduce the rate of vertical transmission.[11]

In the UK, between 1988 and 1996, unlinked anonymous surveys detected 1459 births to HIV infected mothers. Of these only 23% (340 births) were to mothers whose infection had been reported as diagnosed before birth.[12] Combined with the evidence for risk reduction, this has led to widespread calls for routine and even mandatory testing of pregnant women for HIV.[13–17]

Zulueta goes on to suggest that the healthcare professional's duty of care towards her patient is compromised by anonymised HIV testing in pregnancy. Zulueta argues that, "When a patient consents to have a blood test, the implicit assumption is that the test is for information that will benefit the patient. The patient has a right to be informed of the results of the test."[8] Not to inform patients of a positive HIV test, it is claimed, constitutes a failure in the health professional's duty of care and "is a throw-back to the old days when physicians generally did not inform patients of the diagnosis of cancer."[8] The claim is that not to inform patients of a positive test is a clear instance of paternalism and thus unacceptable.

Whilst it is manifestly wrong not to inform a patient of the result of a test she has consented to, this is not the case with anonymised test. No consent has been given for the test, the patient may not even be aware that she has been tested. Thus, it would seem that there is no obligation in this case to inform the patient of results they have not sanctioned. To inform a patient in this way would seem to be an extremely paternalistic course of action, made on the assumption that the healthcare professional knows best what information the patient requires.

Pinching argues that the problem with this argument against anonymous testing of pregnant women is that Zulueta fails to understand a key distinction that:

> [T]he unlinked (anonymised) seroprevalence surveillance (screening) programmes, including that on pregnant women, comprise research studies that are

designed to inform policy and practice, as well as individual decision making. They are not screening for the purpose of clinical care.[18]

Another argument that has some force is that the real focus of Zulueta's argument is not on anonymous testing *per se* but on the fact that pregnant women are not given sufficient opportunity to discover their HIV status by undergoing named testing. What is wrong with anonymous testing of pregnant women for HIV, Zulueta is arguing, is that it leads to neglecting the need of women for information about HIV testing and possible treatments. However, this is a separate issue. Anonymised testing is not the appropriate means for diagnosing HIV infection in named individuals; that role is fulfilled by voluntary named HIV testing programmes that include counselling and support. Informing women of positive HIV test results gained as result of "anonymous" testing would be tantamount to the mandatory testing of pregnant women, something I would argue is not acceptable, for the same reasons that it is not acceptable for any other group in society. Zulueta's worries about anonymous HIV testing, it seems, could be allayed if anonymous testing were accompanied by routine *named* HIV testing, or at least routine offering of a *named* HIV test. (Whether this is actually appropriate for pregnant women is another matter.)[19]

So while objections to anonymised testing based on frustration with the lack of promotion of HIV counselling and named testing may not provide convincing evidence that anonymised testing is ethically unacceptable, such objections do raise valuable and important issues. It may be that there is a need to clarify both the present purpose of anonymous testing and to give more information about HIV and HIV testing.

At present, although no explicit informed consent is required, all centres in the UK involved in anonymous screening are mandated to display posters and leaflets that inform patients that their blood may be anonymously tested for HIV. However, no attempt is made to monitor whether patients actually read these notices or understand what anonymous screening entails. As a result, a recent survey showed that 31.5% of randomly selected UK citizens were aware that blood taken as part of antenatal care, or in general practices, genito urinary medicine (GUM) clinic services and hospitals may be anonymously tested for HIV.[20] According to this survey it would seem that most individuals are not aware of the notices explaining anonymous screening. Further, whilst a considerable proportion *are* aware that screening occurs, this does not necessarily mean that they understand what anonymisation entails. Zulueta points out that:

> The Institute of Medical Ethics accepted the proposal that 'most people do not readily understand what anonymised testing means'. Kahtan gives an example of a patient whose child was later diagnosed as having HIV-related illness after she was tested prenatally, but anonymously. She was bewildered that she was not informed of the result: "… but surely, if they found something wrong they'd tell you, would't they?" … Kahtan's example suggests an ingrained tendency to rely on the medical profession. Patient's cannot grasp the fact that they are being asked to waive their rights, as their trust in health care professionals to protect their interests is so powerful.[8]

Although possible confusion of this kind is worrying, the solution does not lie in informing patients of positive HIV test results gained by anonymous testing, but perhaps in requiring that patients participating in such studies understand the nature of the testing programme involved, i.e. they are required to give informed consent to the anonymised serosurveillance testing.

Requiring informed consent for participation in anonymous serosurveys may be costly in terms of time and resources. It may also mean that high participation rates are no longer guaranteed. However, it could be argued that the cost of informing patients is well spent if it removes confusion about the nature of the anonymous test and also allows provision to discuss HIV and the possibility of named voluntary testing. It could also be argued that there is no reason why participation rates should be severely depleted. If those undertaking the study are confident that anonymity can be maintained and are convinced of the importance of such a study, why could this information not be imparted to potential participants? To assume that either healthcare professionals are unable to explain the study effectively, or that potential participants could not understand what the study entails or would be unwilling to take part in such important research seems at best questionable. Simple reliance on signs and notices in this regard is surely unsatisfactory.

HIV TESTING IN BLINDED CLINICAL STUDIES

HIV testing in blinded clinical studies raises similar issues to those already discussed in the context of anonymised serosurveillance testing. However, there are important differences between the two modes of research. In order to explore these differences in detail we shall use as an example the blinded HIV testing in a South African study exploring the impact of HIV status on the outcome of patients admitted to intensive care units for diseases unrelated to HIV.[21] This was a double-blind study where all patients admitted to a surgical intensive care unit over a 6-month period were tested for HIV. Informed consent was not sought for this testing. The rationale behind the study is explained as follows:

> Limited resources and the high cost of intensive care have compelled clinicians to rationalise the allocation of resources. For example, in our unit it is policy not to admit patients with incurable malignant disease, end stage liver disease, and patients with multiple organ failure who are deemed non-salvageable. The lack of objective data made it unclear whether patients with HIV infection should be treated similarly. To allow rationalisation of the admissions policy with respect to these patients we conducted a prospective study to determine the prevalence of HIV infection among patients admitted to the unit and assess the impact of HIV status (HIV positive, HIV negative, AIDS) on outcome.[21]

Although staff and patients were blinded to the results of the HIV tests while the patient was treated in the unit, on discharge patients were informed that they had been tested for HIV and given the option of knowing the result of this test. The results of the tests were disclosed to the research team after the patient was discharged and removed from laboratory records on conclusion of the study. For the purpose of this paper we shall concentrate on the issue of informed consent in this study and leave aside for others the resource allocation issues it raises.

It was argued that it was justifiable to waive the general prerequisite of informed consent in this particular study. A number of reasons for this were given. It was claimed that in many cases patients admitted to the unit were unable to consent to the study as they were 'critically ill', that the clinical implications of the study were of sufficient importance to justify waiving the patient's right to informed consent and that every effort was made to ensure that indiscriminate disclose of test results did not occur.[22]

There are clearly similarities between this case and the previously discussed case of anonymised HIV testing. The lack of informed consent to participation in this study guaranteed a high participation rate and thus comprehensive results. It was argued that the risk of adverse consequences of testing to the patients was minimal, and the value of the expected results would be significant to counteract any adverse effects. However, whilst there may be compelling reasons to accept the admission of informed consent for anonymised serosurveillance testing, these reasons do not necessarily hold for blinded clinical studies such as the one described here.

It was held that, as samples tested for HIV as part of anonymised serosurveys were coded and could not be traced back to individual patients, there were good reasons for excluding anonymised testing from the usual requirement of informed consent. However, in the case of this blinded study the results of the test were more open to accidental disclosure not only because test results remained linked to named patients, but also because the study included a clear intention to inform the patients of the results of the test.

When others are aware of your HIV status, then there is always not only a chance of unsolicited disclosure but also perhaps equally importantly, compromise in respect for patient autonomy. As Benatar and Benatar point out:

> Knowing that there is an unidentified person who has HIV does not inhibit that person's autonomy or violate his or her privacy. By contrast, obtaining the knowledge that an identifiable person has HIV is an invasion of the person's privacy if he or she has not consented to this information being obtained.[23]

When others are aware of a patient's HIV status then that patient does not have the control over information about him- or herself that true patient autonomy would seem to require. Only by obtaining informed consent to linked HIV testing can patient autonomy be truly respected. If this condition is to be overridden, there would have to be strong evidence to justify this approach.

Further, for reasons related to those given by Zulueta, it appears that the researchers felt it was important that participants have access to their test result, even though they had not consented to potentially receiving this information. The problem with this is that offering voluntary testing is not equivalent to offering to disclose the results of tests already undertaken without consent; if it were, then there would be no ethical problem with testing any patient for a condition without consent but requiring consent for the result. Such a suggestion is clear-

ly not ethically unproblematic. Again, the problem here is with control over information. In both instances patients may choose whether they receive information about their HIV status, but only where testing is informed and voluntary do patients have control over this information, it being up to the patient whether healthcare professionals become aware of their patient's HIV status.

In order to justify a blinded study like the one discussed here, strong arguments to justify infringements of patient autonomy would have to be produced. Now, it may be that arguments offered in support of this trial have some weight. It may well be that the research is of such importance as to justify waiving the patient's right to informed consent and it may even have been the case that as a result of the diligence of the researchers no indiscriminate disclosure of medical records took place. What is not clear is whether these arguments provide evidence so strong that it overrides the need for informed consent. This is especially evident when one considers the possible alternatives to blinded studies like these.

It appears that underlying the South African HIV study was the dual purpose, not only to gain valuable information about HIV but also to provide information about HIV to those who may be infected. If both of these purposes were accepted as valuable and legitimate then they could have both been fulfilled by requiring informed consent. This requirement of informed consent may reduce uptake slightly and perhaps delay publishing of results. On the other hand, insistence on informed consent would have allowed patients access to information about HIV and the power to choose whether they wished to be tested for HIV and to know the results of that test. There seems no strong evidence to prefer blinded research in this instance to participation requiring informed consent.

VACCINE AND TREATMENT TRIALS IN DEVELOPING COUNTRIES

Accessible treatments and vaccines against HIV are potentially crucial weapons in the fight against HIV and AIDS, particularly in poor or "developing" countries where existing antiviral treatments are not generally available. Although clinical trials of HIV vaccines and treatments began in Europe and the USA, an increasing number of trials are now taking place or are proposed to take place within developing countries. The trialing of HIV vaccines and treatments in developing countries raises a great number of ethical problems, but again in this chapter we will concentrate on issues of informed consent.

Vaccine Trials

While the need for research into an effective HIV vaccine is urgent, by 1999 only two phase III efficacy trials of experimental HIV vaccines had begun, one in the USA and another in Thailand.[24] Phase III trials are randomised, controlled, large-scale, efficacy trials, which are only completed after the vaccines have been tested for safety and immunogenicity in human subjects (phase I and phase II trials).

VaxGen, a private biotechnology company based in San Francisco, has begun the first large-scale trial of an AIDS vaccine outside the USA. The vaccine is designed to protect individuals from two strains of HIV prevalent in Thailand; 2500 intravenous drug users will participate in the trial. VaxGen, is also behind the trial of a closely related candidate vaccine to be administered to 5000 volunteers in the USA.[25]

The large-scale Thai vaccine trial is thought to be the first of many that will be conducted in developing countries. There are number of reasons why developing countries are deemed highly appropriate locations for phase III HIV vaccine trials. Phase III trials must be conducted within populations with a high incidence of HIV, and 95% of all infections occur in developing countries. It is important that HIV vaccines be tested in different areas of the world so that their effectiveness against different HIV strains and transmission routes can be gauged.[24]

1999 also saw the instigation of the first AIDS vaccine trial in Africa by the Pasteur Merieux Connaught, a division of France's Rhône-Polenc Group. This is a phase I, and therefore small-scale, trial designed to determine whether the vaccine is safe and can be tolerated by an African population, and if it will generate a significant immune response. The vaccine being used is based on a version of the canarypox virus, which has been genetically engineered to include three HIV genes.[25] Of the 40 participants in the trial, half will get the vaccine, 10 will get a similar canarypox-based vaccine for rabies, and 10 will get dummy injections.

Although this is a small-scale trial, it is an important step in the area of vaccine development. As Dr Jerrold Ellner, one of the researchers involved in the trial points out, "Although small in size, this trial is important symbolically as a first critical step in developing an effective vaccine for Africa."[26] Whilst more than 45 vaccine trials are underway in the USA this is the first in Africa and is likely to pave the way for many more trials in Africa and other developing countries.

Bending the Rules?

It has been argued that because of the devastating scale of HIV in developing countries, the usual research protocols should be relaxed in order that research be completed as quickly as possible. For instance, it was the debate over HIV clinical trials in the developing world that prompted the World Medical Association to begin talks in May 2000 to look at a new draft of the Declaration of Helsinki. It is thought that this may result in individual countries amending guidelines governing clinical trials allowing a relaxation of the usual standards.[27] Marcia Angell describes this trend as a "general retreat from the clear principles enunciated in the Nuremberg Code and the Declaration of Helsinki."[28]

In line with this trend it has been suggested that the usual insistence on individual informed consent should be waived in the case of trials in developing countries. It has been argued that informed consent not only holds up progress towards finding a vaccine but also prevents potential participants from benefitting from trials: involvement in a vaccine trial may be of therapeutic value to participants. There are also those who argue that it is insensitive to local custom to require individual informed consent, claiming that is it more culturally sensitive to gain "group consent" from family members or community elders.[29] Moreover, it has been argued that many citizens of developing countries may be too limited in their education and experience to be able to give informed consent to participation in vaccine trials.[30]

However, despite these arguments, an international consultation process conducted by the Joint United Nations Programme on HIV/AIDS (UNAIDS) unequivocally stresses that:

> Although procedural steps in obtaining consent may vary from one country or region to another, participants in all three regional consultations unanimously concurred that in no circumstances, such as cultures in which women are normally not accorded decision-making authority, may the requirement for individuals to provide voluntary, informed consent on their own behalf be abandoned or weakened.[24]

Although all the examples of research into HIV and HIV vaccines dealt with in this paper are clearly valuable and worthwhile activities, this fact does not conflict with the need to respect individual autonomy. There seems no compelling reason why all efforts should not be made to obtain fully informed consent from potential participants in any HIV study. If researchers intend, as they undoubtedly should, to protect the rights of individual participants in research, then it is not clear whether, if this is explained in an appropriate manner, individuals will refuse to participate. There seems little to be gained from abandoning informed consent in these contexts. Waiving informed consent for HIV research will only increase confusion and mistrust, and misses a vital opportunity to provide information that may or may not be useful to individuals about HIV. If it is felt important that public health policy not only amasses information about HIV but also imparts information to individual citizens, then it seems that the most effective way of doing this is to *require* not abandon informed consent.

Treatment Trials

Marcia Angell, commenting on the ethics of clinical research in developing countries, has drawn parallels with the Tuskegee Study of Untreated Syphilis. This notorious study involved 412 African-American men infected with syphilis who were deliberately left untreated from 1932 to 1972 so that the natural history of syphilis could be determined.[31] Even when penicillin was discovered to be an effective treatment for syphilis they were not offered treatment. This study was clearly ethically unjustifiable. Not only were individuals who were known to be infected not offered the available treatment, but subjects were not informed about the study and did not consent to any of it.

Angell argues that the Tuskegee study is analogous to recent clinical trials of potential HIV treatments undertaken in developing countries. It is suggested that those who defended the Tuskegee study did so for similar reasons to those used in the defence of certain clinical trials of potential HIV treatments. The trials Angell has in mind are those like the ongoing trials of interventions to reduce perinatal transmission of HIV in developing countries.

In 1994 the AIDS Clinical Trials Group protocol 076 (ACTG 076) provided evidence that the use of zidovudine during pregnancy and labour could significantly reduce the rate of vertical transmission of HIV.[9] This use of zidovudine is now routinely recommended for all HIV-positive pregnant women. However, the 076 protocol involves careful monitoring, the use of expensive drugs, and refraining from breastfeeding. For pregnant women in developing countries this protocol is likely to be inaccessible. Estimated at being $800 per mother and infant, the cost of the amount of zidovudine used in the 076 protocol is likely to be prohibitive for pregnant women in developing countries.[32] Researchers therefore are attempting to discover a treatment that is as effective at reducing vertical transmission of HIV but at a fraction of the cost, so that children born to pregnant women infected with HIV in developing countries may benefit.

Lurie and Wolfe give a helpful summary of the trials that were ongoing in 1997 into the reduction of perinatal transmission of HIV:

> Primarily on the basis of documents obtained by from the Centres for Disease Control and Prevention (CDC), we have identified 18 randomized, controlled trials of interventions to prevent perinatal HIV transmission that either began to enroll patients after the ACTG 076 study was completed or have not yet begun to enroll patients. The studies are designed to evaluate a variety of interventions: antiretroviral drugs such as zidovudine (usually regimes that are less expensive or complex than the ACTG 076 regime), vitamin A and its derivatives, intrapartum vaginal washing, and HIV immune globulin, a form of immunotherapy. These trials involve a total of more than 17,000 women.
>
> In the two studies being performed in the United States, the patients in all the study groups have unrestricted access to zidovudine or other antiretroviral drugs. In 15 of the 16 trials in developing countries, however, some or all of the patients are not provided with antiretroviral drugs.[33]

Angell argues that where there is an existing effective treatment it is unethical to compare a potential treatment with a placebo as is the case with the many trials in the developing world of potential HIV treatment, including those aiming to reduce vertical transmission rates. Angell argues that, "It should not be argued that it [a HIV treatment trial involving a placebo group] was ethical because no prophylaxis is the 'local standard of care' ...."[28] Such trials are compared to the Tuskegee Study with the claim that their justifications are similar. Angell claims that the Tuskegee Study was justified on the grounds that the subjects "probably would not have been treated anyway, so the investigators were merely observing what would have happened if there were no study; and that the study was important."[28] Angell suggests that placebo trials into reducing perinatal HIV transmission are justified on similar grounds, i.e. that:

> Women in the Third World would not receive antiretroviral treatment anyway, so the investigators are simply observing what would happen to the subject's infants if there were no study. And a placebo controlled study is the fastest, and most efficient way to obtain unambiguous information that will be of greatest value in the Third World.[28]

Thus, Angell argues, these trials are, analogously as ethically offensive as the Tuskegee Study. However, there are important differences between the two types of study, which are of great ethical significance.

What principally rendered the Tuskegee Study as ethically unjustifiable was that the subjects did not give informed consent to their participation in the study. They were also not provided with local standards of care, as they were not informed of the treatments available to them even when an effective treatment was widely used for others in the USA in their condition. The participant's autonomy was further undermined by deception as to the purposes of some procedures undertaken as part of the study. They were, for example, told that the spinal taps designed to monitor protein levels were a new form of treatment. It was the lack of information and thus respect for individual autonomy that rendered the Tuskegee Study ethically abhorrent.

On the contrary all the trials into interventions to reduce perinatal transmission of HIV have all obtained the informed consent of the participants. There have been reports that while "informed consent" is required for participation in these studies, subjects often did not understand the implications of the trial [see for example, French].[34] This of course means that the informed consent given to these studies was invalid and requires that researchers improve their methods of ensuring that subjects understand the implications of the trial rather than deeming the practice of enlisting subjects who must give informed consent unethical. This is the critical point. It may be that more debate is needed as to whether efforts could and should be made to ensure that placebo-controls are not used where an effective treatment is used for trials elsewhere. However, what is crucial is that fully informed consent is given by trial participants so that their interests may be respected.

INFORMED CONSENT: THE BEST GUARANTOR OF RESEARCH SUBJECTS' INTERESTS

There are many circumstances that pose demanding ethical questions in the area of HIV research. How much risk should subjects be exposed to? Is it ethical to ask subjects to participate in trials to develop treatments when treatments already exist? Should drug companies be obliged to provide treatment to subjects after the trial is concluded? Is it ethically justifiable to ask individuals to participate in a trial for treatment which is unlikely ever to be available to them or their countrymen because of prohibitive cost? These issues must be addressed and every effort must be made to ensure that HIV research is ethically sound. In the mean time a requirement for individual fully informed consent is the best guarantor of research subject's best interest in all research studies. If subjects are fully informed of what participation in a study entails then it is surely unjustifiably paternalistic to deny them a choice whether they should participate. It may be that trials entail some risks or injustices, and these should be addressed, but they should not prohibit subjects from participating as long as they are fully aware of these problems and not coerced into consenting.

Whatever the ethical problems entailed with research into HIV it is paramount that informed consent is not disregarded. It is these ethical problems that make informed consent of research subject essential, not only allowing individuals to make maximally autonomous choices about their participation but also allowing for greater openness and discussion of HIV and AIDS. Just as with the therapeutic and preventative aspects of HIV, the interests of the subjects of HIV research do not seem necessarily to be at odds with the interests of research and public health. Evidence is strong that, if research offers convincing safeguards and benefits to individuals and the wider populations, then there is no reason why participation rates will be significantly damaged by the requirement of informed consent. Equally it can be supposed that insistence on informed consent of research subjects is the best way to protect subjects from exploitation and infringements on their autonomy. Until convincing evidence is provided that requiring informed consent for participation in HIV research is either impossible or imcompatible with public health aims, there should be no question of relaxing the existing guidelines on consent, whether that research is an anonymous serosurveillance study in the UK or an African vaccine trial. Even where such evidence is available, there would, I would argue, be very few cases in which participation in HIV research without consent would be morally defensible.

ACKNOWLEDGEMENTS

I am grateful to John Harris and Len Doyal for helpful comments on earlier drafts of this paper.

REFERENCES

1. UNAIDS, Joint United Nations Programme on HIV/AIDS. *AIDS epidemic update: December 1999*. Available on the Web at http://www.unaids.org/
2. Bennett R, Erin CA, Harris J. *AIDS: Ethics, justice and european policy. Final Report to the European Commission*. Luxembourg: Office of Official Publications for the European Communities, 1998, p. 42.
3. Sherr L. Counselling and HIV testing – ethical dilemmas. In: Bennett R, Erin CA (eds). *HIV and AIDS: testing, screening and confidentiality*. Oxford: Oxford University Press, 1999, pp. 39–60.
4. General Medical Council. *HIV and AIDS: the Ethical considerations*, October 1995.
5. Bayer R. Public health policy and the AIDS epidemic. An end to AIDS exceptionalism? *N Engl J Med* 1991; **324**: 1500–4.
6. De Cock KM, Johnson AM. From exeptionalism to normalisation: a reappraisal of attitudes and practice around HIV testing. *BMJ* 1998; **316**: 290–3.
7. Helsinki Declaration. *BMJ* 1996; **313**: 1448.
8. Paquita de Zulueta. The ethics of anonymised HIV testing of pregnant women: a reappraisal, *J Med Ethics* 2000; **26**: 16–21.
9. Centres for Disease Control. AZT for the prevention of HIV transmission from mother to infant. *Morb Mortal Wkly Rep* 1994; **43**: 285–7.
10. Newell ML, Peckham CS. Risk factors for vertical transmission and early markers of HIV-1 infection in children. *AIDS* 1993; **7**: S591–7.
11. European Collaborative Study. Risk factors for mother-to-child transmission of HIV-1. *Lancet* 1992; **339**: 1007–12.
12. Nicoll A, McGarringle C, Brady AR *et al*. Epidemiology and detection of HIV-1 among pregnant women in the United Kingdom: results from national surveillance 1998–96. *BMJ* 1998; **316**: 253–8.
13. Doctors call for more HIV tests in pregnancy. *The Sunday Times*, 1994: 16th October.
14. Goldberg DJ, Johnstone FD. Universal named testing of pregnant women for HIV. *BMJ* 1993; **306**: 1144–5.
15. Ulanowsky C. Almond B. HIV and pregnancy. In: Almond B (ed). *AIDS: a moral issue*. London: Macmillan, 1990, pp. 41–55.
16. Beder J, Beckerman H. Mandatory HIV screening in newborns: the issues and a programmatic response. *XI International Conference on AIDS*. Vancouver, 1996. Abstract ThC 4613.
17. Rovner J. US specialists object to AMA's call for mandatory testing. *Lancet* 1996; **348**: 330.
18. Pinching J. The ethics of anonymised HIV testing of pregnant women: a reappraisal. *J Med Ethics* 2000; **26**: 22–4.
19. Bennett R. Should we routinely test pregnant women for HIV? In: Bennett R, Erin CA, eds. *HIV and AIDS: testing, screening and confidentiality*. Oxford: Oxford University Press, 1999, pp. 228–39.
20. Kessel A, Watts C, Weiss HA. Bad blood? Survey of public's views on unlinked anonymous testing of blood for HIV and other diseases. *BMJ* 2000; **320**: 90–1.
21. Bhagwanjee S, Muckart DJJ, Jeena PM, Moodley P. Does HIV status influence the outcome of patients admitted to a surgical intensive care unit? A prospective double blind study. *BMJ* 1997; **314**: 1077.
22. Bhagwanjee S, Muckart DJJ, Jeena PM, Moodley P. Commentary: Why we did not seek informed consent before testing patients for HIV. *BMJ* 1997; **314**: 1082.
23. Benatar D, Benatar SR. Informed consent and research. *BMJ* 1998; **316**: 1008–10.
24. Guenter D, Esparza J, Macklin R. Ethical considerations in international HIV vaccine trials: a summary of a consultative process conducted by the Joint United Nations Programme on HIV/AIDS (UNAIDS). *J Med Ethics* 2000; **26**: 37–43.
25. Gottlieb S. AIDS vaccines tested in Thailand and Uganda. *BMJ* 1999; **318**: 626.
26. Anon. Africa's first Aids vaccine trial starts. BBC News Online http://news.bbc.co.uk/hi/english/health/background_briefings/aids/newsid_275000/275411.stm, posted at 19:27 GMT on Monday, February 8, 1999.
27. Anon. Row over medical tests on humans. BBC News Online, http://news.bbc.co.uk/hi/english/health/newsid_736000/736138.stm, posted at 17:35 GMT on Thursday, May 4, 2000.
28. Angell M. The ethics of clinical research in the Third World. *New Engl J Med* 1997; **337**: 847–9.
29. Christakis NA. The ethical design of an AIDS vaccine trial in Africa. *Hastings Centre Rep* 1988, June/July: 31037.
30. Zion D. The Ethics of AIDS vaccine trials. *Science* 1998; **280**(5368): 1329–30.

31. Twenty years after: the legacy of the Tuskegee Syphilis Study. *Hastings Centre Rep* 1992; **22**(6): 29–40.

32. Varmus H, Satcher D. Ethical complexities of conducting research in developing countries. *New Engl J Med* 1997; **337**: 1003–5.

33. Lurie P, Wolfe S. Unethical trials of interventions to reduce perinatal transmission of the human immunodeficiency virus in developing countries. *New Engl J Med* 1997; **337**: 853–6.

34. French H. *New York Times* 1997; October 9: p. A1.

21 · Informed consent and research on assisted conception

Bobbie Farsides and Heather Draper

Infertility treatment is a very special area of medicine. The goal of the treatment is to create a child for the childless individuals involved, and this goal has in recent years led to scientific and medical research of the most ethically challenging kind. The nature of the raw materials of the research, the cost to the individuals involved in the research and the concerns for the welfare of those born as a result of research men that, unlike any other area of medicine, infertility treatment and the research that backs it up is closely regulated and monitored.

In the UK, research into the causes of infertility and means of remedying it fall, for the main part, under the restrictions imposed by the Human Fertilisation and Embryology Act 1990. This Act specifies the parameters of research on the human embryo and governs research into many new forms of infertility treatment because all forms of infertility treatment that involve *in vitro* conception fall under it. The first part of this chapter is, therefore, devoted to an overview of what might be permitted under the Act. It then looks at some of the ethical issues involved in research on infertile patients, and concludes with a brief overview of some of the ethical considerations of infertility research on the human embryo.

It is worth stating at the outset that many types of infertility treatment verge on the edge of therapeutic research, as techniques with relatively low rates of success are applied to new cases, which may differ in some respect to all previous cases. Whilst the cause of much infertility remains a mystery, the application of even well-established therapies retains an element of the experimental. For this reason many of the discussions and considerations that are important in an experimental context already impact upon therapeutic interventions in a non-experimental context. A decision to embark on fertility treatment such as

in vitro fertilisation (IVF) might be shown to be very similar to a decision to embark on an experimental therapy in some other area of medicine. Furthermore, the risks and low promise of benefit of standard therapies might blur the distinction between these and the new and untested; in this area of medicine there might be less reason to instinctively trust the devil you know.

HUMAN FERTILISATION AND EMBRYOLOGY ACT

The Act lays down principles that govern infertility treatment and embryo research in the UK. It also established the Human Fertilisation and Embryology Authority (HFEA) to oversee practice, and it is the HFEA's responsibility to translate the legal principles into guidelines for practitioners. Any intervention or research that requires an *in vitro* human embryo falls under the Act and therefore has to take place in premises licensed by the HFEA. Premises licensed by the HFEA are bound by the Act. Accordingly, if a therapy that does not involve IVF – artificial insemination, for instance – takes place in a licensed clinic, it falls under the Act. All the centres of excellence for infertility in the UK are by necessity licensed and therefore most patients receiving infertility treatment in the UK do so in licensed clinics. It is possible to imagine some kinds of research that do not fall by one means or another under the Act. It is arguable that all infertility therapy *should* be brought under the Act for the protection of patients but, for the purposes of this chapter, it will be assumed that all the research in question is governed by the Act. This does not mean that all possible avenues of research have been anticipated by the Act. In some circumstances, it is left to the HFEA to interpret the spirit of the law and apply this to potential new therapies. The use of ovarian tissue from aborted fetuses, is a case in point.

Schedule 2–3(2) of the Act outlines the only acceptable aims of research using human embryos. It states that research will not be authorised except for the following purposes:

- promoting advances in the treatment of infertility;
- increasing knowledge about the causes of congenital disease;
- increasing knowledge about the causes of miscarriage;
- developing effective techniques of contraception, or
- developing methods for detecting the presence of gene or chromosome abnormalities in embryos before implantation.

The Act forbids certain kinds of activities like some forms of cloning (but, strictly speaking, not the technique used to clone "Dolly", section 3–3[d]), the making of animal/human hybrids (section 4–1[a]), or the use of animals as surrogate mothers for human embryos (section 3–3[b]) or vice versa (section 3–2[a]). Embryos cannot be kept beyond the development of the primitive streak (14 days)(section 3–3[a]), nor can embryos be used in research without effective consent (schedule 2 sections 1–3). In practice, this is taken to mean the specific consent of both parties to its creation.

Research or trials centred on infertility, which involve techniques that may lead to a pregnancy, are also governed by the Act for the reasons outlined above. This means that research, like treatment, has to take account of the welfare of any child who may be created as a result (or, indeed, other children who may be affected)(section 13[5]). Where donated embryos or gametes are involved, consent must have been obtained, and the definitions of legal mother and father outlined in the Act will also apply (sections 27–30). The act does not distinguish between NHS and private patients.

The HFEA, in its *Code of Practice*, reminds researchers that all research on NHS patients must be reviewed by a Local Research Ethics Committee (LREC). Non-NHS clinics must also submit all research to an ethics committee. However, they may either form their own committees, or, subject to prior arrangement, submit to an LREC.[1] In addition, all projects involving human embryos must be peer reviewed by academics chosen by the HFEA.[2]

RESEARCH INVOLVING INFERTILE PATIENTS

For the purpose of this chapter, it is assumed that the research in question involves infertile individuals who are also patients, i.e. actively pursuing infertility treatment, as opposed to healthy volunteers, who will be guinea pigs for the benefit of others.

The Distress of Infertility, Financial Implications and the Risk Too Far

As the Warnock report noted back in 1984,[3] the driving force behind infertility treatment and, accordingly, research into better forms of infertility treatment, is the suffering that infertility brings to those who consider themselves to be infertile. It cannot be assumed that all those who are in fact infertile actually suffer from infertility or even consider themselves to be infertile. For some individuals, the knowledge that they are infertile does not cause suffering, perhaps because in them the desire to have a child is less great, or perhaps it is coincidental to the decision not to have children in any case or perhaps because it is received stoically. There is no doubting the distress that the inability to have children causes in some individuals and couples, nor the psychological difficulties and reduction in well-being, which this distress can generate. This means, however, that at least some of those who might be suitable candidates for research in clinical terms might not be obvious candidates when viewed more holistically. Some will be desperate to have a child by any means possible; indeed, some may already have gone to considerable, but unsuccessful, lengths. This and other facts particular to patients seeking fertility treatment mean that special care needs to be taken when recruiting volunteers for research.

One unusual feature of this patient group is the high proportion that will have to pay for their treatment. Infertility treatment is never cheap and can be very expensive depending upon the amount of intervention required. Experimental therapy, on the other hand, may be offered (wholly or partly) free of charge, which means that there is a financial benefit to infertile participants even though they are not being paid. In ethical terms, this benefit may be analogous with being paid, and thereby introduce the same problems of potential inducement or even coercion. For those who have exhausted all the financial options, or who had no options to begin with, the possibility of participating in research may be the only means open to them of having the child that they desperately want.

Another possible analogy is between those patients who seek to create a life and those who are desperate to save their own lives. In both cases the high stakes might incline potential volunteers to take risks or accept terms that are not in fact in their best interests. Whilst it would be wrong to stereotype all patients in either group as desperate, they are at least vulnerable, and this vulnerability needs to be acknowledged. In Britain, LRECs are very cautious in their approval of clinical experimentation involving terminally ill patients, it is at least possible that equal caution is called for in the case of those undergoing fertility treatment.

It is also worth stating that, even when successful, infertility treatments take their toll on the lives of those who receive them, and, when the treatments fail, the effect can be devastating. It is not simply a matter of considering the physical effects of these therapies, but also the psychological effects of repeated failure, compounded by the fact that patients' lives may revolve solely around their therapy for a significant number of years. Whilst it is important to consider when it is appropriate to call a halt to patients' infertility treatment in their own best interests, it may be even more important to practise restraint when patients are enrolled into research programmes.

Taken together, these points suggest that the participants in infertility research have some very special vulnerabilities, but are these vulnerabilities sufficient to justify paternalism? It could be argued that the participants are all autonomous adults, who should be permitted to decide for themselves what risks they are prepared to take, and when enough is enough. We are all familiar with the powerful arguments in support of respecting patients' autonomy, as these have formed the bedrock of medical ethics for several decades now. It is, however, worth spending some time looking at the possible justifications for paternalism in the context of infertility research.

Most obvious is the obligation of clinicians to protect patients from harm and to act in their best interests (resources and other ethical considerations permitting). A degree of paternalism is standard practice in research. Patients are not approached if the clinician responsible for their care thinks that participation is not in their interests. The possibility of participation is initially decided without the

patient being consulted at all. Likewise, whilst standard consent forms point out to patients that they are free to withdraw from a trial at any point, they also state that the patient's doctor may unilaterally decide to withdraw them. This would not require the patient's consent, although it would be considered good practice to discuss the matter with a patient first.

To our knowledge, these practices have not been condemned despite their potential for undermining patient autonomy, suggesting perhaps that they fall into the category of justified paternalism. Another justification for paternalism might be the claim that a significant proportion of long-term patients, whilst broadly competent, are unable to act autonomously *on this particular issue*. The desire for a child might trump all potentially competing considerations, thus making rational choice impossible. This, combined with the previously mentioned financial benefits of participation, might mean that the moral obligation to uphold patient choice is less forceful here, and the possibility of justifying weak paternalism more clear. Whilst we should not *assume* that desperate or financially pressed patients are unable to make autonomous decisions about participation in research, clinicians need to develop strategies for identifying patients who fall into this category. Having identified them, the clinician might then need to help them confront an uncomfortable truth rather than recruit them into a trial that might further their suffering.

In clinical research the biggest risks are generally justified when they secure the greatest goods, most obviously the saving of a previously unsalvageable life or a substantial improvement in the quality of a life currently characterised by some form of suffering. For an infertile couple the greatest good will doubtless be the birth of a baby. What the arbiters of research need to ask is whether these three goods of saving, enhancing, and creating a life are really equivalent, thereby justifying the bearing of equivalent risk and harms. In objective terms it might be hard to say that they are equivalent, but one then needs to ask whether an objective judgement is appropriate or even possible in this context. Maybe what matters is the value of the good to the potential volunteer, not the value as interpreted by the clinician, or even by society as a whole.

However, one could argue that the clinician is entitled to attempt such an objective evaluation as part of the cost-benefit analysis he or she will engage in, and that society has already done so, as reflected in the differential attitudes to the resourcing of life-saving versus life-creating therapies. Furthermore, as an individual moral agent, the doctor is entitled to "keep their hands clean", in the sense of refusing to be a party to shared projects where the risk involved seems unacceptably high. Whilst it might be true that to the couple receiving infertility treatment the good on offer is worth any price, the clinician should be free to decide whether he or she shares that view as a party to the practices proposed. Of course, a potential obstacle to this type of objectivity might be clinicians' dual role as scientist and doctor, the first of which might incline then to share the subject's enthusiasm for personal reasons, i.e. the desire to advance scientific knowledge and perfect therapeutic interventions. Given that this is so, the involvement of parties beyond the subject and their infertility doctors is to be welcomed.

Not One But Two Patients

A further complicating factor in infertility treatment is that most of it involves couples rather than single patients. Of course, some centres are prepared to treat single women but, even so, such cases remain in the minority; the vast majority of infertility treatment involves couples. The traditional model of consent for research involves just one patient, although there are exceptions such as studies aimed at isolating genes that may involve whole families. In the case of infertility, it is not difficult to imagine a situation where one partner wants to participate but another is reluctant. Strictly speaking, if the clinic was willing to treat single people, either one could proceed alone, provided that donor gametes could be found [and a willing surrogate mother in the case of single men]. This would, however, tend to defeat the original aim of the couple's procreative project, namely to provide *them* with a child. For the purpose of this chapter, we will assume that a scrupulous clinic would not be prepared to carry on in such a case without re-evaluating the whole situation. However, the consent of the reluctant partner remains essential, since the consent of each is required if the gametes of each are to be used. Given that this is the case, it is highly probable that the reluctant partner will be pressured by the willing partner to participate.

In the case of a reluctant woman, this would entail reluctantly taking on considerable physical burdens, and it seems reasonable for a clinician to intervene on the woman's side here. Effectively, a woman's reluctance would make her an inappropriate research participant and her clinician would not seek to enrol her to a study. In the case of reluctant men, the physical burdens of participation are lessened (particularly where frozen gametes are available), but cannot be totally disregarded, and the psychological risks could still be significant. A reluctant man might actually be most concerned about the risks and burdens his female partner will bear for their *shared* project (and this point seems a valid one even though he might not be able to make the same argument about her *own* project). As in the case of the clinician, we might have to say that the man has a right not to become a party to the risks taken by another. One is minded here of the women who choose to continue life-threatening pregnancies against the wishes of their partners. Whilst it might not be justifiable to force a woman to terminate a pregnancy, one might feel that the reasons produced by a man in such cases would have justified his refusal to be a party to *creating* a pregnancy had that been an issue. If a man is convinced of the high risk of harm to his partner, his relationship and himself that further experimental treatment will entail, he is surely entitled to withdraw his consent. In some respects this example is analogous with that of the doctor who decides to withhold or withdraw a patient from a trial, having decided that the costs (physical, emotional, financial, etc.) involved in pursuing the desired for pregnancy by this route are too high, irrespective of what the research subject claims.

The point to be made is this, whereas consent issues are complex enough when only one party's consent is required, the potential complexities increase when two participants are involved. This is particularly true when there is dispute over how much influence each party should have over the decision in question. The role of a potential father is hotly disputed in many areas of reproductive medicine, e.g. abortion, enforced caesarean, or post-mortem delivery, but in this case the law requires that consent be given by both genitors, and therefore differences have to be resolved.

Research with Fuzzy Edges, the Internet and Reproductive Tourism

There may be overlap between experimental and standard therapy in the context of assisted conception. Some aspects of treatment will be standard therapy, whilst others may be experimental. It is important that it is made very clear to the participants those aspects of their care that are experimental and those that are not. In some instances, the experimental aspects of the therapy may be all that is on offer and cannot therefore be replaced with standard therapy, if the subject(s) decline the invitation to participate. This will inevitably place a further strain on the consenting process and require additional care on behalf of the treating clinician to ensure that full informed and voluntary consent is obtained.

We should not assume, however, that patients are passive partners in research. In assisted conception, as in so many other areas of clinical practice, some patients attend clinics armed with the latest research gleaned from the Internet. In such cases it might be the clinician who is put under some pressure to participate in research! Likewise, clinicians may find that they are caring for patients who have travelled abroad to gain some experimental therapy and have now returned to the UK for the remainder of their treatment. In such cases, clinicians have to take account of their own capabilities and balance these against the needs of the patients. It is probably going to be easier to resist the temptation to provide some experimental therapy than it is to refuse to provide continuing care when faced with a *fait accompli*.

And Baby Makes Three

This brings us to the third complication of infertility research. Hopefully the end product of a procedure will be a baby who did not exist at the time the research was undertaken and, even if it had, could not consent to be a participant.

As stated in the first section of the chapter, experimental therapies – like conventional ones that aim to produce a baby – fall under section 13(5) of the Human Fertilisation and Embryology Act. This section states:

> A woman shall not be provided with treatment services unless account has been taken of the welfare of any child who may be born as a result of the treatment (including the need of that child for a father), and of any other child who might be affected by the birth.

Although this section is open to a wide degree of interpretation, there is considerable agreement among clinicians (although not necessary among philosophers[4]) that it is legitimate for them to assess the future welfare of any child whom they help to create. This is not the place to explore this contention further. For the purpose of this chapter, we will assume that clinicians should be bound by the law, but that the law is open to interpretation.

The newer a therapy, the less we know about the potential risks to a baby of being conceived by the method proposed. This being so, the key question is surely how much risk of abnormality is permissible, granted that the main subjects of this risk is not in a position to consent for themselves?

On the one hand, without taking the risk of abnormality the future child will not exist at all. Many children currently existing today would not have been born if the risks involved in creating the first test-tube baby had not been taken. Existence is certainly a precious gift and one that we may think justifies any amount of risk. On the other hand, we might risk creating children who will not thank us for the risk we took, perhaps because their lives are so miserable, or perhaps – and maybe even more seriously – because the lives of their own children are blighted as a result.

In the UK, whilst it is permissible for parents to consent on behalf of their children to participate in research, the level of risk entailed in the research has to be minimal. This has been interpreted by some to exclude relatively risk-free practices such as venepuncture in a non-therapeutic context.[5] If this interpretation of risk is an acceptable one, it would seem to exclude practically all infertility research on infertile patients (because of the risk to potential offspring) and accordingly seem to many people to set the level of risk too low.[6] However, given the requirement to consider the risk to the created child, there is a consequent requirement to set a level beyond which the risks become unacceptable, and this is surely the task of the clinicians and scientists and their regulatory body, the HFEA.

As if the issue of consent and risk was not difficult enough already, there is a further complicating factor. Whilst a child cannot withhold consent to its own creation, it might wish at a later date to withhold consent from procedures consequent upon the special circumstances of his or her conception. However, some might try to argue that those who owe their life to pioneering medical interventions have a special duty to cooperate in the long-term monitoring of those procedures and their after-effects. If we are to be sure of the risk-free nature of assisted reproductive procedures, a cohort of children will need to remain subjects of research for a large part of their lives, even if there are no immediately apparent effects of their assisted conception. This means that the trial their parents initially consented to could continue beyond the stage where the child's conception marks them as different, well into adulthood, when they may wish to avoid medical encounters and adopt a certain anonymity in terms of their unusual beginnings. Being subject to the medical gaze in this way might be considered burdensome by some families, and one must ensure that their consent to continued involvement is genuine and not merely the result of coercive levels of gratitude and beholdeness. Furthermore, one must question the assumption that those who owe their lives to experimental procedures are any more obliged to cooperate in follow-up than those who benefit from more routine procedures.

Summary

This section has isolated at least three senses in which research into infertility relief raises ethical difficulties. The first was that the patient-participants may be particularly vulnerable. The second was that the consent of two patients is required causing difficulties when one person might be willing to participate and the other might not. The third was that the party who is potentially subject to the most risk – the future child – is unable to consent to being part of the research. Even when the future child becomes an actual child, there are questions that need to be raised as to its continued status as a research subject.

BACK TO THE BEGINNING – RESEARCH ON THE HUMAN EMBRYO

All new assisted conception techniques have their origins in embryo research. It is difficult to do justice to the issues raised by embryo research in a small section at the end of a chapter – countless articles and books have been written [7, 8] and there is still no consensus on the issue. All we can hope to do here is to provide an overview of some of the issues for the sake of completeness.

The Human Fertilisation and Embryology Act draws a distinction between embryos up to 14 days (when the primitive streak develops) and those beyond 14 days. Research is only permitted up to the 14-day limit and after this embryos must be allowed to perish. This was somewhat of a legal compromise

between those who hold that the early embryo is nothing but a clump of human cells, and those who hold (to varying degrees) that the embryo has a moral significance in its own right. The only common ground between these many positions is that there is an obligation to protect the person the embryo will become (or already is). Thus, it is agreed that nothing should be done to an embryo that will harm a future person (although we have already explored some of the difficulties of this position in the previous section). It is worth therefore considering the specific issue of experimentation involving embryos that will *not* be implanted as a part of reproductive technology. The issues involved in donating embryos for the use of another couple undergoing infertility treatment will not be discussed here as the primary decision is not related to clinical experimentation.

For those who believe that the embryo has no independent moral status, anything is possible provided that the embryo does not survive (because if it does this may cause harm to some future person), and there might in fact be strong moral arguments in favour of using them as opposed to wasting them. For those who believe that the embryo has moral status in its own right, further considerations must follow.

The first is that embryo research is a form of human research for which the consent of the subject is never and can never be obtained. Some people are prepared to accept the considered consent of the genitors as a reasonable substitute; however this consent is going to be different in type to most other forms of proxy consent, as it will not be guided by a consideration of the best interests of the research subject – the embryo.

For some the idea that parents can consent for their embryo to be researched upon to death does not seem like a reasonable parental judgement, and it is argued that by making such a choice the "parents" indicate that they are inappropriate proxies. Clearly, the upshot of this position has to be that no research is permissible, because anyone giving consent is excluded from being an appropriate proxy by virtue of the fact that they gave consent to something that is against the interests of the subject. However, if one thinks that the embryo has the full moral significance of a human person, this is not an unpalatable conclusion, nor is it unrealistic to expect the genitors to display the characteristics of parents, and therefore refuse consent.

However, those who consent to the use of their

embryos in trials where they know they will not survive can use a number of different justifications. First, they might choose to make a clear distinction between an embryo, which has some but not full moral status, and a child, which has full moral status, and then make a further distinction between their roles as genitors and their role as parents. They may choose to parent those embryos that are implanted, but as genitors they might have different moral criteria for dealing with those that they classify as "spare". If spare, the moral imperative is to make use of the embryo rather than waste it, a goal that can be pursued in the knowledge that the cost to the embryo is high. However, unless implanted, it will either be destroyed or experimented on, and it will be aware of neither fate, and some good will only come of the latter option.

In deciding whether to allow an embryo to be used in research, a genitor should be entitled to know what the research aims will be. A decision to donate embryos for research must surely be based on a positive evaluation of that research, which is the good that replaces any good to the embryo, or the good of producing a child. Although other bodies are also charged with the responsibility of evaluating scientific merit and ethical validity, the genitors are entitled to refuse consent to types of research that they believe to be inappropriate. The Human Fertilisation Embryology Act lays down those aims that are currently legal, but these were not accepted without debate, and individuals will have different views about what ought and ought not to be a subject of scientific enquiry in this area. A true consent will be a specific consent informed by details of what will be done to the embryo and to what purpose.

This is not to say that embryo research divorced from implantation into a woman's body will never count as being in the embryo's interest. As is always the case in this area of medicine, doctors, ethicists, and research subjects need to keep a clear eye on the future. The Act assumes that it is in the best interests of the embryo to be allowed to perish at 14 days but, in terms of the projected development of the artificial womb, this is not obvious. At some point researchers will undoubtedly develop an artificial environment in which an embryo can be gestated from conception to "birth" and eventually there will be pressure to permit human trials. It is not obviously against the interests of an embryo to participate in such a trial, particularly if this embryo is destined otherwise to perish. Even if the chances of success in the initial trials are small, it is potentially inter-

pretable as a piece of therapeutic research by those who consider it to be in the interests of an embryo to develop into a person. It will be interesting to see what the HFEA makes of this possibility when it arises.

Whilst fascinating in their own right, it could be argued that a knowledge of these arguments and debates is also relevant to the proper conduct of infertility research. Recent advances suggest that there will be an increasing need in the near future for embryo research, not only to advance infertility treatments, but also to treat such conditions as Parkinson's disease, dementia, and even spinal injury. Women will be asked to donate their embryos to assist experimentation, and more radical interventions will be attempted at the embryonic stage in order to perfect infertility treatments, particularly for women previously dependent upon egg donorship. The question then arises as to how effectively women can consent to these options without being aware of and explicitly addressing the ethical arguments about the moral status of the human embryo. The clinician then has to decide how and in what manner to test this knowledge and understanding, and how to provide information that is shown to be lacking.

This offers a further challenge to those involved in the counselling that accompanies any attempt at infertility treatment or research. As well as discussing hoped for benefits, potential costs, emotional issues, and relationship factors the counsellor will need to explore a couple's moral attitudes towards the embryos that they propose to use often with little promise of success. This discussion needs to be delicately handled so as to contribute effectively to the consent process, without adding to the burdens of the participants. Consent is a legal and moral requirement but, as always, judgement must be exercised in deciding what goes beyond the information sufficient upon which to base that consent.

CONCLUSION

As stated at the outset, the special features of infertility treatment ensure that many of the issues discussed here are not peculiar to a research setting, nor may the distinction between clinical care and research be as stark as in other areas of medicine. However, it remains important to acknowledge the particular issues raised in the experimental treatment of those whose goal is the creation of a much longed-for child. First, the importance of the goal and its significance to the life of the potential participants makes them particularly vulnerable. Secondly, the high costs associated with standard therapies, combined with the limited hope of success, might cloud the potentially higher costs of the as yet unproven intervention; this could pose very real problems where randomisation is proposed with participants incapable of acknowledging the existence of equipoise. Thirdly, consent is required by not one but two participants in the vast majority of cases, thus making the counselling and negotiation involved potentially more complex. Fourth, consent cannot be given by someone who will necessarily be affected by the research, i.e. the embryo, foetus, or future child. Finally the clinician seeking consent will need to be sure that the participants understand both the clinical and moral implications of their choices, and the way in which this might affect them in the future; during the experimental phase it might be easy to regard an embryo as a means to an end, out if the therapy fails it might not be possible to avoid mourning the loss of the embryo as a being in its own right.

REFERENCES

1. Human Fertilisation and Embryology Authority. *Code of Practice* (4th edn), sections 10.7 & 10.8.
2. *Ibid* section 10.9.
3. Department of Health and Social Security. *Report of the Committee of Inquiry into Fertilisation and Embryology*. London: HMSO, 1984, section 2.4.
4. Harris J. *Clones, genes and immortality*. Oxford: Oxford University Press, 1998.
5. British Paediatric Association. *Guidelines for the ethical conduct of medical research involving children*, 2nd edn. London: BPA, 1992.
6. Gillon R. Research on the vulnerable: an ethical overview. In: Brazier M, Lobjoit M. *Protecting the vulnerable*. London: RKP, 1991.
7. Mulkay M. *The embryo research debate*. Cambridge: Cambridge University Press, 1997.
8. Dyson A, Harris J. *Experiments on embryos*, London: RKP, 1991.

22 · Informed consent for access to medical records for health services research

Brian Hurwitz

> In the nature of things, we visit doctors when we are not well. We may be at our most vulnerable, and confide information which we do not wish to be spread beyond the confines of the consulting room. Tensions are bound to arise when such confidences are not honoured.
>
> Lee R.[1]

> Everyone involved in health care has known for some time that the demise of confidentiality as a viable principle is imminent.
>
> Kennedy I.[2]

A dynamic tension exists between maintaining confidentiality of medical records and permitting access to them for the purposes of research. This has been characterised as a tussle between an "old ethic", seeking to protect the closed secrecies of the consulting room, and a "new ethic", striving after knowledge by asking questions that require data for answers – sometimes from millions of health service records.[3] Though belief in the importance of medical confidentiality, and of sharing information to enable new knowledge to emerge, each claims Hippocratic lineage,[4] strain between these parallel commitments remains apparent in the very title of modern General Medical Council advice on the matter, *Confidentiality: providing and protecting information*.[5]

A chorus of guidance now advises clinicians that in the absence of specific patient consent, clinical information supplied in confidence during medical consultations may be released to third party researchers, so long as certain safeguards can be met.[6–10] Chief among these are that:

- any information supplied be stripped of personal identifiers at the earliest possible stage of data processing, so that identification of individuals in research output is precluded;

- the research proposed be non-intrusive, posing neither inconvenience nor hazard (physical or psychological) to patients;
- information be transferred only to *bona fide* researchers who are "senior professionals" (consultants and principals in general practice are mentioned but non-clinical custodians are also cited) who are subject to discipline by a professional authority for breaches of confidentiality;
- the research protocol be approved by an appropriate research ethics committee and specific exemption from the requirement for consent to disclosure should have been granted to custodians of the medical records.

Twenty years ago, patients who went to see their GP did so in an expectation (not always justified) that they could reveal anything about themselves, assured that details would travel no further without both their knowledge and consent. In today's NHS this expectation has altered: team-based health care, increasing concerns about the sensitivity of medical information and its potential to leak away from the point at which it is supplied, and increased access to records for the purposes of research and audit, have rightly made people more circumspect. It is now not uncommon for patients to pause and ask how confidential medical confidentiality can be, and to request specifically that what they are about to discuss should not be written down in their medical records, and even to decline further investigation because they harbour doubts about medical secrecy.

Until recently, the Royal College of Physicians did not regard independent review by a local research ethics committee as essential for studies proposing access to medical records without explicit patient consent.[6, 8, 11] Though there is some variance between advisory statements offering guidance on confidentiality, the broad focus of this chapter will be to explore the moral foundations of medical commitment to secrecy, and to examine whether disclosure of information without consent of patients – under the conditions set out – can be right.

WHAT IS MEDICAL CONFIDENTIALITY?

Medical confidentiality can be defined as keeping secure and secret from others information given by or about an individual in the course of a professional relationship. Long a principle of medical ethics, it featured within the Hippocratic Oath: "Whatever, in connection with my professional practice or not in connection with it, I see or hear, in the life of men, which ought not to be spoken of abroad, I will not divulge, as reckoning that all such should be kept secret."[12]

Confidence keeping on this formulation admits of an ambiguity; the Oath could be read as meaning that everything heard or seen relating to patients should be kept secret, or, it may mean that not all confidences require the same degree of protection – only those "which ought not to be spoken of abroad," which clearly begs the important moral questions rather than answering them. It is usually assumed that Hippocratic silence did not apply in a blanket fashion to everything seen or heard in the course of clinical work. The Oath's commitment to silence was contingent upon clinicians' intuition and moral judgement, professional secrecy being viewed as a relative (and not an absolute) requirement.[13] Allowing some free rein to clinicians to decide in which circumstances information will be protected appears in later reformulations: "I will do my best to maintain confidentiality about all my patients," runs a modern redraft of the Oath, but "if there are overriding reasons which prevent me keeping a patient's confidentiality I will explain them."[14] Reasons *for* and *against* maintenance of confidentiality are clearly envisaged; whether secrecy should prevail hinges upon the balance of these reasons as perceived by clinicians who today are required to explain the rationale for any unconsented disclosures.

Such relativisim in the application of the duty of medical confidentiality can be found in current National Health Service guidance, which places similar emphasis upon protecting confidentiality as upon meeting the informational requirements of running of a public service efficiently:

A balance needs to be struck between patients' expectation, acknowledged in the Patients' Charter, that information about them will be treated as confidential, and the importance of making patients fully aware that NHS staff and sometimes staff of other agencies need to have strictly controlled access to such information, anonymised wherever possible, in order to deliver, plan and manage services effectively.[15]

How best, in practice, to apply the duty to maintain confidences in the context of a health service embedded in a public institution continues to vex clinicians.[16] Of 24 000 calls made by general practitioners to one of the UK's medical defence organisations in 1999, concerns about confidentiality topped the list of enquiries (alongside those concerning consent).[17]

MORAL UNDERPINNINGS OF CONFIDENTIALITY

One way of looking at confidentiality in the doctor–patient relationship is as a mutual undertaking: secrecy offers patients protection from exposure or embarrassment, and the doctor's role is facilitated by patients who feel at liberty to be candid. Undertaking to protect information gathered during clinical practice acknowledges a right to secrecy; only by consenting to disclosure do patients waive this right. A relationship is thereby created in which intimacy, safety, and truthfulness can flourish, a professional environment likely to encourage trust and optimise effective and efficient health care. Conceptualising the doctor–patient relationship in this way grounds it not only in a rights-based ethic, but upon a consequentialist view, which places the importance of confidentiality not as a good in itself, but as a means to (other) morally desirable ends: "Individuals benefit because it allows them to seek help they might otherwise fear to request. Society gains by doctors being able to offer help to the most vulnerable."[18]

Confidentiality as a professional commitment arises in part from what has been termed the "existential inequality" inherent in doctor–patient relationships.[19] Differences in vulnerability, medical knowledge, and in physical and psychological functioning frequently exist between the two parties to a clinical relationship. Where there is such inequality, the powerful party has moral obligations towards the weaker one – at the very least the negative duty not to take advantage of the weaker party (non-maleficence): not taking advantage includes protecting patients' secrets.

Positive duties also commit health care professionals to the safe-keeping of patients' secrets; the obligation to strive to maximise patient welfare (beneficence) must involve respect for that which one has promised to keep secret.[20] But non-maleficence and beneficence justifications both frame confidence-keeping as a moral requirement of secondary importance, a means by which more fundamental moral ends are striven for, rather than as a good itself.

The obligation to respect confidences also emanates from commitment to respect patient autonomy conceived as an essential aspect of personhood. Based upon respect for the traditional attributes credited to rational agents (self-aware, willing beings, responsible for choices and able to explain them by reference to ideas and purposes[21]) this commitment also finds its foundation in respect for human dignity. Understood in this sense, respect for autonomy places professional secrecy on a par with respecting basic human needs: "human beings want above all to protect the sacred, the intimate, the fragile, the dangerous, and the forbidden. With no capacity for keeping secrets and for choosing when to reveal them, human beings … lose their sense of identity and every shred of autonomy".[22] The self-confidence, dignity, and identity of patients, Sissela Bok argues, depend upon trusting relationships with healthcare professionals. Breaches of confidentiality represent not merely broken promises, but a betrayal of trust, which demotes the human status of the patient, striking at the very core of the doctor–patient relationship.

Although medical confidentiality protects much that may not in fact be secret, maintaining personal secrets lies at its core.[18] Patrolling and guarding boundaries of such shared secrets becomes a particularly difficult and complicated task once such boundaries are considered porous.

TRADITIONAL EXCEPTIONS TO CONSENT FOR DISCLOSURE RULE

A "need-to-know" justification for disclosure of medical information has long been assumed (and is used to justify access by secretarial and other health service staff). Without explicit consent, but based instead upon the assumption of patient understanding and implied consent, clinicians may, some would say *should*, disclose medical information judged essential to enable clinical teams to provide effective healthcare. In the past, sharing patient information for the purposes of education, audit, or research with health professionals lacking clinical responsibility for the patients concerned also found justification, on the grounds that professional obligations of confidentiality guarantee that the circle of confidence will remain unbroken. However, maintenance of one of the characteristics of a shared secret – containment within a circle of those "in the know" – cannot justify the widening of this circle to include other members of the "NHS family."[2]

Disclosure without patient consent, even in the face of specific prohibition, is traditionally justified by compliance with statutory requirements,[23] such as notification of a communicable disease (and here a patient's identity is also revealed), or where serious harm to others is considered likely.[24] In certain circumstances, the GMC speaks of a positive duty to breach confidentiality: where a clinician (who is also a patient), by virtue of his or her medical condition, is placing patients at risk; if a patient continues to drive against medical advice, when unfit to do so; and when disclosure is likely to assist in prevention or detection of terrorism and other serious crime (crimes against persons). Exceptions to the medical duty of confidentiality attempt to be specific, as confidence keeping is held to be "too important a principle to be sacrificed for vague goals or indefinable harms; it should give way only where some 'serious' threat to people looms."[7]

Montgomery argues that primitive commitments to the idea of confidentiality stem from an essentially dyadic notion of private doctor–patient relationships, which is no longer tenable in a modern health service; the modern day commitment to confidentiality, he argues, requires it to be interpreted in data protection terms.[25] Few patients are aware how widely drawn the confidentiality circle in practice can become. In the United States, the medical record of the average hospital inpatient is accessed by some 75 health professionals and hospital personnel.[26] In the UK, NHS financial flows linked to (and triggered by) healthcare provision delivered to identifiable individuals, the development of electronic records, and legal requirements which ensure cooperation between health and social services, have all resulted in a significant shift: from a small circle of people "in the know", to a larger circle whose access to, and routine use of, personal medical information requires to be carefully controlled. In Montgomery's view, the medical profession can no longer be the only (or the principal) guardian of confidentiality; this is now a corporate responsibility involving managers, data processors, and clinical governance leads.[27]

MEDICAL RESEARCH AND DISCLOSURE

Neither the BMA nor GMC accept that release of identifiable patient information for research, audit or education falls within the need-to-know category of acceptable disclosures. Before disclosure for such purposes, they urge patients be given an element of choice:

> Where explicit consent has not been obtained for the use of information or samples in medical research, clinical audit or the education or professional developments of doctors, information should usually be anonymised before it is used by anyone outside the team which provided the patient's care .... The fact that records may be disclosed to persons outside the team which provided the patient's care for the purposes of anonymisation, and that patients have a right to object to such a process, must be made accessible to patients, for example, through practice or hospital leaflets, and in notices in waiting areas.[5]

GMC guidance requires objections to be respected; otherwise lack of dissent by patients counts as permission.[5] What are the moral justifications, in these circumstances, for counting lack of dissent as sufficient moral warranty to disclose anonymised medical information?

The Medical Research Council appeals to a moral obligation upon doctors to paticipate in research in the interests of future patients:

> Medical advance depends on pooling the experience of many doctors. For at least a century clinical and epidemiological research studies have been based upon the systematic collection and analysis of medical information on groups of people; such studies have advanced our knowledge of the causes, nature, course, and outcome of many diseases, and have been invaluable in improving methods of detecting, treating and preventing illness. Advances made in this way are so important that the Council believe that, provided every practicable step is taken, to safeguard confidentiality and to ensure no disadvantage, harm, distress or embarrassment is suffered by any individual as a consequence, there should be no impediment to the use of personal medical information in research.[10]

Harris and Woods (Chapter 27) articulate the moral basis to an expectation we mostly all share, to

have access to effective medical treatment when we need it. For people legitimately to expect best treatment when it is needed, they ought to recognise a reciprocal obligation upon themselves to contribute towards the processes by which effective treatments are determined. On this basis, it is incumbent upon everyone eligible, to participate in medical research; as Chalmers and Lindley indicate (Chapter 26), it is frequently also in patients' own interests to do so. Those who benefit from research in which they themselves refuse to participate act unfairly, Harris and Woods argue, because they are "free riding."

In population-based studies of medical records, where significant patient harm is precluded by appropriate guarantees of confidentiality and anonymisation, everyone eligible for inclusion, in principle, stands to benefit by becoming represented in the distribution of study results. Selective participation resulting from patient refusal will bias research outcomes, and make study samples less representative of the population at large, thereby weakening the potential public health benefit offered by such studies. Participation in research of this sort has been likened to jury service; being a civic obligation for the public good is a sufficient moral basis for overriding rights of refusal to participate (see Chapter 27).

In part this appears to be the rationale behind Wald's refusal to endorse the 1999 Royal College of Physicians' guidance on research based upon archived information (of which he is a dissenting co-author).[8] As an epidemiologist, he takes the view that opt-out rights should not be accorded to patients in these circumstances, because no consent for access to records should be required. Wald believes medical research of this sort to be clearly in the public interest; just as no one can veto notification of certain communicable diseases, so there should be no right for anyone to opt out of contributing archived medical information (suitably anonymised) for purposes of population-based research. On Wald's account, there is no place for leaflet and poster campaigns to inform the public of such studies.[8]

Wald seems to be claiming that failure on the part of individuals to participate in non-intrusive medical records' research disbenefits public health in a manner morally equivalent to failing to notify patients who suffer from notifiable diseases, an omission which breaches the Public Health (Control of Disease) Act 1984. But this Act removes the right of individuals to place the public at risk of specific identifiable diseases, whilst non-compliance with medical records' research results only in (potentially correctable) bias to epidemiological research, together with a potential disbenefit to the non-participants themselves. As one ethicist lawyer has commented: "individuals have a right to resist others imposing ostensible advantages on them".[28]

Like Wald, the MRC envisages situations in which research using medical records' information will be undertaken without explicit patient consent. The Council argues that "making explicit consent a requirement would, on occasion, be likely to vitiate studies which depend on the completeness of samples of information on patients as ... it would not be practicable to seek the consent of each and every person".[10] In these circumstances the MRC supports seeking ethics committee approval and commends campaigns that tell the public that information recorded in medical notes may be used in confidence for the purposes of records based research.[10]

International guidelines for ethical review of epidemiological research are also clear in their recommendations:

> An investigator who proposes not to seek informed consent has the obligation to explain to an ethical review committee how the study would be ethical in its absence ... When it is not possible to request informed consent from every individual to be studied, the agreement of a representative of a community or group may be sought, but the representative should be according to the nature, traditions and political philosophy of the group.[29]

Where individual consent is impractical and risk of patient harm minimal, the role of research ethics committees in the UK (institutional review boards in the USA) may be conceptualised as providing a representative view, a surrogate permission of sorts. Yet arguably, these committees cannot really provide consent on behalf of an entire population, because they cannot presume to know what decision each individual person would make in the circumstances. The ethics committee role here is not one of supplying consent, because the traditional elements making up consent by individuals are lacking (autonomous weighing up of specific information on benefits and risks, together with individual voluntariness and competency). Rather than expressing surrogate consent on behalf of a population, it has been suggested that ethics committee approval offers a "community consensus" that does not obviate a need for further consultation.[30]

According to the GMC, the role of ethics committee deliberations in this situation is one of supplying neither consent nor consensus, but rather it is "to decide whether the public interest in the research outweighs patients' right to confidentiality."[31] The role posited here is assessment of the value of proposed research premised upon unconsented access to confidential medical information; that is, whether this should be allowed to proceed or not.[32]

An alternative formulation has been suggested by Veatch, who also questions the ethical basis for assuming members of review committees can offer consent on the part of others for participation in records-based research, a process he terms "constructed consent". Researchers and members with particular interests in medicine are generally heavily over-represented on these committees, which are in no way representative of the population. In these circumstances, Veatch advocates a new role for such committees: to sample scientifically the views of the eligible population about proposed research, taking (say) 95% approval of participation to be a valid community consent.[33]

This approach, though likely to be expensive, would go some way towards meeting the UK Data Protection Registrar's concerns about unauthorised use of personal data for the purposes of research. The Registrar states that where data users use or disclose personal data "for a non-obvious purpose then, unless the individuals concerned are advised of this intention at the time their personal information is collected," such data are likely to have been obtained unfairly, in breach of the Data Protection Act 1984.[34] Effective (implied) consent to collect personal data should be based upon a consultation process that supplies appropriate information about the reasons and purposes for collection of personal data. Research ethics committees could develop such a role.

THE STATUS OF DATA WITHIN MEDICAL RECORDS

Knox has crystalised two distinct views on the status of the medical record:

> the first that medical records are constructed only for the immediate purposes of the patient–doctor contract and should be seen by no one else, and the second, contrary view, that they should have extended purposes – including communication among doctors, monitoring standards of care, managing health services, and research.[3]

The first view Knox associates with the "absolute

contractual secrecy expressed in the Hippocratic Oath," while the second he associates with the Geneva convention and its reference to a professional duty not only to individual patients but to "humanity" as a whole. Neither viewpoint, he concludes, should be maintained at the total expense of the other.[3]

This tension has emerged in the UK legal arena. The case of *Department of Health* v. *Source informatics* (1999)[35] involved the UK subsidiary of an American company which proposed setting up a scheme to receive information on the prescribing habits of GPs, which it hoped to sell on to pharmaceutical companies for marketing purposes. Without consent from patients, but with the consent of general practitioners (and a £15 donation to the charity of each GP's choice) Source Informatics proposed paying community pharmacists a small fee (£150 per annum), to supply linked information anonymised by patient (GP name, dosage regimen and quantity of medication) abstracted from pharmacy prescriptions.

The Department of Health challenged the lawfulness of the proposed scheme, on the grounds that it would involve pharmacists in a breach of their duty of confidentiality. Source Informatics argued that once pharmacists had extracted and anonymised information from prescriptions, the information would no longer be imprinted with a confidential status. However, the presiding judge in the court of first instance, Mr Justice Latham, approved the Department of Health's view that: "anonymisation (with or without aggregation) does not … remove the duty of confidence towards the patients who are the subject of the data." The Department had argued that "the patient would not have entrusted the information to the GP or the pharmacist for it to be provided to the data company. The patient would not be aware or have consented to the information being given to a data company, but would have given it to be used in connection with his care and treatment and wider NHS purposes."

Mr Justice Latham took the view that pharmacists provide a service to the community as a whole, and in order to retain the trust of the public they must not be seen to breach their patients' confidence for personal gain. He concluded the proposed scheme would "result in a clear breach of confidence unless the patient gives consent," adding that "this may also be the position where doctors and the Health Service itself use anonymous material for the purposes of research, medical advancement or the proper administration of the Service".[35] This last remark he

qualified, saying insufficient argument had been heard during the trial about the use of anonymous patient data for research and administration purposes, for him to come to a firm conclusion on the matter. Nevertheless, the judgement caused considerable alarm amongst epidemiologists, and caused the Medical Research Council and the GMC to become parties to the appeal by Source Informatics for judicial review of this decision by the Court of Appeal.

Despite the commercial context of the case, the High Court judgement was interpreted as threatening to curtail medical research based upon archived information, case control and observational cohort studies, prescription-based research, and studies using computerised databases of medical records. Such studies are of great value not least, as a distinguished group of investigators pointed out, because

> they provide information that is inaccessible to randomised controlled trials, which require ethical aproval and informed consent because they are prospective and experimental. These requirements greatly reduce the inclusion of young children, pregnant women, very old and very sick people, and those unable to give informed consent.[36]

Progress in development of medical treatments for these vulnerable groups could be imperilled, it was contended, by the Source Informatics decision.

Whilst not excluding the possibility that disclosing anonymous information could "necessarily in all circumstances preclude a claim for breach of confidence," the Court of Appeal reversed the decision of the High Court. In doing so it followed in the footsteps of House of Lords decision in *W* v. *Egdell* (1990), which had ruled that disclosure without consent, where appropriate steps to conceal identity have been taken, does not breach confidentiality. However, the Appeal Court accepted that: "even when stripped of anything capable of identifying the patient, the information which the pharmacist proposes to sell to Source is still not in the 'public domain.'"[37]

The Appeal Court drew a distinction between: "use of confidential information in a way of which many people might disapprove, on the one hand, and illegal use on the other." In a judgement that harks back to the relativity of the Hippocratic position on confidentiality (but follows in fact a decision of the High Court of Australia in *Moorgate Co Ltd* v. *Philip Morris Ltd* [No. 2][1984]), the Court formulated the legal obligation of confidentiality as amounting to "an obligation of conscience" arising from the circumstances in which information is communicated or obtained, rather than from whether or not the information is anonymised.

In the leading judgement, Lord Justice Simon Brown held that, in matters concerning disclosure of non-attributable information, the consistent theme that emerges from legal authorities in that

> the confidant is placed under a duty of good faith to the confider and the touchstone by which to judge the scope of his duty and whether or not it has been fulfilled is his own conscience, no more no less. One asks, therefore, on the facts of this case: would a reasonable pharmacist's conscience be troubled by the proposed use to be made of patients' prescriptions? The concern of the law is to protect the confider's personal privacy

and in this case he considered privacy was protected by anonymisation, and ruled: "pharmacists' consciences ought not reasonably to be troubled by cooperation with Source's proposed scheme."[37]

During the hearing, the potential value of medical records based audit and research was emphasised, and the Appeal Judges clearly signalled appreciation of the significance of studies permitting linkage of information back to individual identifiers (required by much clinical audit if the lessons of poor service are to be learned,[38, 39] and by research studies evaluating drug side effects, in which access to specific patient records for the purposes of ascertaining exposures and associated factors can be essential).[40, 41]

HARMS, WRONGS AND PRIVACY

Capron illustrates the moral point of properly informing people about accessing medical records anonymised for purposes of research:

> Suppose that I enter your house (through an unlocked backdoor) while you are away. Suppose that I not only leave everything undisturbed but also that I do not know your identity. Have you suffered a harm? Not in the usual sense – as you would if I took something from the house or if you came home while I was still there and I surprised or, even worse, injured you. But I have wronged you. And that wrong is not overcome if I happen to be a scientist studying dustballs in their native habitat rather than a mere Nosey Parker. The wrong is the invasion of your privacy without your consent. Wrongs of this type may clearly be implicated in epidemiological research. If I have

allowed information to be gathered about me – for example, by my personal physician – and a researcher goes through that information, a wrong has been done even if I do not know about the intrusion ....[42]

Privacy refers to a bundle of rights the invasion of which usually extends beyond matters of keeping confidences, to include vaguer wrongs such as breaching respect for, and protection of, someone's reserve and solitude.[16] The invasion of privacy to which Capron here alludes involves not only unauthorised use of personal information provided and collected for one set of purposes but used (albeit anonymously perhaps with respect for confidentiality) for a quite different set of purposes. Reserve, a state enabling an individual not to reveal aspects of his or her innermost self to others, and solitude, a state in which we are free from observation, were also invaded by the intruder in Capron's story.

Privacy rights imply not only an absence of information about us in the minds of others, but the control we are able to exercise over access to (and communication of) personal data.[43] Several European countries and US states have enacted privacy legislation shifting the requirement for consent for records-based research away from review committees and towards some form of patient informed assent.[44-47] Questions of privacy can arise when data from records are linked in new ways not dependent upon special access to medical records by third parties. The UK Office of National Statistics runs the Longitudinal Study comprising a 1% sample of the population of England and Wales, which allows information on 600 000 individuals from the census and from routinely collected death data to be linked with administrative GP registration records held at the NHS Central Registry. This linkage enables analysis of social mobility between census points to be related to subsequent mortality.[48, 49] On the grounds that they pose no risk of harm to individuals (neither use identifiable patient information nor access data from personal medical records), such studies have hitherto not been deemed to require individual consent (which would be impractical to achieve), or any sort of community-based assent.

Though studies of this sort raise issues of privacy, the UK population at large seems unaware of them. For example, a national survey revealed 68% of the population to be unaware of unlinked anonymous HIV prevalence monitoring within the NHS (in which a proportion of blood samples collected with patient consent for clinically indicated investigations is randomly and anonymously tested for evidence of

HIV infection), though this has been operational for over 10 years. When informed about the programme 26% of survey respondents did not agree with the policy, disagreement being twice as high in those unaware than in those who were aware of the programme.[50] Where ignorance about routine health service activities of this sort remains widespread, privacy rights, ostensibly safeguarded by an ability to opt out from such studies, amount to token rights only.

CONCLUSION

Wide-scale non-intrusive records-based research is predicated upon the belief that harms suffered by individuals as a result of release of anonymised patient data for purposes of research are usually so slight as to be outweighed by the public benefit gained by the research proceeding without consent. However, as we have seen, research that proves harmless to individuals may neither be innocuous ("wrongless")* to them, nor to society at large. Though there appears to be no common law pattern in the UK supporting a general right to privacy,[51] the Source Informatics case indicates that even where data released lacks individual identifiers, allowing medical records to become permeable to the interests of third parties raises questions of privacy, which the courts may be prepared to consider.

Even if it is accepted that no significant breach of confidentiality occurs where unconsented anonymised information is disclosed, in the absence of any general knowledge about it on the part of the patient community, there is insufficient moral warranty for wholesale manipulation of personal health information for purposes quite different from those for which the information was originally supplied. UK poster campaigns advising of the potential for health data transfers in the NHS have so far appeared half-hearted; if undertaken properly, they could help counterbalance the charge that personal information is being collected on a large scale and used for undeclared purposes.

There needs to be much greater public awareness of information flows to third parties within and outside of health services. Information leaflets (in all relevant languages) should be made available at key points in the health service, to inform people of the

integral role of audit in healthcare, and of the value of processing pooled data extracted from personal health records. Better public information about such processes will enable those who wish to restrict use of data about themselves positively to opt out. Privacy and confidentiality will thereby be safeguarded, though not completely, as an opting out system is premised morally not upon informed consent, but upon lack of active dissent. However, because potential harms are minimal or non existent, any slight wrongs are likely to be thought outweighed by the potentially large benefits to be gained from the research taking place. Given other safeguards, such as prospective ethical committee approval (which is not yet a requirement for audit[52–54]), the benefit of research proceeding is likely to outweigh any wrongs and harms that could occur.

There is another morally important reason to undertake public information campaigns: if properly conducted, they would offer people an opportunity positively to identify with medical research conducted on a large scale. A canon of loyalty joining patients and investigators together could thereby be forged, bringing the population into partnership with researchers as "coproducers" of health intelligence and medical research.[55] Such an approach posits patients and potential patients as properly autonomous, and would represent the response of a profession capable of mature and respectful relationships.

ACKNOWLEDGEMENTS

Thanks to Richard Ashcroft, Trisha Greenhalgh, Raanan Gillon, Aziz Sheikh and Helen Watson for offering comments and helpful suggestions on earlier drafts of this chapter.

REFERENCES

1. Lee R. Disclosure of medical records: a confidence trick? In: Clarke L (ed). *Confidentiality and the law.* London: Lloyd's of London Press Ltd, 1990, pp. 23–44.
2. Kennedy I. Between ourselves. *J Med Ethics* 1994; **20**: 69–70, 100.
3. Knox EG. Confidential medical records and epidemiological research. *BMJ* 1992; **304**: 727–8.
4. Bankowski Z. Epidemiology, ethics and 'health for all', *Law, Med Hlth Care* 1991; **19**: 162–3.

*A term coined by Raanan Gillon in commenting upon this chapter.

5. General Medical Council. *Confidentiality: providing and protecting information*. Draft 17. London: GMC, 1999.

6. Working Group of Royal College of Physicians of London. Independent ethical review of studies involving personal medical studies. *J Roy Coll Phys Lond* 1994; **28**: 439–43.

7. British Medical Association. *Confidentiality, disclosure and justified breaches – ethical guidance from the British Medical Association*. London: BMA, 1999.

8. Committee on Ethical Issues In Medicine of the Royal College of Physicians. Research based on archived information and samples. *J Royal Col Phys Lond* 1999; 264–6.

9. Anonymous. Position statement by representatives of the Royal College of Surgeons of England, Royal College of Physicians of England, the General Medical Council, the British Medical Association, the Central Consultants and Specialists Committee (BMA), the Committee of Public Health Medicine and Community Health (BMA) and the General Medical Services Committee (BMA). London: 1995.

10. Medical Research Council. *Responsibility in the use of personal medical information for research*. London: MRC, 1994.

11. Royal College of Physicians. *Guidelines on the practice of ethics committees in medical research involving human subjects*. London: Royal College of Physicians, 1996.

12. *The genuine works of Hippocrates*. Translated by Adams F. London: Sydenham Society, 1849 (Republished: Birmingham, AL. Classics of Medicine Library, 1985; pp. 778–9).

13. Gillon R. *Philosophical medical ethics*. Chichester: John Wiley, 1985, pp. 106–12.

14. British Medical Association. Revision of Hippocratic Oath. In: *Annual report of the council of the BMA*. London: BMA, 1997, pp. 26.

15. NHS Executive. *The protection and use of patient information*. NHSE: London 1996.

16. Francis HWS. Of gossips, eavesdroppers, and peeping toms. *J Med Ethics* 1982; **8**: 134–43.

17. Anonymous. Calls grow to GP legal defence helpline. *Gen Practit* 2000 (February 4th): 8.

18. Bok S. The limits of confidentiality. *Hastings Center Rep* 1983; 24–31.

19. Pellegrino ED, Thomasma DC. *The virtues in medical practice*. Oxford: Oxford University Press, 1993.

20. Bok S. *Lying*. London: Quartet Books, 1980, p. 149.

21. Berlin I. *Two concepts of liberty*. Oxford: Clarendon Press, 1958, p. 16.

22. Bok S. *SECRETS*. Oxford: Oxford University Press, 1982, pp. 281–2.

23. Darley B, Griew A, McLoughlin K, Williams J. *How to keep a clinical confidence*. London: HMSO, 1994.

24. Kennedy I, Grubb A. *Medical law: text with materials*. London: Butterworths, 1994, pp. 644–7.

25. Montgomery J. Confidentiality in the modernised NHS: the challenge of data protection. *Bull Med Eth* 1999; (March): 18–20.

26. Siegler M. Confidentiality – a decrepit concept. *New Engl J Med* 1982; 1518–21.

27. Department of Health. *Report on the review of patient identifiable information*. London: DoH, 1997 (Caldicott report).

28. Dickens NM. Issues in preparing ethical guidelines for epidemiological studies. *Law Med Hlth Care* 1991; **19**: 175–83.

29. Council for International Organisations of Medical Sciences. *International guidelines for ethical review of epidemiological studies*. Geneva: CIOMS, 1991. Republished in *Law Med Hlth Care* 1991; **19**: 247–58.

30. Gostin L. Ethical principles for the conduct of human subject research: population-based research and ethics. *Law Med Hlth Care* 1991; **19**: 191–202.

31. General Medical Council. *Confidentiality*. London: GMC, 1995, p. 7.

32. Biros MH, Lewis RJ, Olson CM, Runge JW, Cummins RO, Fost N. Informed consent in emergency research: consensus statement from the coalition conference on acute resuscitation and critical care researchers. *JAMA* 1995; **272**: 1283–7.

33. Veatch RM. Consent, confidentiality and research. *New Engl J Med* 1977; **336**: 869–70.

34. British Medical Association. *Draft Guidance for the NHS on confidentiality, use and disclosure of personal health information. Comments from the Data Protection Registrar* (Manuscript) London: BMA, 1996, pp. 1–8.

35. *Department of Health* v. *Source Informatics Ltd*. [1999] 4 All ER 185, 197.

36. Lord Walton, Doll R, Hurley R et al. Consequences for research if use of anonymised patient data breaches confidentiality. [Letter] *BMJ* 1999; **319**: 1366.

37. Source Informatics. Application for judicial review. Court of Appeal (Civil Division) (Manuscript). London: Royal Courts of Justice, 1999, pp. 18–19.

38. Beresford NW, Evans TW. Legal safeguards for the audit process. *BMJ* 1999; **319**: 654–5.

39. Dyer C. BMA's patient confidentiality rules are deemed unlawful. *BMJ* 1999; **319**: 1221.

40. Anonymous. The ethics of learning from the patient [Editorial]. *Lancet* 1994; **344**: 71–2.

41. Lynge E. European directive on confidential data: a threat to epidemiology. *BMJ* 1994; **308**: 490.

42. Capron AM. Protection of research subjets; do special rules apply in epidemiology? *Law Med Hlth Care* 1991; **19**: 184–91.

43. Fried C. Privacy. *Yale Law J* 1968; **77**: 482.

44. Vandenbroucke JP. Maintaining privacy and the health of the public. *BMJ* 1998; **316**: 1331–2.

45. Melton LK III. The threat to medical records research. *NEJM* 1997; **337**: 1466–70.

46. Snider DE Patient consent for publication. *JAMA* 1997; **278**: 624–6.
47. Westrin C-G, Nilstun T. The ethics of data utilisation: a comparison between epidemiology and journalism. *BMJ* 1994; **308**: 522–3.
48. Fox AJ, Goldblatt PO. *Socio-demographic mortality differentials: Longitudinal Study* 1971–75. Series LS 1. London: Her Majesty's Stationery Office, 1982.
49. Blane D, Harding S, Rosato M. Does social mobility affect the size of the socioeconomic mortality differentia?: evidence from the Office of National Statistics Longitudinal Study. *J R Statist Soc* 1999; **162**: 59–70.
50. Kessel A, Watts C, Weiss HA. Bad blood? Survey of public's views on unlinked anonymous testing of blood for HIV and other diseases. *BMJ* 2000; **320**: 90–1.

51. Chalton S, Gaskill S. *Data protection law*. London: Sweet and Maxwell, 1988, p. 1001.
52. Wilson A, Grimshaw G, Baker R, Thompson J. Differentiating between audit and research: postal survey of health authorities' views. *BMJ* 1999; **319**: 1235.
53. Warlow CP, Al-Shahi R. Undue protection of patient confidentiality jeopardises both audit and research [Letter]. *BMJ* 2000; **320**: 713.
54. Scott PV. Clinical audit is research [Letter]. *BMJ* 2000; **320**: 713.
55. Tudor Hart J. What evidence do we need for evidence based medicine? *J Epidem Comm Hlth* 1998; **51**: 623–9.

23 · Informed consent, medical research, and healthy volunteers

SM Louise Abrams and GA Browning

After a new compound with therapeutic potential has been synthesised, it is extensively investigated in animals. These data are used to predict the likely beneficial effects in man, as well as the toxicity, both short term and long term. Animal studies will also be done on pregnant females, and their offspring studied. Finally, the pharmacokinetics (drug absorption and elimination) of the new compound must be studied. Animal experimentation is subject to strict legal controls and registration.

Ultimately, however, any new drug must be tested in humans. Animal data are not adequate to enable us to predict therapeutic doses or pharmacokinetics in man. Before a drug can be given to patients, the compound must be tested in normal volunteers. Is it ethical to conduct clinical research on healthy volunteers, and are there any legal constraints?

BACKGROUND

What is a normal volunteer? A cynic might reply that it is a person who has not been adequately investigated. Originally, normal volunteers were associates of the investigator, often working in the same laboratory, or even students of the experimenter who had a certain amount of moral pressure exerted on them to help "push back" the frontiers of science. The Declaration of Helsinki[1] addresses the issue of non-therapeutic research: "The subjects should be volunteers – either healthy volunteers or persons or patients for whom the experimental design is not related to the patient's illness." The key elements in defining a normal volunteer are that:

- the individual cannot be expected to derive therapeutic benefits from the proposed study;
- they are not known to suffer any significant illness; and
- they freely give valid consent to the proposed study.

The first condition is easy to define. The issue of whether the volunteers suffer from any significant illness will be discussed below. The validity of consent is not unique to normal volunteers, but is a problem encountered with patients for therapeutic research and therapies in general. The situation is complicated in normal volunteers because payment is usually involved, and this is likely to affect their willingness to undertake research.

Experimental or other procedures that may cause an animal pain, suffering, distress, or lasting harm are regulated by the Animals (Scientific Procedures) Act 1968. Such animals would in no way benefit from these procedures and could be considered the animal equivalent of human normal volunteers. The rules are very rigorous and precise. Both the person undertaking the research and the individual project must be licensed by the Secretary of State. (The personal licence must be reviewed every five years.) The premises on which the research is conducted must also be approved, and a veterinary surgeon or other suitably qualified person must be specified to give advice. Inspectors are appointed to monitor the Act and they have the right to inspect the premises. Statistics are published every year about this research.

There is, surprisingly, no equivalent law or safeguards (such as inspection of premises) covering research on healthy human volunteers. It would not be illegal for any member of the public to conduct a drug trial in healthy volunteers and to pay them for their services. Consent to research is governed by common law. If an injury occurs as a result of failure of care by the investigator, the volunteer will have to pursue a claim for negligence or breach of contract. Even that would not stop the experimenter continuing his "research".

In 1969 the Association of the British Pharmaceutical Industry (ABPI) set up a committee to advise on medical experiments involving pharmaceutical company staff acting as normal volunteers. Their *Guidelines* have subsequently been revised, most recently in 1994.[2] As a set of *Guidelines*, it has no legal standing and, in theory, only applies to members of the ABPI. In practice, these *Guidelines* are also used as a standard by which to judge the integrity of research that is not conducted under the auspices of the ABPI, for example in academic institutions.

ABPI *GUIDELINES*

The ABPI *Guidelines* state that any research undertaken on normal volunteers should be expected to produce good quality and important data and that the risks involved in obtaining this data must be considered. It therefore follows that research in normal volunteers can only occur after extensive animal research.

Recruitment and reward of volunteers is addressed. A direct personal approach is not approved, but posters and advertisements may be displayed provided that payment is not mentioned.

The issue of the safety of the volunteers is addressed. There are three areas to be considered. There should be minimal risk associated with giving the compound and any procedures involved with the experiment. The *Guidelines* state that such studies should only be conducted after appropriate pre-clinical biological studies have been undertaken. Secondly, risk to the subject will also be minimised if the study is conducted in an appropriate environment by personnel with the relevant training (see below).

The third aspect of volunteer safety is to ensure that the volunteers are indeed healthy: so called volunteer screening. In the light of many of the submissions to one of the authors' local research ethics committee, colleagues assume that if someone is young and not obviously labelled as being sick, e.g. a medical student on a ward round, they must be healthy. Until fairly recently many submissions to the ethics committee were received that did not even address the issue of volunteer screening. The *Guidelines* make it quite clear that this is not acceptable. They insist that the subjects should be screened by "a clinician who should take an appropriate medical history, including reference to allergies, smoking, alcohol or consumption of other medically active substances." This would therefore mean questioning the volunteers about illicit drugs. They also mention that a medical examination should be carried out and, again, state that this should be appropriate to the nature of the planned research. It should include "blood, urine or other tests". In practice most

pharmaceutical research would include a physical examination including measurement of the blood pressure, and urine testing for protein, glucose, cells, and drugs of abuse. Pregnancy testing is usually done on urine. The volunteers would normally be expected to have an ECG and blood tests to check for anaemia, liver and kidney function. The *Guidelines* also comment about timing: "this screening must take place shortly before the study begins." The *Guidelines* explicitly state that any abnormalities found that could increase the risk to the subject should preclude that person from entering the study. Subjects should also not enter the study if there is any evidence of drug abuse, including alcohol.

The *Guidelines* do not talk about routinely screening the personality of the volunteers, although that might be done in special circumstances, e.g. in a psychiatric study. There is some evidence that volunteers may not be psychologically normal. Several authors have administered personality questionnaires to their subjects.[3–5] Whilst some authors suggest that the volunteers are substantially balanced and reliable, two of the studies suggest a higher than normal level of extroversion.[4, 5]

The issue of screening should be explicit in the consent form, especially when screening is made for drugs of abuse. There is a dilemma here. Whilst some volunteers may be happy to have a full health check (commercial value around £250), many have not considered the implications of health screening. Singh and Williams performed a retrospective analysis of the medical notes of 1293 subjects who had volunteered for studies at Zeneca.[6] As a result of screening, 11 % of the volunteers were rejected for medical reasons: 42 of the volunteers had a previously diagnosed chronic medical condition; eight volunteers were found to have excess ethanol intake (with normal liver function); 16 of the volunteers were anaemic. Pancytopenia (absence of red and white blood cells and platelets) and a breast lump were also found as a result of this screening. The screening may reveal that the subject has a chronic health problem for which there is inadequate treatment. Sometimes counselling is offered prior to screening, as was the case in testing a potential HIV vaccine. Clearly all subjects required an HIV test prior to entry to the study, and appropriate arrangements were made. The East London, City & Hackney Health Authority ('ELCHA') Research Ethics Committee (of which one of the present authors is a member) will usually insist that the screening investigations are mentioned in the consent form with particular attention being paid to pregnancy tests and screening for drugs of abuse.

When taking a medical history, the physician is relying on both the memory and the honesty of the subject. Some data from Germany cause concern.[7] In a retrospective survey of 440 volunteers, 3% admitted to incorrectly answering the recruitment questionnaire regarding their medical history: six out of the 13 made a mistake; six deliberately gave incorrect information, but did not expect this to result in a serious risk; and one wanted to be sure of getting into the study. In order to improve the reliability of the medical history, permission should be sought to approach volunteers' general practitioners to confirm suitability for the research project. Many volunteers, however, are travelling students from abroad, particularly Australia or South Africa, or even UK citizens who cannot remember their GP's name; and not all GPs read all their correspondence, so this safety net is not fool-proof.

The GP also provides one of the three methods suggested by the ABPI *Guidelines* for monitoring, and hence preventing, excessive exposure to drug-based research. The volunteers should be given a record card documenting drugs and radiation, counselled on the dangers of excessive volunteering, and the research institution should also keep a record. From personal experience one of the authors' research nurses recognised a volunteer from her previous place of work, where he had been an experimental subject within the previous six weeks. He had filled in a health questionnaire stating that he had not participated in a clinical trial for the past three months and initially denied the previous recent research experience when questioned. It is hard to see how this can be avoided without the setting up of a national register of volunteers. A national register would also address the problem of long-term follow-up. It is possible that in 30 years' time a volunteer may present with an illness that may be related to previous drug exposure. Will subjects even remember that they participated in a study, let alone the name or dose of the drug? The GP may no longer have the relevant documentation.

The ABPI *Guidelines* give explicit recommendations about the conduct of the trial. Prior to commencement, the protocol must be approved by a research ethics committee constituted according to the *Guidelines of the Royal College of Physicians*. There are instructions concerning the qualifications of the medical and nursing personnel conducting the study and the suitability of the premises, for example full resuscitation facilities and staff who undergo regular training in their use. This is a huge improvement from the days when research might be conducted in a corner of an ill-equipped laboratory by non-medical personnel on students studying in that laboratory.

A crucial part of any ethics committee submission is the consent form. The outline of the study and possible hazards will usually have been explained to the subject prior to this. It is difficult to ensure that volunteers adequately comprehend the implications of being research subjects and do not only remember the volunteer fees. Should they be informed that there have been some volunteer deaths? If a drug has never been administered to man, can one predict all likely hazards?

What should happen if something does go wrong? Normally the injured person would have to prove that the doctor had not demonstrated the standard of care that competent doctors would normally have shown. That may be very difficult, particularly where a new procedure is involved, and it is difficult to prove what other competent doctors would have done. The ABPI *Guidelines* therefore state that a contract should be made that accepts liability for injury, without the subject having to prove there was any negligence ("no fault compensation"). The ELCHA Committee has fought a long battle to ensure that non-commercially funded research carried out by the hospitals and medical college in its area also offers the same protection to its research subjects.

In summary, the ABPI *Guidelines* have improved the safety of research conducted by the pharmaceutical industry and shown the rest of the profession how to improve its standards.

INTERNATIONAL HARMONISATION

Much research involving normal volunteers is sponsored by the pharmaceutical industry. The manufacturer must produce the results of the research when applying for a product licence in order for the compound to be prescribed. Most companies are multinational and will want to market their products internationally.

From January 1997 clinical trials carried out in Europe should comply with ICH-GCP (Good Clinical Practice). This refers to the International Conference on Harmonisation of Technical Requirements for Registration of Pharmaceuticals for

Human Use. It was sponsored by the European Commission, the US Food and Drug Administration, and the Japanese Ministry of Health and Welfare and their associated pharmaceutical associations. Like the ABPI *Guidelines*, it covers research on healthy volunteers as well as patients. It specifies the duties of an ethics committee reviewing a protocol and contains detailed instructions about the conduct of clinical trials. It was adopted by the European Union in 1997. A European Directive has made this mandatory and will provide a legal basis for inspection of the sponsors, investigators and facilities by the regulatory authority. However, like the ABPI Guidelines, it will only apply to the pharmaceutical industry when they submit the results of research in an application for a product licence, and not to academic research.

THE ISSUE OF INFORMED CONSENT

Informed consent is a crucial factor in therapeutic treatments where the patient may be expected to benefit. It should be an even more important issue for research on normal volunteers where no benefit is likely, and only harm can occur.

Obtaining genuinely informed consent is not easy. The strong impression that money is the major consideration for volunteering for a study is confirmed by a questionnaire from Germany.[8] An anonymous questionnaire was sent out to 440 subjects: 76% of the volunteers indicated financial motives as a reason for undertaking the research; social responsibility was a reason in 18% of the subjects; other motives included a free medical check-up! Van Gelderen also asked the question "Why?" In a survey of 153 volunteers, 144 of whom filled in a questionnaire, 96% of younger subjects (aged 18–30) gave financial reasons for participation. Of those over 61, 83% claimed to be participating for the benefit of others.

The ABPI *Guidelines* do acknowledge, however, that volunteers do not necessarily volunteer for altruistic reasons and that payment is acceptable, but should not be excessive. The payment should be reasonable and related to the degree and nature of the inconvenience and discomfort involved.

The basis on which the level of payment is decided must be made clear. It must not reflect the level of risk to the volunteer. A decision about the safety of a piece of research should be made before any consideration of how much to pay. It is clearly unacceptable to increase volunteer fees because a study

is a bit risky. Where research in normal volunteers involves significant risk, it should not be undertaken. The ABPI *Guidelines* suggest that the level of payment should reflect only the "nature and degree of inconvenience and discomfort involved." In practice a major consideration will be the length of the study and the restrictions placed on the volunteers whilst they are participants. Studies involving compulsory residence in a clinical trials unit would attract a much higher fee than a similar study where the volunteers were only required to make a 20-minute daily visit. There may be dietary restrictions, compulsory exercise testing, tedious or even painful investigations to be undergone and it seems reasonable that these should be factors in deciding the level of the fees.

Even if the amount paid per day is reasonable, researchers should remember that an experiment continuing over a lengthy period may lead to a large sum that may override the volunteers' judgement. It is not uncommon for experiments to require volunteers to 'live-in' for a month. The considerable, and entirely reasonable, resulting payment may affect the validity of the consent of, for example, unemployed people or students during a vacation.

Financial motivation may well be such a strong inducement that the volunteer may not pay enough attention to the detail of the consent form. An ingenious solution to this problem has been suggested by the Centre for Vaccine Development at the University of Maryland.[9] Volunteers were solicited by means of newspaper advertisements. Following successful screening, each subject underwent a lengthy explanation from two investigators about the illness. This explanation included slide demonstrations and was given on the research ward over one to two days. The volunteers then had to pass a written multiple choice examination with an arbitrary pass mark of 60%. There were also 10 questions dealing with the conduct of the study. Only two out of 91 volunteers failed and neither was allowed into the study. It is interesting to note that most volunteers obtained better marks than members of the medical faculty specialising in that illness! This demonstrates that, with an obvious reward, normal non-medical subjects can be made correctly to assimilate knowledge about a study and its conduct, which is a major part of obtaining informed consent.

However, minimal or no payment can itself lead to problems relating to the consent. The concept of informed consent implies that the subject was well informed about the study and genuinely agreed to participate. The question of "moral coercion" needs to be considered even today. In an academic institution there are frequently financial constraints to the funding of research, and volunteers are asked to participate without any financial inducement. This may be as problematical as excessive financial inducement. If no reasonable payment is offered, people may not volunteer and colleagues and friends may feel obliged to participate.

One of the authors has been a volunteer for a fairly uncomfortable 6-hour experiment that was not dangerous but was certainly unpleasant and for which no payment was made. It involved taking a day of annual leave and the author agreed to do it only because no one else would. The author was then asked to find other volunteers, but refused because it was unreasonable to expect people to give up a day and feel unwell for no recompense, just a desire to help a colleague.

There may be very real pressure from a senior member of the department (possibly an implied threat of a poor reference) if volunteers from the department are not forthcoming. Colleagues may also feel under a moral obligation. Several years ago one of the authors was asked to become involved with a study for which no volunteer payments were to be made. She was asked to conduct the volunteer screening for this study to make sure that all the subjects were genuine volunteers. Two of the subjects really did not want to do the study but knew the researcher was having difficulty recruiting subjects and had difficulty saying "no" to him because "he was such a nice chap." An independent researcher to undertake volunteer screening thus helped to remove moral pressure from colleagues and this would be one safeguard that could be applied. This situation would not have arisen if volunteer fees had been available: reasonable remuneration would have ensured an adequate supply of normal volunteers.

THE RISKS INVOLVED

Informed consent must always include an assessment of the risk involved. Many normal volunteer studies involve new compounds, which necessarily makes risk assessment difficult. There is clearly no benefit to the subject to offset against any risk. There have been three documented deaths of normal volunteers with a varying degree of certainty between whether the death was directly attributable to participation in the study.

In 1996 a healthy 19-year-old female volunteer underwent a research bronchoscopy.[10] Topical lignocaine was used. She left the unit 60 minutes later, although she was complaining of chest pain. She was noted by her boyfriend, just over one hour later, to be having an epileptic fit. She had suffered a cardiac arrest by the time she arrived in the emergency room and was declared dead two days later. It appears that lignocaine toxicity was the cause of death. On reviewing the procedures, it appeared that the lignocaine solution used was of a higher concentration than was specified in the protocol. The lignocaine concentration in her blood was measured 3 hours after the procedure and from this it is possible to calculate approximately the dose of lignocaine used. This was four times the maximum dose specified in a previous protocol for a different study. However, the protocol for the study in question did not specify an upper dose limit of lignocaine for the procedure at all (nor did professional guidelines). This case shows us that an ethics committee has to be obsessional when reviewing protocols and that investigators must adhere strictly to the protocol. This was a preventable death.

In April 1985, *The Times* announced: "Drugs offers cash after open verdict on 'guinea-pig' student." A 21-year-old medical student took part in a drug study in Wales. The drug midazolam was already on the market. Nine months later he died owing to aplastic anaemia (lack of blood cells in his blood). This is a rare but documented side effect of midazolam. It may also occur spontaneously, hence an open verdict was recorded by the coroner. If we accept the premise that it is ethical to do normal volunteer studies, it is hard to see how this death could have been avoided.

Earlier in the same year, *The Lancet* carried a report of the death of a normal volunteer in Dublin.[11] Following a dose of eproxinidine, a new antiarrhythmic agent (a drug to stabilise the heart rhythm), the volunteer went into astystole and resuscitation was impossible. It subsequently became apparent that this particular volunteer had received an injection of a psychiatric drug on the same day he had received the research drug. His death was almost certainly related to receiving both drugs concurrently. Prior to being accepted into the study the volunteer had undergone a very thorough medical examination and a battery of investigations. At no time did this volunteer admit to having received any medication or to any past medical history that would have precluded him from taking part in the study.

Had the history of psychiatric disease or medication been known, according to the ABPI *Guidelines* this subject would not have been accepted into the study. Could this death have been prevented? It is possible, although not certain, that the subject's GP might have known about the psychiatric history. Clearly the volunteer knew and chose not to disclose this information. This raises the whole issue of the necessity and validity of volunteer screening.

Several authors have tried to estimate the total risk of adverse events occurring in normal volunteers. In 1985, Royle and Snell[12] published the results of a survey of 43 companies (who were members of the ABPI) undertaking research in non-patient volunteers. Adverse events are usually categorised as a) major: death or life-threatening; b) minor: trivial or transient such as a rash or headache; and c) serious: events that are neither minor nor life-threatening. They found the incidence rate of serious adverse events as 0.27 per 1000 subject exposures and of minor adverse events as 31 per 1000 exposures. There were no major adverse events.

In 1989 Orme published a similar survey.[13] It found an incidence of 6.9% of minor adverse events and an incidence of 0.55% of moderate adverse events, postural hypotension and abdominal pain being the most common. There were three serious adverse events: severe skin irritation requiring hospitalisation, anaphylactic shock (severe allergic reaction) after an oral vaccine, and perforation of a duodenal ulcer after multiple doses of a non-steroidal anti-inflammatory drug (aspirin-like). In all cases a full recovery was made. The above survey was sent to clinical pharmacology units who would not necessarily conform to ABPI *Guidelines*.

The ABPI conducted its own survey of five years' research ending in December 1994.[14] It reported 21 claims for compensation. This gives an incidence rate of 0.005%, but may well not reflect the true adverse event rate.

In Germany 433 volunteers filled in questionnaires about their study experiences[7]: 17% had occasionally had an adverse event and 2% reported that they had frequently had an adverse event, the most common being headache and fatigue. This figure may seem to be very high but some subjects would have participated in several studies, and some of the adverse events would have occurred whilst the subject was on placebo. More worrying is what the subjects said they did when they had an adverse event: 14% did not report it promptly; 20% first sought advice from other volunteers; only 63% reported them immediately to the medical staff, whilst 1% reported them to their family physician. This survey would suggest that there may well be an under-reporting of adverse events. All the data so far refer to adverse events in the short term. The present authors are not aware of any long-term follow-up of normal volunteers who have participated in research.

CONCLUSIONS

It would be extremely difficult, if not impossible, to create and develop new drugs without the use of normal volunteers. If we are going to continue to use such volunteers in research, we must ensure that the risk to them is minimised. There clearly is a risk, as some of the above surveys have shown.

In view of the strict legislation governing experimentation in animals, it is suprising that there is no legislation to protect human volunteers. Many such subjects are not medically qualified and would not be in a position to assess the safety of the premises or the qualifications of the staff involved, let alone the safety of the experiments. In this country there is at least a set of *Guidelines* that is voluntarily adhered to by ABPI members. This only applies to the pharmaceutical industry and researchers in universities, and hospitals are not obliged to follow them. The new EU Directive will also not apply to academic research.

The law assumes that normal volunteers are not in need of protection because they sign a consent form voluntarily, but we question whether such consent is necessarily properly informed and given for non-financial motives.

Research ethics committees can play a policing role by denying permission if they are not satisfied about the protection afforded to the volunteers. How often, for example, do they inspect the premises where the research is being undertaken? In any case, researchers are not obliged by law to abide by the decision of an ethics committee or even to submit their study to one. It has been suggested that the ultimate sanction is in the hands of the publishers: a study that is deemed to be unethical will not be published. Surely this is too late and will the publisher know the details of how the research was conducted?

Should all research be carried out according to the ABPI *Guidelines*? This would be a huge step forward. However, there would still be some serious omissions.

In our view there needs to be a central registry of subjects. This should prevent volunteers participating in more than one study simultaneously, and would make long-term follow-up easier. We also consider that no study should commence without the written approval of the subject's GP.

We should like to see volunteers offered at least similar protection to that which animals in this country receive. Nothing will change we suspect until there are serious adverse events.

REFERENCES

1. Declaration of Helsinki.
2. ABPI Guidelines.
3. Berto D, Milleri S, Squassante L, Baroldi PA. Evaluation of personality as a component of the healthy condition of volunteers participating in phase I studies. *Eur J Clin Pharmacol* 1996; **51**: 209–21.
4. Ball CJ, McAllen PM, Morrison PJ. The personality structure of 'normal' volunteers. *Br J Pharmacol* 1993; **36**: 369–71.
5. Pieters MSM, Jennekens-Schinkel A, Cohen AF. Self-selection for personality variables among healthy volunteers. *Br J Clin Pharmacol* 1992; **33**: 101–6.
6. Singh SD, Williams AJ. The prevalence and incidence of medical conditions in healthy pharmaceutical company employees who volunteer to participate in medical research. *Br J Clin Pharmacol* 1999; **48**: 25–31.
7. Herman R, Heger-Mahn D, Mahler M *et al*. Adverse effects and discomfort in studies on healthy subjects: the volunteer's perspective. *Eur J Clin Pharmacol* 1997; **53**: 207–14.
8. van Gelderen CEM, Savelkoul TJE, van Dokkum W, Meulenbeit J. Motives and perception of healthy volunteers who participate in experiments. *Eur J Clin Pharmacol* 1993; **45**: 15–21.
9. Woodward WE. Informed consent of volunteers: A direct measurement of comprehension and retention of information. *Clin Res* 1979; **27**(3): 248–52.
10. Day RO, Chalmers DRC, Williams KM, Campbell TJ. The death of a healthy volunteer in a human research project: implications for Australian clinical research. *Med J Aust* 1998; **168**: 449–51.
11. Darragh A, Lambe R, Kenny M, Brick I. Sudden death of a volunteer. *Lancet* 1985; **1**: 93–4.
12. Royle JM, Snell. Medical research on normal volunteers. *Br J Clin Pharmacol* 1986; **21**: 548–9.
13. Orme M, Harry J, Routledge J, Hobson S. Healthy volunteer studies in Great Britain: the results of a survey into 12 months activity in this field. *Br J Clin Pharmacol* 1989; **27**: 125–31.
14. Wells F. Clinical trials compensation. *Lancet* 1995; **346**: 1164.

Part 4

The limits of informed consent in medical research: rights, duties, skills

24 · Informed consent and human rights in medical research

Ann Sommerville

THE INTERFACE BETWEEN HUMAN RIGHTS AND MEDICINE

Rules to protect widely-agreed values are crucial to every society. Among the modern values so defended is a set of fundamental human rights, central to which are concepts of liberty and self-determination. Over the past 50 years, attempts have been made to incorporate these core values into all spheres of activity, including medical research, where they have often sat uneasily with fundamental research goals. In crude terms, the priority for research is to benefit populations rather than individuals. Human rights activity, on the other hand, attempts to ensure that individuals' rights are not sacrificed even if that benefits the group. The scope for tension between the two priorities is clear. Modern research ethics look to the concept of informed subject consent to resolve the conflict but dilemmas still occur. Throughout its history, "a utilitarian ethic [has] continued to govern human experimentation".[1] Increasingly, the rights and needs of individuals claim priority, but this may make some vital research virtually impossible. The gradual incorporation into research ethics of the key concept of informed consent can be seen as major consequence of international human rights activity. Nevertheless, this chapter examines how the goals of research and of human rights activity can remain discordant.

While both research and human rights activity aim to promote human flourishing, many examples exist of profoundly abusive research. Invasive, risky and non-consensual research is frequently seen as typifying the tension between the priorities of research and those of the human rights community. To some extent, however, this is a predominantly western or Eurocentric perspective, shaped largely by awareness of the experiments conducted by the Nazi doctors[2] or in Tuskegee[3] and the US radiation experiments.[4] For the developing world, the right to be *included* in responsible research poses a bigger challenge.

Modern regulatory ethical codes are only beginning to adjust to the fact that ethical and human rights concerns for the majority of the world's population have shifted from trying to protect people from the hazards of experimental interventions towards campaigning for their right to be included in some such interventions. In Africa and Asia, for example, where HIV infection continues to pose a major health threat, participation in research is increasingly viewed as "an opportunity or even a benefit to which people are entitled, rather than a burden from which they must be protected".[5] Claiming entitlements to benefits is as much part of human rights as protecting people's liberty and autonomy. Nevertheless, invoking human rights' instruments in support of a right to be included in research represents a significant departure from the way in which human rights and research ethics are generally perceived to interact.

ABUSE OF HUMAN RIGHTS IN RESEARCH

Liberty Rights

Examining the interface between medicine and human rights, research is inevitably identified as one sphere of medical endeavour where human rights are most consistently and repeatedly at risk. Historically, the most abusive research focused on particularly vulnerable or dependent groups, such as prisoners, who were selected partly because their liberty and choices were already seriously compromised. That is to say that they represented groups for whom the human rights community has particular concern.

The key benchmark of modern human rights standards is the Universal Declaration of Human Rights, adopted by the United Nations General Assembly in 1948. The declaration sets out two specific categories of rights: civil and political rights, and social and economic rights. Among rights potentially relevant to research are the right to equality and freedom from discrimination (articles 1, 2 and 7); the right to life, liberty, and security of the person (article 3); the right to freedom from cruel, inhuman, and degrading treatment (article 5) and the right to basic medical care (article 25). These principles are further developed in international human rights conventions, such as the European Convention and in some national legislation.* Even if governments have not enacted domestic legislation, they are bound to respect human rights if they have ratified international instruments such as the International Covenant on Civil and Political Rights, and the International Covenant on Economic, Social, and Cultural Rights.

The most familiar category of human rights, in western societies, is that of individual civil and political rights. These focus on liberty, personal autonomy, and informed consent. Early statements of human rights were of this kind. Civil and political rights centre on individuals' right to be free from external interference, including medical research and experimentation, unless informed and voluntary consent to participation is given. The same values are also reflected in modern codes of medical ethics and guidelines for the conduct of medical research.

Article one of the UN's Universal Declaration of Human Rights emphasises that "all human beings are born free and equal in dignity and rights." The principle of equality and the right of protection from discrimination are reinforced in articles 2 and 7 of the Declaration, which emphasise that all individuals are equal before the law and are entitled to the same freedoms. It is well recognised that institutionalised discrimination infringing the liberty of some groups may be the start of a general erosion of rights. Human rights literature warns of the dangers inherent in any suspension of the normal rules that protect individual autonomy in pursuit of other values. Routinely elevating other social goals above respect for the individual holds a risk, even when those other social goals are intrinsically desirable. Human rights reports show, for example, how suspension of civil liberties to reduce crime or counter a threat of terrorism can lead to the systematic use of torture by law enforcement agencies and signal the beginning of wider political repression. The slide towards an erosion of basic human rights often

*The Human Rights Act 1998 incorporates into English law the provisions of the European Human Rights Convention.

begins with the identification of some "victim" group within society: some population seen as different or threatening. Such a group may be gradually disenfranchised, excluded from the full panoply of normal human rights, imprisoned, "ethnically cleansed", or physically eliminated. In the past, in extreme cases, research abuse occurred because it was assumed that some people were expendable and that discovering information was more important. Much wartime human experimentation, for example, relied on this justification.[1]

The overwhelming majority of medical research, however, represents the polar opposite of this mind-set. Rather than exploiting or marginalising vulnerable populations, its entire focus is on providing benefit for those who are sick and drawing them back into the mainstream of society. Problematic for the modern researcher is the fact that some of the conditions that most urgently require research, such as mental illness, brain damage, and conditions affecting the very young and the very old, also reduce the possibility of obtaining patients' informed consent. Awareness of past abuse means that there has been a reluctance to carry out any research on groups who may be subject to pressure, such as prisoners, even though they could benefit by increased knowledge about particular conditions more prevalent in the prison population. In other cases, there is no doubt about the desirability of obtaining consent, but debate rages about how detailed and rigorous the process should be. Indeed, past awareness of the crimes committed in the name of research can result in modern researchers being almost hypersensitive about consent issues. This may be an inevitable part of the intellectual baggage that underpins modern research.

It is undeniable that in the past, however, some of those selected for research were particularly vulnerable to coercion, infringing the human rights principles of non-discrimination and the universality of rights. It is notable that much of the most abusive research was carried out on individuals that contemporary society considered burdensome, less valuable and therefore more expendable than others. "When I began my experiments with black smallpox pus," said Swedish researcher Dr Carl Janson in 1891, "I should perhaps have chosen animals for the purpose but the most fit subjects, calves, were obtainable only at considerable cost."[6] The high cost of calves led Dr Janson to experiment on 14 orphans provided by the head doctor of a Stockholm foundlings' home.

Prisoners, members of the armed forces, institutionalised patients, handicapped children, and orphans provided the most accessible pools of subjects for research without consent.[1] In his 1966 seminal paper on unethical research in the US, Henry Beecher cited 22 unethical experiments, which endangered people without their knowledge or consent.[7] As Rothman points out, in "almost all the 22 protocols, the subjects were institutionalized or in some other situation that compromised their ability to give free consent," such as the charity patients with typhoid fever from whom therapy was withheld as part of a research project. The subjects were a disenfranchised population without choices. Similar patterns emerge from the 1996 report of the US Presidential Advisory Committee on Human Radiation Experiments concerning three decades of radiation research. Among those irradiated to discover, for example, the dosage necessary to induce sterility were inmates of Oregon and Washington State Prisons and mentally retarded teenagers. In other cases, part of the researchers' justification was that only patients considered "terminal" were chosen: the implication being that they were expendable.[4]

In such extreme cases, where research involves significant risk, subjects' human right to life is jeopardised, in breach of article 3 of the UN Universal Declaration of Human Rights. Non-consensual research, involving pain or suffering may breach article 5 of the same UN Declaration, which prohibits cruel, inhuman or degrading treatment. In the most notorious cases, research projects clearly qualify as such treatment. Nazi research[8] and similar contemporaneous research projects – notably that of Dr Ishii of Unit 731 in the Ping Fang centre in wartime Manchuria[9,10] – violated both the right to life and the right to freedom from torture. At Unit 731, prisoners were infected with virulent pathogens, and some were bled to death without anaesthetic. Japanese army researchers experimented on around 12 000 prisoners, some of whom were dissected while still alive. Commentators have demonstrated how the notorious Nazi and Japanese wartime research differed from that carried out by other nationalities, mainly in terms of its scale and ruthlessness.[2,3] The same fundamentally utilitarian ethos regarding the expendability of some groups permeated research in many countries. During the same period, the Australian army authorities deliberately infected Australian troops and Italian and German internees with malaria and dengue fever as part of drug trials.[11]

Entitlement Rights

As potentially important as "freedom" rights is the category of human rights, which exerts positive claims to services. These can also mean the difference between life and death, and are reflected in international instruments, including the Universal Declaration of Human Rights. This covers the right to medical care and the special protection owed to children and mothers (article 25). Similar "claim rights" are reiterated in article 12, para 2 of the UN Convention on Social, Economic, and Cultural Rights, which recognises the right to the enjoyment of the highest attainable standards of physical and mental health. It mandates measures to ensure the fulfilment of these rights, including the creation of conditions that ensure medical attention to all in the event of sickness.

Governments that permit research that deprives participants of remedies known to be beneficial could be in breach of the UN Convention. Such research occurs in order to test out new therapies or to gauge the full effects of non-treatment. Again, extreme examples exist, such as the Tuskegee Syphilis Study,[3] whereby 400 African-Americans suffering from syphilis were deliberately left untreated even after penicillin was known to be effective. More recently, much of the debate concerning drug trials in developing countries has focused on this issue of non-provision of a known therapy. Either a proven treatment may not be extended to all trial participants or it may only be provided for the limited period of the trial, subsequently leaving subjects without the benefit of the drugs whose efficacy they help to prove.

Polarisation around the issues was highlighted in 1997 by allegations that some HIV drug trials to reduce transmission from mother to child were unethical.[12] Commentators focused predominantly, however, on the ethical duties of the researchers and trial sponsors rather than the human rights perspective. Debate revolved around the fact that, in industrialised countries, antiretroviral regimes were standard for HIV-infected pregnant women, and reduced transmission to the child. Western companies carrying out trials in developing countries, however, restricted this option on grounds of cost, using placebos, which would inevitably result in some preventable HIV infections in infants. As article 25 of the Universal Declaration of Human Rights makes clear, this particular research population of infants and mothers are entitled to "special care and assistance" as well as having a general human right to medical care.

Arguably, therefore, governments who condone a failure to provide proven therapies could be contravening the Universal Declaration of Human Rights. The sponsors themselves are not bound in the same way by the human rights conventions and treaties that apply to states' parties but, by applying a lower standard of care to overseas participants, they may be seen as discriminative. They might also be in contravention of other standards, such as the international ethical guidelines laid down by the Council of International Organisations of Medical Sciences (CIOMS), which specify that the same standards of care should be provided in developing as in sponsoring countries. From the patient's perspective, it also breaches that person's right to the highest attainable standards of health.

Bitter debate rages around this issue. From a research perspective, placebo-controlled studies provide answers about the safety, value and feasibility of sustainable interventions in particular settings. If successful, the research contributes to the "right to health" in the developing world by providing appropriate and affordable products. From a human rights perspective, however, this is just a small part of a much larger debate about the parameters of a right to "health" and to healthcare. Problematic for the human rights community is the fact that although the right to health (and therefore logically to healthcare) is delineated in various international instruments, consensus about the scope and content of the right is lacking.

Another complication is that claims to services could also be made under interpretations of the "right to life", which is central to any statement of human rights. The 1998 Human Rights Act, for example, includes the right to life, which can be interpreted as a right to receive medical services essential to maintain life or health. We have already seen how abusive research can focus on some vulnerable or dependent groups. Human rights concerns also arise when populations are completely excluded from research that could benefit them. Women, for example, have sometimes been excluded from research. This could constitute a violation of their right to life if it resulted in a lack of effective therapies being developed for them. In South Africa under the apartheid regime, the health system centred on the needs of white patients. Research neglected conditions that predominantly affected non-whites,[13] such as diseases of the respi-

ratory system, enteritis, and other diarrhoeal diseases that were major causes of premature death for the black population.

OTHER CAUSES OF DISSONANCE BETWEEN RESEARCH AND HUMAN RIGHTS

Some resources of tension between research and human rights goals have been identified. A further source of dissonance stems from the fact that the human rights discourse is essentially *modern*. Ideas about universal human rights only really developed in the second half of the twentieth century. Medical experimentation has a long history, for most of which notions of individual rights were absent. Rather, research drew its moral grounding from the traditional concept of the doctor's ethical duty to benefit patients and the Hippocratic dictum of avoiding harm. Because of the relatively recent nature of notions of human rights, much research that is repeatedly quoted as flagrantly breaching those rights pre-dates awareness of them. Until very recently, protection of the research subject was thought to be best ensured by the emphasis on the duties of careful researchers rather than the involvement of patients as consenting partners. Beecher, in his exposure of unethical human experiments in 1966, for example, perceived the solution to bad practice as lying in better self-regulation and the conscience of the responsible investigator.[7] One problem with this is that doctors' views and societal views about what constitutes responsible practice change and evolve. That social, cultural, and political values play an integral part in shaping medical practices and notions of rights has long been acknowledged.[14] Braslow, for example, points out how doctors in every era generally believe that their therapeutic practices are based on the firm bedrock of contemporary science, whereas, in reality, they rely partly on the vagaries of sociocultural context.[15]

A further problem at the interface between research and human rights is that, even now, there is generally little expectation within the medical profession that human rights have much to do with medicine or research. Human rights are seen as preoccupied with the protection of political rights, such as free speech rather than with the conduct of randomised controlled trials. In addition, until recently the paternalistic notion of "therapeutic privilege" permitted doctors to withhold information from patients about the experimental nature of procedures.

Allegations of paternalism were also made against researchers who tried to control US HIV drug trials of the late 1980s and 90s, which were strongly influenced by the consumer movement. An articulate, informed patient population volunteered for research but on its own terms. Arguably, under the fundamental human right to life, patients can claim the best available treatment. They may also claim early access to drugs that are only available in clinical trials. With AIDS, the conflict between the research goal of improving knowledge for all and the human rights focus on individual rights came into sharp relief. Volunteers argued for the wide availability of new, unlicensed treatments and mixed experimental pharmaceutical products with other therapies. Some, anxious to ensure that they received active treatment and not placebos, had their medication analysed. Such focus on individual rights and personal control of medication made verification of the drugs' efficacy impossible. The fact that drug availability was restricted to trial participants was perceived as infringing patients' autonomy, since their consent was not unpressured but the result of desperation. Some argued, however, that pressure does not infringe choice but merely reflects the limitations of everyday life.[16]

The arguments rehearsed in these drug trials focused on the rights of current HIV sufferers rather than the notion of a duty to benefit future patients. Human rights instruments speak mainly about *rights* and entitlements rather than about individuals' *duties*. Only governments ("states parties") are charged under the international conventions and treaties with clear obligations in respect of human rights. From a moral standpoint, it can be argued that patients have some duty to assist research since treatment that they themselves receive has been developed through knowledge gained at the expense of previous patients. At an even more basic level, all citizens might be held to have a moral duty to contribute to the societal goal of increasing useful knowledge. Indeed, such arguments were made in the past to legitimise research on non-consenting prisoners or institutionalised people. As Rothman points out, particularly in wartime, "using mentally incompetent inmates as research subjects accorded closely with popular ideas about the sacrifices appropriate to the home front."[1] However, articulating such individual duties flies in the face of the notion of personal liberty and autonomy which

underpin the edifice of international human rights instruments.

On the other hand, can there be a moral duty to refrain from research? Relevant to the human rights discourse is the fact that some research advances knowledge not only on how to heal but also on how to damage people. Genetic research offers potentially useful data both for developing therapies and for the development of genetically-targeted weapons. Among the evidence given to the Truth and Reconciliation Commission in South Africa, for example, was information about research conducted during the 1980s to identify a germ or bacterium capable of infecting and killing only black people. Other allegations concerned the development of products capable of rendering black women infertile.[17] Medical research also looks at the effects of weapons. Data about the type of wounds caused by landmines or various projectiles contribute to better medical care of the injured. Clearly, however, such data are also useful to weapons manufacturers. As the World Health Organisation points out, this research has a humanitarian focus but "the knowledge obtained through the research is used also ... to inflict more suffering more efficiently."[18]

A COMMON CONCERN FOR RESEARCH AND HUMAN RIGHTS: INFORMED CONSENT

Having considered how research and human rights can be in tension, it is important also to consider where they coincide. Common ground exists between human rights discourse and the modern development of effective regulation of research. At the centre of this common ground is the concept of informed consent. Just as international concern with human rights is a relatively recent phenomenon, so is international interest in the concept of informed consent in research. Chronologically, the history of international human rights instruments coincides with the first international recognition of the importance of informed consent in medical research. Although some national legislation on civil rights and international agreements on humanitarian issues pre-date the World War II, the current international system of human rights protection only came into being in 1945 with the implementation of the UN Charter.[19] This coincided with the development of the Nuremberg Code following the Nazi doctors' trial. Shuster argues that the "key contribution of Nuremberg was to merge Hippocratic ethics and the protection of human rights into a single code".[20] The Code not only requires the researcher to protect the welfare of the subject – a traditionally articulated duty – but also says that subjects can protect themselves by informed consent and the right to withdraw. "By replacing physician-centred Hippocratic ethics with subject-centred human rights, the judges at Nuremberg gave the subjects as much autonomy as the physician-researcher."[21]

The first principle, the very essence of the Code, is the indispensability of the voluntary and informed consent of the human subject, which clearly accords with the fundamental liberty principles articulated in the Universal Declaration of Human Rights. The Code claims to be derived from the "natural law" of all people.[22] Human rights claim the same antecedent. Both came into being through the medium of the law, although the Nuremberg principles stemmed from judge-made law, and the human rights conventions were enshrined in international law.

Unfortunately, the rights set out in the UN Declaration and in the Nuremberg Code have often proved more theoretical than real. Whilst it is true that the end of the World War II marked the formulation of a widely agreed set of rights, many of these rights – both in the civil and political sphere, and in the social and economic arena – remain unfulfilled. In the research world, as Rothman points out, World War II marked a turning point in human experimentation and "practices established during these years profoundly influenced researchers' behaviour in the postwar era."[1] He goes on to emphasise that this was not a benign influence since practices established during the exigencies of wartime conditions positively undermined a sensitivity to the need to obtain the consent of subjects or respect their rights.

The charge of exploitation is avoided where individuals can choose to give or withhold consent. "If patients expect to be personally worse off by being in a trial but nevertheless give their consent, they would be altruistic in a strong sense, meaning that they expect to sacrifice clinical benefit for the psychological satisfaction of helping others".[23] Consent is put in doubt when research subjects have no option. For medical conditions which currently lack effective therapy, research may only theoretically be a matter of free choice. In developing countries, lack of any choice obliges patients to participate in research to obtain any treatment. Minogue makes

this argument, emphasising that offering potentially lifesaving treatment only within the confines of a trial can infringe patient autonomy.[24] Consent has little moral value when subjects are desperate. When the trial ends, care and treatment also usually ends. As Mary Warnock has pointed out, the key moral principle in the research debate is often referred to as the principle of autonomy, but a more precise title is the principle of non-exploitation.[25]

The principle of informed consent is emphasised in every ethical code and guideline; although it is not invariably reflected in practice.[23] Research in developing countries raises particular concerns in this respect. On the one hand, non-industrialised countries may appear more attractive to research because of the manner in which human rights are generally less rigorously monitored. On the other hand, however, they can present acute difficulties to the conscientious researcher because of the population's sometimes desperate desire to obtain western medicine and their overconfidence in the efficacy of whatever product is on offer.

Arguments are sometimes made for lesser standards of informed consent in such contexts on the grounds that the complexities involved cannot feasibly be explained to research subjects or that the achievement of important knowledge supersedes individual rights. Many recent examples of such reasoning exist. In 1997, for example, a controversial South African study was published. This research involved HIV testing, without the patients' prior knowledge or consent, of all patients admitted to intensive care units in Durban for diseases unrelated to HIV.[26] Part of the researchers' rationale was that it was essential not to inform the patients since "patients who were likely to be at risk for HIV infection would also be inclined to refuse the study, which would seriously limit its value." Also in 1997, a cervical cancer research study in India, commissioned by the Indian Council of Medical Research, excluded any requirement for informing the participants of their risk of developing cancer. The researchers argued that the women participating in the study were illiterate and obtaining informed consent would be impossible.[27]

Although they may seem simply to reiterate the spurious justifications for non-consensual research carried out in past decades, many commentators agree that research in the developing world can pose particular challenges to the concept of informed consent. In some cases the subjects' understanding about the benefits of experimental drugs is overly dependent on their trust in western research or in their government which promotes it. It is said that "informed consent in the context of HIV preventative trials in Thailand does not afford the kind of protection that it does in developed countries owing to the differences between the cultural and ethical backgrounds of the investigators and subjects."[28] Similarly, in HIV drug trials in Côte d'Ivoire in 1997, it became clear that participants poorly understood the implications of participating, even though they gave apparent consent.[29] Whilst efforts must be made to overcome such problems by better communication, there is no easy solution.

CONCLUSION: CAN ENDS JUSTIFY MEANS?

Human rights and research ethics coincide in emphasising the pivotal role of informed subject consent to participation in research. Nevertheless, it has long been recognised that usual civil liberties and human rights can legitimately be infringed in some cases in order to secure a greater goal, such as the maintenance of public health. The rights of individuals must be balanced against the reasonable health needs of the population as a whole. This is an argument periodically revisited when researchers deem a project too important to be held up by the vagaries of individual patient choice. Throughout the twentieth century, however, a litany of examples of abusive research testifies to how fragile that balance is and how easily it can be lost, with the result that human rights are unjustifiably sacrificed in pursuit of scientific knowledge. The moral and human rights arguments for obtaining informed consent stem from the fact that "patients who volunteer for medical research can face risks over and above those normally encountered in their everyday lives. The degree of such risks can often be known only after the research has been completed."[30] As Len Doyal points out, to deny research volunteers information is a clear breach of their moral rights. It also constitutes a lack of respect of their fundamental human rights.

Whether the ends can ever justify the means depends in part on the relative value society places on achieving various goals. Respect for human rights is increasingly seen as a key goal that should not be compromised because of the risk of the slippery slope and further erosion of moral standards. Hans Jonas has argued that medical research is an optional goal of relative rather than absolute value. Research, he argues, risks objectifying individuals for purposes that are not their own.[31] Ethically, they may be asked to relinquish voluntarily some rights in order to further the common good but, without that informed consent, research subjects are simply the means of fulfilling the goals of others. As Mary Warnock reminds us, to treat someone merely as a means is widely agreed to be a moral evil and, in Kantian theory, breaches the very foundations of morality.[25]

The indispensability of informed subject consent has been the key moral issue in research since 1947 but remains one upon which unanimity still appears sometimes elusive. Continuing debate indicates the difficulties of translating the ideal into practice and raises questions about whether genuinely informed consent is practically feasible or merely a shibboleth. Studies repeatedly show that the public does not understand the concept of risk or randomisation but persists in expecting some benefit from participation in research. Research in the developing world raises yet other ethical and human rights concerns. This is particularly the case when expensive therapies are pioneered in countries whose annual expenditure on basic healthcare would be clearly incapable of meeting the cost of new drugs, once they are proven effective.

It is clear, however, that researchers are attempting to address some of the dissonance between the aims of research and those of human rights. In 1990, for example, an innovative trial began in which subjects could choose whether they wanted to join the arm of the trial comparing a particular drug with other active treatments or the arm comparing it to a placebo. Such a very tiny minority, however, chose the latter option that the trial was statistically impossible to complete.[32] Offering choice, whilst clearly at odds with the goal of research may, nevertheless, be the way forward. It may be "the price we pay for living in a society which is morally worth preserving, one where we treat each other with respect and where we take human rights seriously".[30]

DISCLAIMER

The views expressed in this chapter are those of the author and do not necessarily reflect those of the BMA.

REFERENCES

1. Rothman DJ. Ethics and human experimentation: Henry Beecher revisited. *N Engl J Med* 1987; **317**: 1195–9.

2. Annas GA, Grodin MA, eds. *The Nazi doctors and the Nuremberg Code*. Oxford: OUP, 1992.

3. Katz J. The concentration camp experiments: their relevance for contemporary research with human beings. In: Michalczyk JJ, ed. *Medicine, ethics and the Third Reich: historical and contemporary issues*. Kansas: Sheed and Ward, 1994.

4. McCally M, Cassel C, Kimball DG. US Government-sponsored radiation research on humans 1945–1975. *Med Global Survival* 1994; **1**: 4–17.

5. Grady C. *Review of the search for an AIDS vaccine: ethical issues in the development and testing of a preventive HIV vaccine*. Bloomington: Indiana University Press, 1995.

6. Lederer SE. *Subjected to science: human experimentation in America before the Second World War*. Baltimore: Johns Hopkins Press, 1995, p. 51.

7. Beecher H. Ethics and clinical research, *N Engl J Med* 1966; **274**: 1354.

8. Taylor T. Opening statement of the prosecution, December 9, 1946. In: Annas GA, Grodin MA, eds. *The Nazi doctors and the Nuremberg Code*, 1992, OUP, pp. 67–93.

9. Harris SH. Japanese biological warfare research on humans: a case study of microbiology and ethics, *Ann NY Acad Sci* 1992; 21–52.

10. Harris SH. *Factories of death*. London: Routledge, 1994.

11. Kenyon G. Australian army infected troops and internees in second world war. *BMJ* 1999; **318**: 1233.

12. Lurie P, Wolfe SM. Unethical trials of interventions to reduce perinatal transmission of HIV in developing countries. *N Engl J Med* 1997; **337**: 847–9.

13. Chapman AR, Rubenstein LS, eds. *Human rights and health: the legacy of apartheid* (joint report from the American Association for the Advancement of Science (AAAS), Physicians for Human Rights, the American Nurses Association and the Committee for Health in Southern Africa). Washington: AAAS, 1998.

14. Rosenberg CE, Golden J. eds. *Framing disease: studies in cultural history*. New Brunswick (NJ): Rutgers University Press, 1998.

15. Braslow J. Therapeutic effectiveness and social context: the case of lobotomy in a California state hospital, 1947–1954. *West J Med* 1999; **170(5)**: 293–6.

16. Logue G, Wear S. A desperate solution: individual autonomy and the double-blind controlled experiment. *J Med Philos* 1995; **20**: 57–64.

17. Report of the Truth and Reconciliation Commission. Chemical and biological warfare. In: *Human rights report*, Human Rights Committee, South Africa, June 1998.

18. Prokosh E. *The technology of killing. A military and political history of antipersonnel weapons*. London: Zed Books, 1995, p. 11.

19. Davidson S. *Human rights* (in the series Law and Political Change). Buckingham: Open University Press, 1993.

20. Shuster E. Fifty years later: the significance of the Nuremberg Code. *N Engl J Med* 1997; **337**: 1436–40.

21. Shuster E. The Nuremberg Code: Hippocratic ethics and human rights. *The Lancet* 1998; **351**: 974–7.

22. Grodin MA. Historical origins of the Nuremberg Code. In: Annas GJ, Grodin MA, eds. *The Nazi doctors and the Nuremberg Code*. Oxford: OUP, 1992, pp 121–44.

23. Edwards AJL, Lilford RJ, Hewison J. The ethics of randomised controlled trials from the perspectives of patients, the public, and healthcare professionals. *BMJ* 1998; **317**: 1209–12.

24. Minogue BP, Palmer-Fernandez G, Udell L, Waller BN. Individual autonomy and the double-blind controlled experiment: the case of the desperate volunteer. *J Med Philos* 1995; **20**: 43–55.

25. Warnock M. Informed consent – a publisher's duty. *BMJ* 1998; **316**: 1002–3.

26. Bhagwanjee S, Muckart DJ, Jeena PM, Moodley P. Does HIV status influence the outcome of patients admitted to a surgical intensive care unit? a prospective double blind study. *BMJ* 1997; **314**: 1077–81.

27. Trust us, we're doctors. *New Scientist* 1998 (28 March): 20.

28. Zion D. Ethical issues in international HIV/AIDS vaccine trials. Monash University (unpublished paper), 1998.

29. French H. AIDS research in Africa: juggling risk and hopes. *New York Times*, 9 October 1997.

30. Doyal L. Informed consent in medical research. *BMJ* 1997; **314**: 1107–11.

31. Jonas H. Philosophical reflection on experimenting with human subjects. In: Freund PA, ed. *Experimentation with human subjects*. New York: George Braziller Inc, 1969, pp. 1–31.

32. Medical Research Council. HIV-trials and controversies. *MRC News* 1998; (news bulletin no. 79, p 21).

25 • 'Fully' informed consent, clinical trials, and the boundaries of therapeutic discretion

Raanan Gillon

As a long-standing advocate of adequately informed consent and opponent of medical paternalism, I had enormous sympathy with the intentions underlying my friend and colleague Len Doyal's advocacy of a very tough approach to obtaining "fully informed consent" for clinical research.[1] Like him I do not subscribe to the view that patients have a moral duty to participate in medical research (I believe it is morally admirable, though supererogatory – above the call of duty – when they do). Like him I do not accept the crude utilitarian argument that if abolishing accepted norms of research ethics can be expected to save lives by, for example, getting scientifically valid life-saving results faster, then those accepted norms should be over-ridden. Nonetheless I cannot agree with Len Doyal that all medical research requires "fully informed consent" with the exceptions of certain sorts of research on mentally incompetent patients, certain sorts of records research, and certain sorts of research on stored tissue.

In this chapter, I first argue that **no** medical research requires or can possibly obtain "fully informed consent" and I continue my personal quest to replace the use of this misleading term, by accepting as the proper moral standard for consent in both medical treatment and medical research on human subjects, the concept of "adequately informed consent."[2-4] (In his *BMJ* paper Doyal calls for both "fully informed consent" and "adequately informed consent" – adequately informed consent is all we need for the standard – and different degrees of "fullness" of information will be required for adequacy of information in different circumstances.) However, accepting that, in certain categories of medical research on human subjects, those subjects routinely ought to be given a substantial amount of written information before their consent to participate is

sought (paradigmatically all possibly harmful non-therapeutic medical research carried out on volunteers not for their benefit but for the possible benefit of others), I propose the term "extensively informed consent" to replace the term "fully informed consent" in those contexts where the latter term is used to indicate that extensive and written information is needed. I then argue that there are differences between non-therapeutic and therapeutic research that in some circumstances justify less than such extensive information as being sufficient for adequately informed consent in certain cases of therapeutic clinical research.

Such cases justify the addition of two other and substantial exceptions to Doyal's own list of exceptions to the need for "fully informed consent" (or, as I would like to call it, "extensively informed consent"), whilst still requiring adequately informed consent. The first exception – in the area where good research and good therapy may be difficult to distinguish – covers the whole range of clinical therapeutic research that compares two or more standard medications for the patient's condition. The second exception, again in the area where good research and good therapy may be difficult to distinguish, is clinical research that compares a standard medication with a new and "promising", potentially better (but also, of course, potentially worse), medication for the patient's condition, where the standard treatment is not very effective and where the doctor has some justifiable reason to believe that it is in the patient's interests to participate in the trial. In both types of exception the doctor must also have reason to believe that the patient does not wish to receive *extensive* information either about his or her condition or about the clinical trial, but is nonetheless willing to participate in the trial, having been given initial basic information about the research, with the offer of more extensive information if he or she would like it. I then urge, briefly, that discretion should also be left available for research ethics committees to accept other possibly justified exceptions to the need for "extensively informed consent" – exceptions currently unthought of – provided they conform to the principle of "adequately informed consent", where adequacy of information is at least in part determined by the patient's own view of how much information he or she wishes to have. Finally, I propose, again *pace* Doyal, that medical journals should not normally override decisions of *bona-fide* research ethics committees about the ethical acceptability of particular research projects by refusing to publish research that has been approved by such a committee.

LET'S ABANDON "FULLY INFORMED CONSENT" AS A MORAL STANDARD AND REPLACE IT BY "ADEQUATELY INFORMED CONSENT"

I have long advocated use of "adequately informed consent" as the appropriate moral standard for consent to medical interventions.[2–4] Why reject the standard of "fully informed consent"? The first reason is that there can be no such thing – "fully informed consent" is a mirage – simply because it is always possible, whatever information one has given and continues to give about a treatment or research proposal, to give additional information about it. Thus the information given is never, and can never be, "full" because "full" means that no more can be added. If fully informed consent is thus in fact impossible to achieve, then it is misleading and wrong to pretend that it can be achieved, and the term ought to be abandoned for a more accurate term or terms.

The second reason for rejecting the standard of "fully informed consent" as a moral standard for information is that I think it would be wrong even if one could achieve it. For even if one could obtain and impart full information about a proposed treatment or research project, it would not necessarily be morally required or relevant for the patient's ethically valid consent, and its very fullness might – in many cases would be likely to – diminish rather than enhance its moral usefulness. Think, for example, of the "small print syndrome" found in so many agreements to purchase or hire equipment, in which information relevant to the customer is buried in reams of irrelevant information, printed in almost illegibly

small print itself purportedly justified by the necessary extensiveness of the information to be imparted. (Think too of the vogue, now increasingly discredited, in America for consent documents the size of medical textbooks, largely unread by patients or doctors.) As Internet explorers increasingly discover, there are vast quantities of information sources on most subjects, but they require sorting both for relevance and reliability. If fully informed consent were in fact a possible target it would involve near infinitely large sources of information that would require vast amounts of time and effort to be similarly sorted for relevance and reliability.

The relevant moral standard for consent is surely not this mythical "fully" informed consent, but rather "adequately informed consent", in which the notion of adequacy is deliberately evaluative and unspecific. Why unspecific? Because the adequacy of information is context-specific, being related primarily to adequacy as perceived by the particular patient and/or subject who is giving or withholding consent; but also to adequacy as perceived by others; adequacy as perceived by the doctor offering the treatment and/or proposing the research project; adequacy as perceived by the medical profession collectively; adequacy as perceived by other relevant ethical scrutineers, for example research ethics committees; and adequacy as perceived by lawmakers on behalf of their societies. Adequacy is also context-specific in relation to the intervention being proposed and the underlying norms for such interventions.

ADEQUACY OF INFORMATION IN THE NORMAL THERAPEUTIC RELATIONSHIP – THE "HIPPOCRATIC COMMITMENT"

In the normal therapeutic relationship between doctor and patient there is a long-established norm that a treatment will be proposed by the doctor only if, in that doctor's professional and expert assessment, that treatment is likely to produce net benefit to the patient with minimal harm. This "Hippocratic commitment" has been at the heart of medical ethics for at least 2500 years when it was incorporated into the Hippocratic Oath,[5] and has been accepted ever since by doctors as a fundamental ethical commitment and obligation to their patients. Importantly it has also been accepted by patients and public alike as part not only of this self-proclaimed commitment of the medical profession to its patients but also as part of the duty of the profession – both the moral duty of the profession and in many jurisdictions also part of the profession's legal duty of care.

Given trust by a patient that this "Hippocratic commitment" will be honoured, then that patient may well feel that he or she does not need to check out a doctor's proposal for treatment in the thorough way that a prudent person is likely to check out, for example, a travelling salesman's proposal that the person buy his commercial product. There simply is no equivalent among commercial salesmen to the medical Hippocratic commitment such that a commercial product will be offered to a customer only if, in the salesman's expert assessment, that product is needed by the customer and is likely to produce for that customer net benefit with minimal harm. On the contrary the widely accepted norm for good salesmanship is to sell as many items as possible. To protect the customer there are the relevant laws and institutions plus the widely accepted common-sense rule of *caveat emptor.*

In ordinary therapeutic medical practice, however, there is, in addition to legal protection and *caveat emptor*, the additional protection for patients of the Hippocratic commitment which promises that the doctor will propose an intervention only if, in the doctor's professional assessment and judgement, that intervention will be in the patient's interests. Given the patient's acceptance that the norm will be honoured, then when a doctor prescribes a medicine adequate information may be quite properly synoptic ("You have such-and-such an infection, and I'd advise you to take this antibiotic at this frequency for such-and-such a time" – the doctor already having ascertained that there is no history of dangerous reactions to the particular medication proposed!) The patient may wish to ask questions about the treatment and the alternatives, which the doctor should of course answer. However, there is no need either morally or legally to hand over a lengthy document detailing the anticipated benefits, all possible harms (with any substance one ingests there is a lengthy list of possible harms), all available alternatives (with infections there is often a wide range of alternative antibiotics, and no treatment at all may nonetheless be followed by the body curing itself – though no treatment may also be followed by more or less dangerous deterioration), assurance that the proposed treatment has been found acceptable by an ethics committee, and finally for the doctor to request a signature from the patient confirming that he or she understands the treatment and its alternatives, and consents to take the treatment.

Even in the case of serious disease, for example cancer, although we have long known that most patients wish to know their diagnoses and to discuss at some length the available treatments and the anticipated course of events,[6,7] they will often prefer to assimilate information over a period of time, not all at once. Furthermore, a minority of patients positively do not wish to be told the details of their condition or its prognosis and prefer to leave treatment decisions entirely to their doctors.[7] Even in the majority of cases where information is wanted, the provision of such sensitive information, relating as it must to the risks of impending mortality, should, it is surely uncontroversial to assert, be done in a way that responds to the needs and wishes of the particular patient in the particular context.

WHY MEDICAL RESEARCH IS ETHICALLY DIFFERENT FROM MEDICAL TREATMENT – THE PARADIGM CASE OF NON-THERAPEUTIC RESEARCH

Of course, medical research is not the same as medical treatment and much medical research does not involve treatment at all, or any other attempt to benefit the participant in the research – the "research subject". Indeed the fundamental morally relevant difference between medical treatment and "pure" medical research is just the presence or absence of the Hippocratic commitment that is at the heart of the doctor–patient relationship in the ordinary therapeutic context. In treatment the doctor is committed to try to make the treated patient better. In "pure" medical research – typified by non-therapeutic research on healthy volunteers – there is, by definition, no Hippocratic commitment to the "subject" and the doctor/researcher's intention is to discover generalisable knowledge, with the intention ultimately of benefitting the health of others. (If this intention is missing from any scientific research, then I can discern no justification for calling it medical research – it is simply scientific research.)

This difference in the doctor's intention is obviously of crucial moral significance for the patient. For where the doctor's intention is not to benefit the patient (even though it is to benefit other people by the production of potentially useful medical knowledge), then the Hippocratic commitment clearly does not and cannot apply to that patient, and the underlying basis for the patient's trust, that the doctor will propose only what is in the patient's interest cannot exist. In those circumstances a prudent patient will wish to scrutinise in considerable detail the interventions proposed by the doctor especially for any harms entailed or even risked, including high probability minor harms (such as inconveniences, needle jabs, minor side-effects, etc.) and low probability major harms (for example, dangerous and even possibly fatal idiosyncratic reactions to the substance being tested).

Moreover, the medical profession collectively has wished in recent times to distinguish very clearly between its non-therapeutic research activities where its Hippocratic commitment by definition does not and cannot apply (but to which it is nonetheless committed by its continuing obligation to develop more effective and less risky ways of benefitting patients), and its therapeutic activities in which the Hippocratic commitment does apply. Similarly society generally has had an interest in clearly distinguishing non-therapeutic research carried out by doctors from ordinary medical treatment. The outcome of these joint concerns, massively stimulated by the notoriously outrageous behaviour of the Nazi doctors (and others since) has been the establishment of highly protective norms for medical research. Stemming from the judgements of the Nuremberg war trials[8, 9] and the World Medical Association's Declaration of Helsinki,[9] these protections are based on informed consent and the acceptability of no more than very low levels of additional risk to subjects where these risks are not taken for the subjects' own intended overall benefit.

These protections are overseen by research ethics committees who scrutinise all proposals for medical research on human subjects and ensure, among other objectives, that non-therapeutic research is not carried out unless the risks are minimal – usually equated to risks no greater than those acceptable in everyday life[10–12] (though which interventions are to be regarded as of "minimal risk" in this sense remains a matter of controversy[12, 13]) and the establishment of a variety of procedures designed to protect all subjects of medical research.[14–16] Among the norms established for non-therapeutic research (medical research carried out with no intention or likelihood of benefitting the subjects of that research – for example in the early development of new medications in which volunteers are administered the new agent in order to discover, say, concentrations in the blood achieved by different doses) has been a requirement for extensive information about the research project, its hoped-for results, details of the desired involvement of the volunteer, and details of any known inconveniences, side effects, and risks (though not any express requirement to explain that there may be *unknown* risks, even though these must have been minimised by previous research including animal and toxicology assessment). A written information sheet and a signed agreement from the subject, confirming that he or she has understood the information and agrees to participate, are also required as standard.[10, 17]

MEDICAL RESEARCH COMPARING TWO OR MORE STANDARD TREATMENTS

The rationale that justifies different information requirements for implementing the single common standard of adequately informed consent in the two contexts of ordinary medical treatment and non-therapeutic research is thus clear enough – the presence or absence of the Hippocratic commitment to the individual is what makes the moral difference. However, much medical research is carried out on patients to compare a standard treatment for the patient's condition either with some other standard treatment (to discover which is better) or with some new medication for which early developmental research has shown promise that the new agent will be better than the standard treatment or treatments. In these circumstances the researchers have both the Hippocratic commitment to do their best for the patient, and the medical research commitment to discover new knowledge that will be beneficial to patients in the future.

Take for example the case of research into cancer treatments, which are often still only moderately effective whilst being substantially toxic and having unpleasant side effects. The clinician who is not involved in medical research may have a choice of two standard treatments, neither of which is clearly superior to the other. Each of that clinician's individual patients will have different needs and wishes concerning the amount of information about the disease and its treatment, and about the timing of such information. Some, probably a large majority, as indicated above, will wish to be given extensive information, though perhaps over a period of time rather than all at once. A minority will not want much information, especially unpleasant information, such as written details indicating a high probability that they will soon die and that available treatment for their condition is both toxic and often not very effective.

The clinician will wish to be able to respond to each patient as an individual with individual preferences and needs and to give information in a way that matches those preferences and needs. At the same time the clinician will wish to provide the best treatment to each patient and, if there are a variety of standard treatments many clinicians would prefer to find out (in the interests of the particular patient quite apart from the interests of future patients), which of the available options is best.

Often the way to find out is to ask the patient to participate as a subject of medical research in a well-designed randomised controlled trial of the alternatives. Must all such patients/subjects be required to give "fully informed consent" as Doyal proposes (assuming that he or she is competent to do so)? Since, as argued above, there can be no such thing as "fully informed consent", let us understand this term to mean "extensively informed consent", with the information needed being comparable to that needed for adequately informed consent for non-therapeutic research. Must all patients suffering from potentially fatal cancer be given comparably extensive information before they can be enrolled as research subjects in a comparison of two standard treatments for their cancer, even if the patients themselves do not want such extensive information, or do not want it all before they start treatment within the trial?

It seems clear to me that patients themselves should be allowed to choose to have as much or as little information as they prefer and still be allowed to participate in trials of standard treatments for their condition. In order to respect such patient choice, the doctor's basic approach would be similar to that in the ordinary therapeutic context, eliciting first the amount of information and involvement in treatment decisions that the patient wants, and passing on the information that in any case would be necessary if the treatment were to be given (for example, likely side effects plus an indication that the treatment could itself be risky). Then, as in the ordinary therapeutic context, delicate negotiations between doctor and patient establish how much or how little information the patient wishes to be given, at least at that stage. If the patient makes clear that he or she does not want much information or involvement, then this should be respected. The physician could explain that there were two or three standard treatments for the patient's condition and that it was impossible at present to know which was better for the patient. The doctor could either sim-ply choose a treatment, without good reason to make such a choice, or the patient could participate in a research study to try to find out which treatment was better. This would involve the patient being allocated at random to one or other of the standard treatments without either the patient or the doctor knowing which, to avoid any bias, and then comparing the overall results. The doctor would be happy to give as extensive information as the patient would like about the study, now or later, but would also be happy to accept the patient's preference to leave it at that, leaving the offer of further information "on the table" should the patient want it later on.

Something along those lines – and it would be for the clinician to judge how exactly to offer the information to each individual patient in a way that most closely matched that patient's wishes – should surely, for patients who did not want further details but accepted participation in the trial, constitute adequate information, just as it would, appropriately modified, be adequate information in ordinary therapy. Treatment with either standard medication would be in the patient's interests, but finding out which was the better treatment would be even more in the patients' interests. Thus such a trial is a paradigm example of "therapeutic research", in which the Hippocratic commitment to intervening only if the doctor believes that the intervention is in the patient's interests, is maintained. Given that in ordinary therapy patients may give adequately informed consent for a treatment on the basis that they want little information and simply wish the doctor to do what the doctor thinks is best for them, it seems clear that they should similarly be allowed to reject extensive information, while accepting participation in a clinical trial of standard treatments for their condition, and that their consent based on the relatively little information outlined above would nonetheless constitute adequately informed consent. Equally clearly such consent would not be extensively informed, let alone fully informed. Such cases therefore constitute a morally legitimate exception to Doyal's requirement for fully informed consent for patient participation in medical research, even if this term is understood as extensively informed consent.

COMPARING STANDARD TREATMENT WITH A NEW TREATMENT

The argument just offered concerned comparison of

two or more standard treatments, already accepted as standard and potentially beneficial for the particular patient's condition. What about trials comparing a newly developed potentially therapeutic agent with a standard treatment? Must "fully informed" (understood as extensively informed) consent always be obtained if a patient is to be enrolled in such a trial? Here I think the answer will depend on how effective and safe the existing standard treatment is, and therefore the extent to which participation in a trial is likely to be beneficial to the patient (as distinct from how beneficial it is likely to be for others). If there is already a very effective and safe treatment (for example an effective antibiotic that works well against the patient's infection), and this is being compared with a new antibiotic as part of the general development of new antibiotics needed in the continuing battle against bacterial resistance to antibiotics, then it seems that extensively informed consent is required. Any patients who do not wish to have the standard and extensive information routinely given in such a trial should not be enrolled in the trial and simply be given the standard treatment. My reasoning here is that it is unlikely to benefit the patient to participate in such a trial, or at best only very remotely likely (if, for example, the new antibiotic were found to be effective, and on a future occasion the patient suffered a further infection with an organism resistant to the standard antibiotic but sensitive to the newly developed one). So while development of new antibiotics is likely to be of benefit to future patients, participating as a subject in such a trial – in the absence of special features that would make it more likely to benefit the patient – is more akin to being a volunteer participating in non-therapeutic research for the potential benefit of others than to being a patient in a trial to ascertain which of two standard treatments is better for the patient as well as for others.

Let us assume that the doctor asks the standard question required by the Hippocratic commitment: which available intervention is likely to produce optimal benefit for my patient with minimal harm? Then, in the case of the trial outlined of a new antibiotic, the answer is surely "I don't know, but I have better reason to think that the standard antibiotic is likely to do so than the new antibiotic, and I have good reason to think that the standard antibiotic *will* produce optimal benefit with minimal harm for this patient." There may not be much in it, and there is no particular reason to reject the trial of the new antibiotic, and good reason to pursue it, provided the

patients involved (or their proper surrogates) are properly aware that their participation will be for the potential benefit of others rather than themselves. In the absence of such awareness (i.e. in the absence of extensively informed consent), then my duty to my patient – my Hippocratic commitment – requires me to use the standard antibiotic treatment rather than enrol the patient into the trial.

Suppose, however, that the standard treatment of the patient's condition, while somewhat effective and certainly better than nothing, is not very effective. It might, for example, be a standard anticancer "cocktail" of three or four medications, with a success rate as measured by five-year survival of 20% whereas five-year survival of untreated patients was previously (say) 2–8%. Now suppose that a patient is ready to participate in a trial of this standard treatment against the standard treatment plus a new agent, but does not want all the associated trial information including details of his or her condition and its prognosis. Must the doctor in such a case insist on extensively informed consent or exclude the patient from the trial and use the standard treatment? Here the answer seems to be "No!", not if the patient does not want such extensive information but is nonetheless ready to participate in the trial.

Again, of course, the initial requirement as usual will be for the doctor sensitively to find out how much the patient wishes to be informed about his or her condition and its standard treatment/management, and to pass on in any case whatever minimal information would be necessary for the standard treatment to be given; i.e. even if the patient would prefer no information at all, professional and legal minimal standards would require information to be given on the likely efficacy, and any substantial side effects and risks, with an offer to answer any questions. For the patient who did not want further information (or at least not at that stage), if this basic minimal information constituted adequate information for the patient's adequately informed consent to have the standard treatment, what about enrolling such a patient into the postulated trial? Given that the standard treatment does not have a high success rate, it might well be in the patient's interests to participate in such a trial. Suppose, for example, that the doctor, having reviewed the trial information, is persuaded that *prima facie* the new agent is promising: there have been promising *in vitro* results and promising animal model results. Furthermore, pharmaceutical firms tend not to invest in the substantial costs of developing and trialling a new medication unless they have initial results that indicate that it is at least as effective and as safe as existing standard medications and has a reasonable prospect of being better.

Let us further imagine that, if the doctor himself or herself had the cancer concerned and were given the option of the standard treatment or the standard treatment plus the new agent, the doctor would choose the combination. Thus, whilst the doctor might accept that there was only slender evidence at this stage favouring the new agent and that the trial was needed to support or refute this initial evidence before the new agent could be recommended as an effective and preferred treatment for the cancer, nonetheless the doctor would, if given the option, choose the standard treatment combined with the new agent. Of course the doctor is aware that the results of the trial might show this preference to be mistaken; that is why the trial is necessary. In the meantime the doctor considers a slight bias in favour of the new agent to be justified. The doctor also realises that others, with different risk perceptions might well be biased *against* the new agent, reasoning that, until there was good scientific evidence to the contrary, it would be safer to avoid the new agent and stick with the tried-and-tested standard therapy, even if it were only moderately effective; the new one might prove even less effective or have worse adverse effects. So, normally, the doctor would wish patients to be thoroughly, extensively, informed about the pros and cons of participating in such a trial and make their own decisions. However, given a patient who did not want extensive information but was happy – perhaps positively wished – to participate in such a trial, and given also the doctor's marginal but justifiable bias in favour of the new treatment, it seems morally acceptable for the doctor to enrol such a willing patient in the trial without "fully informed" (understood as extensively informed) consent. This would respect the patient's autonomy by *not* forcing him or her to have unwanted information; it would avoid inflicting unnecessary distress,[18] and it would increase the chance of the patient receiving treatment that the doctor *suspected* to be more beneficial than the existing standard treatment.

In rejecting this position, some might argue that the doctor is irrational to have even a *prima facie* preference for the new medication prior to the trial being carried out. Such a view of "rationality" is surely too rigid. While I have no doubt that positive results from a well-designed clinical trial favouring the trial agent would provide *good* evidence in its favour, whereas

the pre-trial toxicology and animal model results, along with evidence of the pharmaceutical firm's readiness to invest in the clinical trial, produce only *slight* evidence in its favour, nonetheless acceptance of slight evidence to choose one way rather than another can be quite "rational" especially in life-threatening circumstances when better evidence is not available. Such disagreement about the case outlined is much more likely to stem from people's different levels of risk aversiveness than from their different degrees of "rationality". (It would also be foolhardy to respond that "rationality" correlated either directly or inversely with "risk aversiveness".)

CONCLUSIONS

To generalise from the examples given, it seems clear to me that clinical research – so-called therapeutic research (as distinct from non-therapeutic research, in which there is and can be no intention to benefit the participant subjects of that research) – always has two components: a component of pure research intended to produce generalisable medical knowledge, and a component of therapy, where the intention is to benefit the particular patient/subject's own health. There is no way that I have been able to discover of quantifying, with any precision, the relative strength of each of these components in a given trial. However, as argued, at one end of the scale (comparison of two existing standard treatments for the patient's condition when the clinician has no good reason to prefer one over another), a clinical trial may have a very large component of ordinary therapy; at the other end of the scale (e.g. comparison of a new medication with a standard medication when the existing standard therapy is known to be highly effective and safe for existing patients), the trial is essentially "non-therapeutic" in being highly unlikely to benefit the patient/subjects, and designed almost entirely to produce generalisable knowledge that it is hoped will benefit other patients in the future. The more a clinical trial is consistent with the Hippocratic commitment of ordinary therapy, whereby interventions are only offered if they are in the interests of the particular patient, the more it is justifiable for patients and doctors to rely on that Hippocratic commitment and to treat the trial as an aspect of ordinary therapy. The less a trial shares in that Hippocratic commitment, i.e. the less it is intended and likely to benefit the individual patient subject, the more it should be treated as non-therapeutic research aimed at benefitting others and not the participant subjects, and therefore the more such a trial should incorporate the safeguards appropriate to non-therapeutic research, including the need for extensively informed consent.

Because of the variable extent of the "Hippocratic commitment" that exists in different clinical trials, and because of the difficulty in many trials of precisely assessing the relative strengths of therapeutic benefit to individual patient/subjects versus non-therapeutic benefit to others, many are inclined to treat all clinical research involving patients as though it were non-therapeutic research, and to require the same rules, including the need for extensively informed written consent, for all clinical research. There is also the converse danger of treating all clinical research that has a therapeutic element as though it were simply medical treatment conforming to the Hippocratic commitment. I have given arguments for rejecting such blanket approaches in favour of a more nuanced assessment, in which the preferences of some individual patients for less information can be respected, whilst still also respecting their willingness to participate in certain sorts of clinical trials. Given the tension that to some extent necessarily exists in all clinical research between the Hippocratic commitment to the individual patient and the scientific commitment to reliable generation of new knowledge independently of such a commitment, I have no doubt that the presumption in favour of extensively informed consent for participation in all clinical trials should remain, including the presumption towards providing patient participants with extensive written information. I have argued that this presumption can be overridden, where the patient does not want such extensive information yet accepts participation, provided that the patient's involvement in the trial would, in the doctor's assessment, also be in his or her interests.

Finally, to respond briefly to Doyal's additional claims in the paper[1] that prompted this book, let me assert, but in the interests of space not argue, that discretion should be left to research ethics committees to accept other examples, *should they arise*, of research projects in which patients may give consent to participation while rejecting standard extensive information. I can't think of other examples, but am wary in ethics of inflexible requirements that preclude the possibility of unanticipated but justified counter examples. Similarly let me also assert but not argue that I personally would be reluctant to see medical journals and their editors override decisions by research ethics committees by refusing to publish studies that the journals consider unethical, but that the committees have accepted as ethical. While again I can think of rare justifications for such moral censorship, generally I would argue, had I the space, that if a journal or its editor disapproves of a research project that has been approved by a *bona fide* research ethics committee (and there's a subject for further analysis), then the proper action is to publish it (assuming it meets the other criteria for publication) along with an ethical critique plus responses from those criticised.

REFERENCES

1. Doyal L. Journals should not publish research to which patients have not given fully informed consent – with three exceptions *BMJ* 1997; **314**: 1107–11.
2. Gillon R. Adequately informed consent. *J Med Ethics* 1985; **11**: 115–16.
3. Gillon R. *Philosophical medical ethics*. Chichester: Wiley, 1986, pp. 113–18.
4. Gillon R. Medical treatment, medical research and informed consent. *J Med Ethics* 1989; **15**: 3–5, 11.
5. British Medical Association. *Medical ethics today*. London: BMJ Publishing Group, 1993.
6. McIntosh J. Patients' awareness and desire for information about diagnosed but undisclosed malignant disease. *Lancet* 1976; **VII**: 300–3.
7. Thorpe G. Experiments on the dying. In: Williams CJ. *Introducing new treatments for cancer–practical, ethical and legal problems*. Chichester: Wiley, 1992, p. 219.
8. The Nuremberg Code. Reprinted in: Reiser SJ, Dyck AJ, Curran WJ, *Ethics in medicine – historical perspectives and contemporary concerns*. Cambridge, Massachusetts; London, England: MIT Press, 1977, pp. 272–3.
9. 50th Anniversary Papers concerning the Nuremberg doctors' trial in the *BMJ*, 1999; **313**: 143–75.
10. Royal College of Physicians of London. Research on healthy volunteers. London RCPL, 1986, p. 5.
11. Nicholson R, ed. *Medical research with children: ethics, law and practice*. Oxford: Oxford University Press, 1986; pp. 76–124 (esp. 104–6); 231–43 (esp. 232–3).
12. Macklin R. The ethical problems with sham surgery in clinical research. *New Eng J Med* 1999; **341**: 992–5.
13. Freeman TB, Vawter DE, Leaverton PE *et al.* Use of placebo surgery in controlled trials of a cellular based therapy for Parkinson's disease. *New Engl J Med* 1999; **341**: 988–92.

14. Department of Health. *Local Research Ethics Committees* (Health Service Guidelines (91) 5). London: Department of Health, 1991.

15. Royal College of Physicians of London. *Guideline on the practice of ethics committees in medical research involving human subjects* (3rd edn). London: RCPL, 1996.

16. Council for International Organisations of Medical Sciences. *International ethical guidelines for biomedical research involving human subjects*. Geneva: CIOMS in collaboration with the World Health Organisation, 1993.

17. Association of the British Pharmaceutical Industry. *Guidelines for medical experiments in non-patient human volunteers*. London: ABPI, 1988.

18. Tobias JS, Souhami RL. Fully informed consent can be needlessly cruel. *BMJ* 1993; **307**: 1199–201.

26 · Double standards on informed consent to treatment

Iain Chalmers and Richard I Lindley

I need permission to give a drug to half of my patients, but not to give it to them all.

Richard Smithells[1]

The clinician who is convinced that a certain treatment works will almost never find an ethicist in his path whereas his colleague who wonders and doubts and wants to learn will stumble over piles of them.

Lancet[2]

More than three decades have passed since the publication of Maurice Pappworth's book *Human guinea pigs: experimentation on man*[3] provoked a proper concern to expose and prevent unjustifiable medical experimentation. One expression of this concern has been the professionalisation of the subject of medical ethics. There are now centres, institutes, departments, and programmes identified with the field. Many individuals are now paid to think and write about medical ethics, and they often refer to themselves as medical ethicists or bioethicists. These developments are reflected in an increasing number of books and specialist journals on medical and bioethics: *Ulrich's International periodicals directory* contains 24 journal titles that include words referring to healthcare ethics or bioethics; all have been initiated during the 31 years since Pappworth's book was published, and there is an International Association of Bioethics.

Against the background of this burgeoning of professional ethicists and the institutions with which they are associated, it is remarkable that so few of them have seriously confronted an issue that was raised very soon after publication of *Human guinea pigs*. The then President of the Royal College of Physicians pointed out the problems that faced anyone wishing to define "experiment"[4]: as Claude Bernard had noted more than a century earlier: "physicians make therapeutic experiments daily on their patients".[5] This issue was raised many years ago by the ethicist Robert Levine,[6–9] but, as Evans and Evans[9] have shown more recently, the fundamental problem has not gone away: clinical research and routine clinical practice are simply much more similar than many acknowledge.

This is no mere sophistry: over 20 years ago, prompted by an article by Pappworth[10] in which he used the terms "experiment" and "experimentation", one of us challenged him to clarify what he meant by these words, as follows[11]:

I am not as sure as Dr Pappworth seems to be that the clinical world can be divided as neatly as his writings imply into a minority of clinical experimentalists, who should be required to submit their proposals for clinical practice to ethics committees, and a residual majority of other doctors, who need not subject their proposed practice to such scrutiny.

The matter at issue can be illustrated with an example. In the 1940s, poorly conducted research in the United States led to claims that diethylstilboestrol was beneficial in treating a wide range of conditions in pregnancy. Broadly, there were two responses to these claims. A tiny minority of obstetricians conducted well controlled research that failed to show any benefits of the treatment, and so they abandoned it. Most clinicians accepted uncritically claims made about the drug by manufacturers and others and used it on a wide scale for the next thirty years; and we know now that this policy had important adverse effects on women and men who were exposed to diethylstilboestrol as fetuses.

Now it so happens that informed consent was not obtained from the pregnant women who participated in one of the randomised trials that suggested that the drug was useless. But which groups of obstetricians behaved more ethically: the handful of clinical researchers who, by conducting a randomised trial, ensured that at least half their patients would avoid the side effects of the drug, and then gave up using it when no benefit was shown; or the thousands of less questioning clinicians who involved millions of pregnant women in the poorly controlled experimentation of 'accepted clinical practice'?

Pappworth did not respond to this challenge in 1978; nor did he do so 13 years later when it was put to him again[12] in response to his article entitled "*Human Guinea Pigs: a history*".[4]

"Guinea pigs" is an emotive epithet to describe patients receiving treatment, as is the demeaning term "subjects", which is used more or less routinely when referring to patients receiving treatment within the context of controlled experiments.[13-15] But who are the guinea pigs in healthcare? Beverley Beech, a consumer advocate in the field of maternity care, has emphasised the widespread application of a double standard on informed consent to treatment. "Unfortunately," she notes, "the only people interested in giving out medical (information) leaflets are those involved in *controlled* trials. We have yet to formulate a means of dealing with those who are happily conducting *uncontrolled* trials, and by so doing are using pregnant women and their babies as guinea pigs in *uncontrolled experimentation*."[16] As a way of promoting a single standard on informed consent to treatment, she proposed that notices with the following text should be drawn to the attention of patients:

> Doctors at this and every hospital will come to a decision about what types of care to offer you in a variety of ways. Sometimes there will be good evidence of the effectiveness and relative safety of the treatments recommended. More often, doctors will be influenced by tradition, prejudice, fashion or bad evidence in making their recommendations. Occasionally, doctors who want to ensure that they maximise the chances of you having whichever turns out to be the best of alternative treatments will select your treatment at random from the likely best alternatives.
>
> If you want to know anything about the basis on which your treatment has been selected; or about the alternatives and their relative merits and disadvantages; or what doctors here are trying to do to minimise their unintended mistakes and protect their patients from them, then do not hesitate to ask for this information.

As hinted by Beech, other double standards are lurking in this field. For example, it is often noted that "physician-researchers may find that their interest as researchers in enrolling subjects [*sic*] brings them into conflict with their obligation as physicians to do what is in the best interest of their patients,"[17] and that "research transforms the doctor-patient relationship into something other than a fiduciary relationship in which the physician's sole concern is the wellbeing of the individual patient."[18]

This emphasis implies that the conflicts facing clinicians participating in controlled experiments (many of whom, especially in multicentre trials, would not actually regard themselves as researchers) are cause for greater concern than the conflicts that exist outside the context of controlled experiments.[19] In the light of the observations of Molière, George Bernard Shaw and numerous other commentators on some of the less creditable drivers of decisions in healthcare, this is astonishing. These influences range from pecuniary greed, through inappropriate speciality allegiances, to ignorance as a result of difficulties in accessing reliable research evidence to guide practice. All of these influences, and many others, may conflict with the interests of patients. Indeed, at the most basic level, because every doctor has many patients and most doctors practice within healthcare systems, "no adequate healthcare ethics can think only of the 'sacred dyad' of 'one doctor, one patient'."[20]

Although people have been drawing attention to these double standards for over quarter of a century,[1, 2, 21-61] a recently published systematic review,[19] which involved extensive searches for relevant evidence, confirmed that professional medical ethicists have only very rarely acknowledged them.[9]

More than a decade ago, for example, one of us co-authored an article with William Silverman entitled "Public and professional double standards on clinical experimentation", which was published in the journal *Controlled Clinical Trials*.[62] Our hope had been that the title of the piece and its place of publication would have provoked some interest among professional medical ethicists. A search of the *Science Citation Index* 11 years later yielded 17 citations by people other than the authors: 14 of these referred to articles authored by clinical researchers.[32-37, 42, 44, 50, 52-54, 61, 63] Two of the remaining three articles were editorials in medical journals which referred explicitly to double standards.[2, 49] Only one of the 17 citations, however, referred to an analysis of the issue by a medical ethicist – John Lantos, of the Center for Clinical Medical Ethics at the University of Chicago.[64]

IDENTIFICATION OF "A CONFUSED ETHICAL ANALYSIS"

Lantos' thoughtful piece was based on a talk that he gave at a National Institutes of Health workshop on "Bone marrow transplantation for haemoglobinopathies."[64] He noted that:

If a clinician tries a new therapy with the idea of study-ing it carefully, evaluating outcomes, and publishing the results, he or she is doing research. The subjects [*sic*] of such research are thought to be in need of spe-cial protection. The protocol must be reviewed by an Institutional Review Board (IRB). The informed con-sent form will be carefully scrutinized and the research may be forbidden. On the other hand, a clin-ician may try this new therapy without any intention of studying it, merely because he believes it will be of benefit to his patients. In that situation, trying the new therapy is not research, the trial does not need IRB approval, and consent may be obtained in a manner governed only by the risk of malpractice litigation.

It would seem that the patients in the second situ-ation (nonresearch) are at much higher risk than are the patients in the first situation (being part of formal clinical research). Furthermore, the physician in the first situation seems more ethically admirable. The physician in the first situation is evaluating the ther-apy, whereas the physician in the second situation is using the therapy based on his or her imperfect hunches. Nevertheless, because ethical codes that seek to protect patients focus on the goal of creating gen-eralizable knowledge, they regulate the responsible investigator but not the irresponsible adventurer.

This analysis echoes Chalmers' and Silverman's[62] observation six years earlier that:

> … a mischievous view has been promoted that the interests of the vast number of patients involved in the poorly controlled experiments of informal medical 'tinkering' are less in need of protection than are those of the relatively small number of patients who are involved in planned, properly controlled clinical experiments.

Predictably, we agree with Lantos' conclusion that, "This confusing real world situation seems to reflect a confused ethical analysis," and that "Guidelines for the evaluation of innovative therapy cannot simply try to apply the principles that govern nonthera-peutic research." We would add only that his con-clusion applies with equal force to inadequately evaluated "established" therapies. Acquiescence in and promotion of this double standard by profes-sional medical ethicists is reflected in statements such as the following by physician researchers:

> After formal discussion with this hospital's drug com-mittee and informal discussion with its ethics com-mittee, it was decided that the usage [of buserelin] that we report was merely an extension of the drug's reg-ular use and that formal ethical approval was not nec-essary as our study was not a randomised trial.[65]

There is no shortage of examples of treatments that have come into widespread use without rigor-ous evaluation and have subsequently been shown to be useless or harmful. One dramatic recent exam-ple is the "prophylactic" use of antiarrhythmic drugs during myocardial infarction: at the peak of their use in the late 1980s it has been estimated that these drugs were causing between 20 000 and 70 000 deaths every year in the USA alone,[66] a yearly total of the same order of magnitude as the total number of Americans who died in the Vietnam war.

Prior to the discovery of the lethal potential of these drugs, professional ethicists might well have regarded their widespread use as evidence that this massive and poorly controlled global experiment reflected "a standard intervention whose risks and benefits (were) well understood."[17] Their attention would have been focused on protecting the interests of the tiny minority of patients who participated in the placebo controlled trials of these drugs. The best estimate[67] suggests that, worldwide, less than 100 deaths attributable to antiarrhythmic drugs occurred among patients participating in controlled trials, and that allocation to placebo in these trials meant that premature death was avoided in approximately the same number.

To the extent that professional medical ethicists have failed to confront double standards on informed consent to treatment and the widespread use of poor-ly controlled experimentation in healthcare, we sug-gest that, by default, they have promoted both of these. We think that the way that the professional medical ethics community has ignored repeated calls by others to address these double standards is a scan-dal, and that it is high time that it started to deal with the "confused ethical analysis" that Lantos has iden-tified.[64]

FOUNDATIONS FOR AN IMPROVED ETHICAL ANALYSIS: THE NEED TO CONSIDER THE INTERESTS OF *ALL* CURRENT PATIENTS

For those professional medical ethicists who decide to take up this longstanding challenge, we raise a question that seems to us to be fundamental. Are the interests of *current patients* served more effectively by active promotion of well controlled experimentation, or by passive acquiescence in poorly controlled experimentation?

Although it is widely agreed that promoting con-trolled experiments should benefit *future* patients, many medical ethicists appear to think that *current* patients who participate in controlled trials of treatments face risks over and above those that they normally encounter, and that they run these risks "in the public interest".[68] In 1970, for example, Jonas suggested that individuals are "conscripted" to "sacrifice" themselves in the service of the "collective" (Jonas 1970, cited in ref.25). This attitude is still prevalent.[9, 68] A medical ethicist contributing to a conference on controlled trials in 1998, for example, referred to patients being "sacrificed" in controlled trials for the benefit of future patients. He went on to say that if his general practitioner invited him to participate in a controlled trial addressing an area of clinical uncertainty about antibiotic therapy, he would look for another doctor.[69]

The ethical basis for controlled experimentation is uncertainty among well-informed healthcare professionals and patients about which of alternative treatments to prefer.[21, 70–73] The criteria used by patients and professionals as a basis for their uncertainties about the relative merits of alternative treatments are likely to vary,[13] but these judgements should be informed by systematic assessments of whatever evidence is judged to be relevant and valid. It is clearly undesirable, if not unethical, for clinicians to involve patients when faced with justified uncertainty in the poorly controlled experimentation that characterises much routine clinical practice.[74–76]

Optimism about the effects of treatments, particularly new treatments, often leads to an assumption that those assigned in controlled experiments to receive "standard" treatments will be "denied" the hoped-for beneficial effects of new treatments. For example, Ashcroft maintains that "the principle holds that the researcher (and a respectable body of professional opinion) must believe that the new treatment will turn out to be at least no less effective (that is beneficial) than any alternative treatment we could offer."[77]

Frequently used language such as this ignores the empirical evidence that new treatments are as likely to be worse as they are to be better than existing treatments.[78–87] Furthermore, even for those new treatments that do turn out to be better than existing alternatives, the extent of the benefit is frequently overestimated.[88]

As illustrated by the randomised trials of diethylstilboestrol and antiarrhythmic drugs presented above, random allocation to alternative treatments in the face of uncertainties about their relative merits provides an efficient hedging strategy for patients.[62] A 1:1 randomisation ratio maximises the likelihood that patients will receive whichever of the two treatments, including placebo treatment, turns out to be superior, and protects patients from a pervasive "optimism bias", which, although understandable, is unsupported by evidence.

Table 26.1 *How does treatment given within a randomized controlled trial differ from treatment given in routine clinical practice?*

Stage	Controlled trial	Routine Practice
Protocol	Externally reviewed	Not usually reviewed
Diagnosis	Systematic, protocol-driven	Often haphazard
Patient information	Detailed, written	Often rudimentary, verbal
Consent procedure	Formal process	Haphazard process
Treatment allocation	Random	Often haphazard
Treatment	Protocol-driven, often after systematic review of all the relevant data; care often provided by local or national experts	Considerable variation; care often provided people at varying levels of expertise
Record keeping	Planned; standard minimum; often archived retrievably	Often haphazard; no standard minimum; often destroyed
Treatment response	Often monitored independently, using prespecified criteria	Haphazard, inconsistent
Accumulating evidence	Monitored; inferior treatments discontinued when evidence accumulates against them	Often not examined; inferior treatments often continued because evidence ignored
Continued professional development	Often through collaborators' meetings in multicentre studies	Haphazard
Dissemination of results	Likely to be published	Rarely collated or published
Impact on future practice	Can be influential	Unlikely to be influential

Hedging one's options in the face of uncertainty and optimism bias is not the only advantage to current patients of participating in well-controlled clinical experiments. Table 26.1 lists some ways in which treatment given within the context of randomized controlled trials is likely to differ from treatment given as part of usual clinical practice. Given the many safeguards and quality checks involved in controlled experiments, it should not come as a surprise that a systematic review of 15 studies comparing patients treated in the context of controlled trials with apparently similar patients treated outside trials showed that, on average, the prognoses of the former are better than those of the latter.[19] This conclusion is strengthened by the results of at least seven other studies[89-95] that were not identified for possible inclusion in the systematic review (which is currently being updated for publication in *The Cochrane Database of Systematic Reviews* (Sackett, personal communication).

The authors of the systematic review[18, 19] have noted that these differences may be explained in a number of ways, including selection bias, placebo effects, and adherence to well-defined protocols. Lantos goes on to note, however, that the phenomenon of "inclusion benefit", if real, raises a profound challenge to the current framework governing medical research, which currently begins from the assumption that research is a risky endeavour.[18] "What if," he asks "instead of creating increased risk, clinical research creates increased benefit? Perhaps we should include, as part of the informed consent process for clinical research, a statement to the effect that participation in a research protocol has been shown to lead to better outcomes than non-participation." (This is an interesting suggestion, particularly in the light of the fact that one of us [RL] was told by an ethics committee recently that it was "unethical" to inform potential participants in a controlled experiment that this evidence exists!) Ashcroft, also, has noted that the emphasis on risks rather than benefits in research ethics may be "a somewhat misleading or distorting emphasis", and has begun to make explicit the lack of a clear analysis of what should be regarded as experimentation in healthcare.[77]

Further suggestive evidence to support more routine use of randomised controlled trials (to base treatment decisions) is provided by the series of interlocking leukaemia treatment trials in the United Kingdom.[96] A high proportion of patients with leukaemia have participated in controlled trials, thus ensuring that they received either the state of the art treatment, or a treatment that appeared to hold promise of being even better. This way of organising treatment for leukaemia has been associated with a dramatic increase in survival rates.

Some people who have thought about the implications of the evidence referred to above and are thus aware of the potential advantages of participating in controlled experimentation have made clear that they wish to be invited to participate in controlled trials when they are patients.[18, 97] We are not referring here to the advantages of gaining access to treatments that are only available within the context of controlled experiments, for which some AIDS activists, for example, have lobbied.[98, 99] Rather, we refer to those who have considered the empirical evidence cited above and concluded that seeking involvement in controlled experiments is an effective strategy for protecting their interests.[12, 13, 100, 102-105] One of us (IC), for example, carries a medical emergency card inscribed with the instruction, "Invite me to participate in all randomised controlled trials for which I am potentially eligible."[106] The other (RL) has proposed that a "randomised controlled trial card" be introduced, to be carried by people who understand randomised controlled trials, including those who have already participated in trials, and wish to be considered for future studies.[107]

Those who have expressed these views are all healthcare professionals, so they can hardly be regarded as typical patients. As far as we are aware, however, no medical ethicist has ever tried to explore and document why these people are so clear that, as patients, they would wish to be invited to participate in well controlled experiments. Perhaps it is because ethicists find it difficult to understand that this could simply be an expression of naked self-interest by people who realise that the alternative is usually participation in poorly controlled treatment adventures. In his contribution on selection of "subjects" (*sic*) to the *Encyclopedia of Applied Ethics*, for example, Ashcroft assumes that people enrol in research "for no reason other than altruism, curiosity, or an interest in playing a part in scientific progress."[77]

CONCLUDING REMARKS

Some of those from whom we sought comments on earlier drafts of this chapter, including the editors, urged us to clarify whether we think that the single standard on informed consent to treatment for which we have called should be reflected in a relaxation of the requirements of those engaged in controlled experimentation, or an extension of such requirements to those involved in the poorly controlled experimentation that characterises much routine health care.

We have not attempted to extend our analysis to address this question, mainly because we are confident that other contributors to this book have presented a variety of views on what should be regarded as "informed consent to treatment". We predict that their contributions will note that different patients in different cultures have different expectations on this issue,[108] and that, in this respect, the notion of a single standard for informed consent to treatment is at best illusory[20, 25, 109, 110] and at worst a reflection of cultural imperialism.[111]

To have discussed the lack of a single standard on informed consent – whatever that standard might be – in these terms would have served only to distract attention from an aspect of informed consent to treatment that we believe has been ignored for too long. This is the double standard, within cultures, on the requirements for consent to treatment in well-controlled treatment experiments on the one hand, and consent to treatment in the poorly-controlled experiments of routine clinical practice on the other.

We could have laid the failure to address this double standard at the door of any one or more of the variety of people who are involved in some way in seeking, giving, requiring, analysing or commenting on informed consent to treatment. We have concentrated our attention on professional medical ethicists because they have become a very influential force in therapeutic research, and, in principle, they should have few vested interests other than to promote the interests of patients, and of the public more generally. We believe that those professional medical ethicists who have failed to confront this double standard when they should have addressed it[112, 113] are failing in their special responsibility to current and future patients.[2, 72, 114–119]

Claude Bernard's injunction to medicine to "apply the experimental method systematically"[5] will continue to present substantial practical challenges. Although we are clear that well-controlled experimentation is preferable to poorly-controlled experimentation in clinical practice, we recognise that there are many perverse incentives to do clinical research, and that this will sometimes lead patients to become involved in badly designed or irrelevant studies.[120] Indeed, these incentives will sometimes

result in unethical studies being endorsed by research ethics committees[121] and in patients being invited to participate in studies in which a majority of clinicians would not wish themselves or their relatives to participate.[71, 122, 123] Although these issues are certainly relevant in the context of controlled experiments, they are much more relevant in routine clinical practice, if only because of the vastly greater numbers of patients who are being offered care that is of dubious value, if not already known to be actually harmful.

Relatively uncontrolled experimentation remains the dominant mode of professional practice,[29] and for a number of reasons this seems likely to continue. In particular, the immense power of market and professional forces seems certain to oppose attempts to increase regulation and extend the use of controlled experimentation by the minority of professionals and lay commentators who are convinced by empirical evidence and logic that this would protect the interests of people using the health services.

Indeed, in our view, the most hopeful catalyst for stimulating movement in the direction that our analysis implies is greater public awareness of the evidence and arguments that we have considered. As the public becomes increasingly aware of uncertainties about the effects of healthcare and how controlled trials of treatment can help to deal with these, it seems likely that they will come to appreciate that well-controlled experimentation is preferable to the poorly-controlled experimentation that characterises much healthcare. As Hazel Thornton, chair of the Consumers' Advisory Group for Clinical Trials, has noted:

> To make a useful contribution, patients will need to face unpleasant realities; learn to appreciate uncertainty; be educated to understand the dilemmas and problems of clinical research and the dilemmas of obtaining consent; understand the need for trials to evaluate new treatments and assess the value of established ones; demand quality; be aware of the diversity of opinion within the profession and be prepared to work hard to acquire understanding of all aspects of research activity, preferably when they are well, so that they may effectively participate in the shared responsibility and debate.[124]

Greater involvement by patients and other members of the public in all stages of research on the effects of treatment should indeed help to improve matters.[13, 125–128] As David Roy, of the Centre for Bioethics in Montreal observed more than a decade ago, new alliances are required, and a "shift from a

---

Key messages

- Double standards on informed consent to treatment have been ignored by most professional medical ethicists for more than a quarter of a century.
- Some medical ethicists have realised that this has resulted in "a confused ethical analysis".
- The prognosis of people who participate in controlled clinical research is better than the prognosis of apparently similar people receiving treatment outside controlled trials.
- The foundation for an improved ethical analysis is a recognition of the need to consider the interests of *everyone* currently receiving treatment, not just the tiny minority who participate in controlled trials.
- Relatively uncontrolled experimentation remains the dominant mode of professional practice.
- Greater participation in randomised controlled trials within routine healthcare should improve standards of care, by accelerating the identification and adoption of treatments more likely to do good than harm.
- Greater involvement by patients and other members of the public in all stages of research on the effects of treatment should help to improve matters.

---

previously necessary emphasis on the need for protection against scientific abuse to a more mature emphasis on the co-responsibility of patients, citizens, and medical-scientific professionals for the common good of current and future generations."[75]

Professional medical ethicists have an important role to play in these developments,[129] but they must begin to sort out the "confused ethical analysis" identified by Lantos.[64] The possible implications for the workload of research ethics committees cannot be accepted as a legitimate reason for dismissing this challenge, as some have suggested.[9] Indeed, we conclude by noting the encouraging evidence that some professional ethicists are beginning to get to grips with the challenge we have posed to them. As one of them has observed:

> If ethicists and others want something to criticise in clinical trials, they should look at scientifically inadequate work, reinvention of wheels, and above all, unjustifiable exclusions and unjust and irrational uses of resources. The present debate is flawed by a failure to take notice of what trials are for – to make sure that

the treatments we use are safe, and do what they do better than the alternatives. There are no short cuts in ethics – no more than in trials.[130]

ACKNOWLEDGEMENTS

We thank Phil Alderson, Doug Altman, Richard Ashcroft, Thurstan Brewin, Jan Chalmers, Rory Collins, Benjamin Djulbegovic, Ann Greer, Jayne Harrison, Andrew Herxheimer, Tony Hope, John Lantos, Richard Lilford, Dave Sackett, Bill Silverman, Hazel Thornton and the editors for comments on previous drafts of this chapter.

REFERENCES

1. Smithells RW. Iatrogenic hazards and their effects. *Postgrad Med J* 1975; **15**: 39–52.
2. Editorial. Medical ethics – should medicine turn the other cheek? *Lancet* 1990; **336**: 846–7.
3. Pappworth MH. *Human guinea pigs: experimentation on man*. Boston: Beacon Press, 1968.
4. Pappworth MH. Human guinea pigs: a history. *BMJ* 1990; **301**: 1456–60.
5. Bernard C. *An introduction to the study of experimental medicine* [first published 1865] (translated by Henry Copley Greene). New York: Henry Schumann, Inc. 1949, p.18.
6. Levine RJ. The impact on fetal research of the report of the National Commission for the Protection of Human Subjects of Biomedical and Behavioral Research. *Villanova Law Rev* 1977; **22**: 367–83.
7. Levine RJ, Lebacqz K. Ethical considerations in clinical trials. *Clin Pharmacol Therapeut* 1979; **25**: 728–41.
8. Levine RJ. *Ethics and regulation of clinical research*, 2nd edn. New Haven: Yale University Press, 1988.
9. Evans D, Evans M. *A decent proposal: ethical review of clinical research*. Chichester: John Wiley and Sons 1996, pp. 51–61.
10. Pappworth MH. Medical ethics committees: a review of their functions. *Wld Med* 1978 (Feb 22): 19–78.
11. Chalmers I. Medical experimentation. *Wld Med* 1978 (Apr 5): 18.
12. Chalmers I. Human guinea pigs. *BMJ* 1991; **302**: 411.
13. Chalmers I. What do I want from health research and researchers when I am a patient? *BMJ* 1995; **310**: 1315–18.
14. Boynton PM. People should participate in, not be subjects of, research. *BMJ* 1998; **317**: 1521.
15. Chalmers I. People are "participants" in research. *BMJ* 1999; **318**: 1141.

16. Beech BL. *Who's having your baby?* London: Bedford Square Press, 1991, pp. 89–90.

17. Brody BA. *Ethical issues in drug testing, approval, and pricing: the clot dissolving drugs*. Oxford: Oxford University Press, 1995, pp. 139–142.

18. Lantos J. The inclusion benefit in clinical trials. *J Ped* 1999; **134**: 130–1.

19. Edwards SJL, Lilford RJ, Braunholtz DA, Jackson JC, Hewison J, Thornton J. Ethical issues in the design and conduct of randomised controlled trials. *Hlth Technol Assess* 1998; **2**(15): 16.

20. Ashcroft RE. Ethics and health technology assessment. *Monash Bioethics Rev* 1999; **18**: 15–24.

21. Bradford Hill A. Medical ethics and controlled trials. *BMJ* 1963; **2**: 1043–9.

22. Chalmers TC. Randomization of the first patient. *Med Clin N Amer* 1975; **59**: 1035–8.

23. Brewin TB. Consent to randomised treatment. *Lancet* 1982; **2**: 919–21.

24. Chalmers I, Baum M. Consent to randomized treatment. *Lancet* 1982; **2**: 1050–1.

25. Levine RJ. Informed consent in research and practice: similarities and differences. *Arch Intern Med* 1983; **143**: 1229–31.

26. Chalmers I. Scientific inquiry and authoritarianism in perinatal care and education. *Birth* 1983; **10**: 151–66.

27. Chalmers I, Grant A. Informed consent. *BMJ* 1983; **286**: 1279.

28. Brewin TB. Truth, trust and paternalism. *Lancet* 1985; **2**: 490–2.

29. Chalmers I. Minimizing harm and maximizing benefit during innovation in health care: controlled or uncontrolled experimentation? *Birth* 1986; **13**: 155–64.

30. Challah S, Mays NB. The randomised controlled trial in the evaluation of new technology: a case study. *BMJ* 1986; **292**: 877–8.

31. Bradford Hill A. Clinical trials and the acceptance of uncertainty. *BMJ* 1987; **294**: 1419.

32. Keller MB, Lavori PW. The adequacy of treating depression. *J Nerv Mental Dis* 1988; **176**: 471–4.

33. Baum M, Zilkha K, Houghton J. Ethics of clinical research – lessons for the future. *BMJ* 1989; **299**: 251–3.

34. Grimes DA. Evaluating tri-phasic oral contraceptives – the rationale for a randomised trial. *Am J Obstet Gynecol* 1989; **161**: 1390–2.

35. Chalmers TC. Ethical implications of rejecting patients for clinical trials. *JAMA* 1990; **263**: 865.

36. Chalmers TC. A belated randomized controlled trial – Commentary. *Pediatrics* 1990; **85**: 366–8.

37. Chalmers TC, Frank CS, Reitman D. Minimizing the three stages of publication bias. *JAMA* 1990; **263**: 1392–5.

38. Chalmers I. NZ medicine after Cartwright. *BMJ* 1990; **300**: 1199.

39. Buyse M. Randomized clinical trials in surgical oncology. *Eur J Surg Oncol* 1991; **17**: 421–8.

40. Segelov E, Tattersall MM, Coates AS. Redressing the balance – the ethics of not entering an eligible patient on a randomized controlled trial. *Ann Oncol* 1992; **3**: 103–5.

41. Chalmers I. Ethics, clinical research, and clinical practice in obstetric anaesthesia. *Lancet* 1992; **339**: 498.

42. Grimes DA. Laparoscopic surgery – experiment or expedient? *Am J Obstet Gynecol* 1993; **168**: 1333–4.

43. Thornton H. Clinical trials – a brave new partnership. *J Med Ethics* 1994; **20**: 19–22.

44. Tobias JS, Houghton J. Is informed consent essential for all chemotherapy studies? *Eur J Cancer* 1994; **30A**: 897–9.

45. Tauer CA. The NIH trials of growth hormone for short stature. *IRB: Rev Human Subjects Res* 1994; **16**: 1–9.

46. Lantos J. Ethics, randomization and technology assessment. *Cancer* 1994; **74**: 2653–6.

47. Baum M. The ethics of randomized controlled trials. *Eur J Surg Oncol* 1995; **21**: 136–9.

48. De Deyn PP. On the ethical acceptability of placebo application in neuropsychiatric research. *Acta Neurol Belg* 1995; **95**: 8–17.

49. Goodare H, Smith R. The rights of patients in research. *BMJ* 1995; **310**: 1277–8.

50. Altman DG, Whitehead J, Parmar MKB, Stenning SP, Fayers PM, Machin D. Randomised consent designs in cancer clinical trials. *Eur J Cancer* 1995; **31A**: 1934–44.

51. Irwig L, Glasziou P, March L. Ethics of n-of-1 trials. *Lancet* 1995; **345**: 469.

52. Tyson JE. Use of unproved therapies in clinical practice and research – how can we better serve our patients and their families? *Sem Perinatol* 1995; **19**: 98–111.

53. Shaw WC. Commentary on ethical issues in the case of surgical repair of cleft palate. *Cleft Palate-Craniofacial J* 1995; **32**: 277–80.

54. Mant J, Dawes M, Graham Jones S. Randomised trials in general practice. *BMJ* 1996; **312**: 779.

55. Hutton JL. The ethics of randomized controlled trials: a matter of statistical belief? *Hlth Care Anal* 1996; **4**: 95–102.

56. Bland M. Informed consent in medical research: let readers judge for themselves. *BMJ* 1997; **314**: 1477–8.

57. Stewart-Brown S. Informed consent in medical research: clinicians are being disingenuous with themselves. *BMJ* 1997; **314**: 1478–9.

58. Counsell CE, Sandercock PAG. Informed consent in medical research: failure to publish completed randomised controlled trials is unethical in itself. *BMJ* 1997; **314**: 1481.

59. Frosh AC, Hanif J. Informed consent in medical research: in routine practice the consent form is a request from and informed consent is informed choice. *BMJ* 1997; **314**: 1482–3.

60. Barer D. Informed consent: respect for autonomy may conflict with principle of beneficence. *BMJ* 1997; **315**: 254.

61. Rogers CG, Tyson JE, Kennedy KA, Broyles RS, Hickman JF. Conventional consent with opting in versus simplified consent with opting out: an exploratory trial for studies that do not increase patients' risk. *J Pediat* 1998; **132**: 606–11.

62. Chalmers I, Silverman WA. Professional and public double standards on clinical experimentation. *Controlled Clin Trials* 1987; **8**: 388–91.

63. Chalmers TC. Design of clinical trials the need for early randomization in the development of new drugs for AIDS. *J Acquired Immune Defic Synd Human Retrovirol* 1990; **3**: S10–S15.

64. Lantos J. Ethical issues – how can we distinguish clinical research from innovative therapy? *Am J Pediat Hematol Oncol* 1994; **16**: 72–5.

65. Rutherford AJ, Subak-Sharpe RJ, Dawson KJ, Magara RA, Franks S, Winston RML. Improvement in in vitro fertilisation after treatment with buserelin, an agonist of luteinising hormone releasing hormone. *BMJ* 1988; **296**: 1765–8.

66. Moore T. *Deadly medicine*. New York: Simon and Schuster, 1995.

67. Teo KK, Yusuf S, Furberg CD. Effects of prophylactic anti-arrhythmic drug therapy in acute myocardial infarction. *JAMA* 1993; **270**: 1589–95.

68. Doyal L. Informed consent in medical research: journals should not publish research to which patients have not given fully informed consent – with three exceptions. *BMJ* 1997; **314**: 1107–11.

69. Holm S. What is informed consent and who gives it? Paper presented at *BMJ* meeting on "50 years of clinical trials: past, present and fixture", London, 29/30 October 1998.

70. Paterson R. Clinical trials in malignant disease. *Proc Roy Soc Med* 1965; **58**: 625–6.

71. Atkins H. Conduct of a controlled clinical trial. *BMJ* 1966; **2**: 377–9.

72. Collins R, Doll R, Peto R. Ethics of clinical trials. In: Williams CJ. ed. *Introducing new treatments for cancer: practical and legal problems*. Chichester: Wiley, 1992, pp. 49–66.

73. Lilford RJ, Jackson J. Equipoise and the ethics of randomization. *J Roy Soc Med* 1995; **88**: 552–9.

74. Bradford Hill A. The clinical trial. *New Engl J Med* 1952; **247**: 113–19.

75. Roy DJ. Controlled trials: an ethical imperative. *J Chronic Dis* 1986; **39**: 159–62.

76. American Medical Association. *Code of medical ethics: current opinions and Annotations*, 1996 (http://www.ama-assn.org/ethic/pome.htm).

77. Ashcroft R. Human research subjects, selection of. In: Chadwick R, ed. *Encyclopedia of applied ethics*, Vol. 2. San Diego: Academic Press, 1998, pp. 627–39.

78. Gilbert JP, McPeek B, Mosteller F. Progress in surgery and anaesthesia: benefits and risks of innovative therapy. In: Bunker JP, Barnes BA, Mosteller F, eds. *Costs, risks and benefits of surgery*. New York: Oxford University Press, 1977, pp. 124–69.

79. Bailar JC, Smith EM. Progress against cancer? *New Engl J Med* 1986; **314**: 1226–32.

80. Buyse M, Dalesio O. Paper presented at the Colloquium on Long Term Clinical Trial Strategies, Radcliffe Infirmary, Oxford, 15–17 December 1989.

81. Berlin JA, Begg CB, Louis TA. An assessment of publication bias using a sample of published clinical trials. *J Am Statist Ass* 1989; **84**: 381–92.

82. Colditz GA, Miller JN, Mosteller F. How study design affects outcomes in comparisons of therapy. I: medical. *Statist Med* 1989; **8**: 441–54.

83. Miller JN, Colditz GA, Mosteller F. How study design affects outcomes in comparisons of therapy. II: surgical. *Statist Med* 1989; **8**: 455–68.

84. Gøtzsche PC. Bias in double-blind trials. *Dan Med Bull* 1990; **37**: 329–36.

85. Gøtzsche PC. Meta-analysis of NSAIDs: contribution of drugs, doses, trial designs, and meta-analytic techniques. *Scand J Rheumatol* 1993; **22**: 255–60.

86. Machin D, Stenning SP, Parmar MK *et al.* Thirty years of Medical Research Council randomized trials in solid tumours. *Clin Oncol* 1997; **9**: 100–14.

87. Chalmers I. What is the prior probability of a proposed new treatment being superior to established treatments? *BMJ* 1997; **314**: 74–5.

88. Yusuf S, Collins R, Peto R. Why do we need some large, simple randomised trials? *Stat Med* 1984; **3**: 409–20.

89. Clemens JD, van Loon FF, Rao M *et al.* Nonparticipation as a determinant of adverse health outcomes in a field trial of oral cholera vaccines. *Am J Epidemiol* 1992; **135**: 865–74.

90. Van Bergen PFMM, Jonker JJC, Molhoek GP *et al.* Characteristics and prognosis of non-participants of a multi-centre trial of long-term anticoagulant treatment after myocardial infarction. *Int J Cardiol* 1995; **49**: 135–41.

91. Hancock BW, Aitken M, Radstone C, Vaughan Hudson G. Why don't cancer patients get entered into clinical trials? Experience of the Sheffield Lymphoma Group's collaboration in British National Lymphoma Investigation studies. *BMJ* 1997; **314**: 36–7.

92. King SB III, Barnhart HX, Kosinski AS *et al.* Angioplasty or surgery for multivessel coronary artery disease: comparison of eligible registry and

randomized patients in the EAST trial and influence of treatment selection on outcomes. *Am J Cardiol* 1997; **79**: 1453–9.

93. Skrutkowska M, Weijer C. Do patients with breast cancer participating in clinical trials receive better nursing care? *Oncol Nurs Forum* 1997; **24**: 1411–16.

94. Albert SM, Sano M, Marder K *et al.* Participation in clinical trials and long-term outcome in Alzheimer's disease. *Neurology* 1997; **49**: 38–43.

95. Schmidt B, Gillie P, Caco C, Roberts J, Roberts R. Do sick newborn infants benefit from participation in a randomized clinical trial? *J Pediat* 1999; **134**: 151–5.

96. Galloway J. Game plan for cancer care. *Lancet* 2000; **355**: 150.

97. McNamee D. Public's perception of RCTs. *Lancet* 1998; **351**: 772.

98. Merigan TC. You can teach an old dog new tricks. How AIDS trials are pioneering new strategies. *N Engl J Med* 1990; **323**: 1341–3.

99. Epstein S. Activism, drug regulation, and the politics of therapeutic evaluation in the AIDS era: a case study of ddC and the 'surrogate markers' debate. *Social Stud Sci* 1997; **27**: 691–726.

100. Chalmers I. Research needed into the process of ethical decision making. *NCBHR Communiqué* 1991; **2**: 5–6.

101. Chalmers I, Chalmers TC. Randomisation and patient choice. *Lancet* 1994; **344**: 892–93.

102. Harrison J. Patients should not be discouraged from entering trials. *BMJ* 1996; **313**: 1488.

103. Harrison J. Clinical trials: a patient's views. *MRC News* 1998; **79**: 22–3.

104. Lees KR. If I had a stroke... *Lancet* 1998; **352**(Suppl. III): 28–30.

105. De Takats P, Harrison J. Clinical trials in stroke. *Lancet* 1999; **353**: 150–1.

106. Chalmers I. Randomized clinical trials. *N Engl J Med* 1991; **325**: 1514.

107. Lindley RI. Thrombolytic treatment for acute ischaemic stroke: consent can be ethical. *BMJ* 1998; **316**: 1005–7.

108. Holmes W. Informed consent in medical research: minimum ethical standards should not vary among countries. *BMJ* 1997; **314**: 1479.

109. Christakis NA. Ethics are local: engaging cross-cultural variation in the ethics for clinical research. *Soc Sci Med* 1992; **35**: 1079–91.

110. Ashcroft RE, Chadwick DW, Clark SRL, Edwards RHT, Frith L, Hutton JL. Implications of socio-cultural contexts for the ethnics of clinical trials. *Hlth Technol Assess* 1997; **1**(9)

111. Cullinan T. Informed consent: other societies have different concepts of autonomy. *BMJ* 1997; **315**: 248.

112. Woodward B. Challenges to human subject protections in US medical research. *JAMA* 1999; **282**: 1947–52.

113. Ellis GB. Keeping research subjects out of harm's way. *JAMA* 1999; **282**: 1963–5.

114. Chalmers I. Empirical evidence and authoritarian ethicists. *BMJ* 1987; **294**: 247–8.

115. Chalmers I. The promotion of poorly controlled experimentation on children by medical ethicists. *Paediat Perinat Epidemiol* 1988; **2**: 104–6.

116. Goujard J, Bréart. Risk related to methodologically disputable studies: the example of vitamin therapy for the prevention of neural tube defects. *Rev Epidemiol Santé Public* 1994; **42**: 444–9.

117. Meade TW. The trouble with ethics committees. *J Roy Coll Phys Lond* 1994; **28**: 102–4.

118. Resch KL, Ernst E. The ethical type II error. *Lancet* 1996; **347**: 62–3.

119. Sackett DL. Challenges to human subject protections in US medical research. *JAMA* 2000; **283**: 2388.

120. Chalmers I. The perinatal research agenda: whose priorities? *Birth* 1991; **18**: 137–45.

121. Savulescu J, Chalmers I, Blunt J. Are research ethics committees behaving unethically? Some suggestions for improving performance and accountability. *BMJ* 1996; **313**: 1390–3.

122. Mackillop WJ, Palmer MJ, O'Sullivan B, Ward GK, Steele R, Dotsikas G. Clinical trials in cancer: the role of surrogate patients in defining what constitutes an ethically acceptable clinical experiment. *Br J Cancer* 1989; **59**: 388–95.

123. Brundage MD, Mackillop WJ. Locally advanced non-small cell lung cancer: do we know the questions? *J Clin Epidemiol* 1996; **49**: 183–92.

124. Thornton H. Patients' role in research. In: *Health Committee Third Report: Breast Cancer Services*. Vol II. London: HMSO, 6 July 1995, pp. 112–14.

125. Thornton H. Clinical trials: a "ladyplan" for trial recruitment? Everyone's business. *Lancet* 1993; **341**: 795–6.

126. Pfeffer N, Alderson P. Informed consent: The central problem is often poor design and conduct of trials. *BMJ* 1997; **315**: 247.

127. Ashcroft R, Toth B. Informed consent: research suffers if patients suspect that their rights may be breached. *BMJ* 1997; **315**: 252.

128. Standing Group on Consumers in NHS Research. *Involvement works*. 2nd report. Leeds: NHS Executive, 1999.

129. Miké V. Ethics, evidence and uncertainty. *Controll Clin Trials* 1990; **11**: 153-6.

130. Ashcroft R. Giving medicine a fair trial. *BMJ* 2000; **320**: 1686.

27 · Rights and responsibilities of individuals participating in medical research

John Harris and Simon Woods

It might seem initially that the proper moral concern of medical research is with the *rights* of the research participant and not their *obligations*. This sentiment certainly seems to be broadly at one with the *World Medical Association Declaration of Helsinki*, which advances the principle that: "Concern for the interests of the subject must always prevail over the interests of science and society."[1] These are two powerful reasons to prioritise the claims of research subjects. Moreover, it is important to bear in mind that clinical trials are impossible without the participation of patients – indeed the whole purpose of such studies in the longer term is to benefit future patients. As Heather Goodare claims "patients should be at the forefront of researchers' minds when they design, conduct and report clinical research."[2]

At a second glance, however, the claim that researchers must have the interests of the research subjects to the fore is not the same exacting requirement as that made by the *Declaration of Helsinki*. We shift to talking of "research subjects" because of course not all participants in research are "patients". There is something supererogatory in the *Declaration of Helsinki*, which is not sufficiently implied by the assertion that researchers ought to be concerned for the best interests of the research subjects. What is supererogatory in the *Declaration of Helsinki* is the claim that the interests of the research subject are *paramount*. This is quite simply an error of reasoning since becoming a research subject is not something that could conceivably augment a person's moral status. It should be clear that this is emphatically not to detract from the moral importance of human research subjects and their welfare as the quite proper, central concern of researchers. *All* people are morally important and each has an equal claim to respect and consideration. The researcher's duty to safeguard the interests of the research subject are sufficiently met by the general duty of care each person has to prevent harm coming to others through their acts or omissions – the researcher's duty of "non-maleficence".

In recognising this error of reasoning in the Helsinki prescription, we are required to think again about the ethics of medical research and consider the balance between the *rights* and the *responsibilities* of research subjects. This paper will argue that a person's expectation to receive the best medical treatment ought to be premised upon the recognition of an obligation to contribute to the processes by which effective treatments are determined. What this amounts to, as we shall see, is a moral obligation (perhaps of modest force) to participate in medical research. This obligation is founded on a number of considerations:

- It is part of the general duty that we all have to refrain from harming one another.
- It is in everyone's interests.
- It seems only fair.

MEDICINE, HEALTH, AND THE BEST INTERESTS OF INDIVIDUALS

The perhaps controversial claim that persons have any such obligation obviously requires more detailed justification, since it is not intended as a licence to ride roughshod over the interests of the potentially vulnerable research participant. First it is important to recognise that there is a distinction between a person's interests proper and a person's preferences or wishes. What is or is not in someone's interests is an objective matter. Whilst it is true that, as medical researchers, we do not have exhaustive knowledge of people's interests, this merely reinforces our assumption that individuals usually have a special role to play in determining these, but not that they have an *exclusive* role in so doing. We know, for example, that human beings are apt to act against their own interests, having such self-harming preferences as smoking and participation in dangerous sports. Even reckless acts of selfless altruism are not entirely unknown. It is, however, important to note that an individual's preferences are not necessarily reliable indicators of their interests. A person may have a very strong preference to avoid the unpleasant iatrogenic effects of a course of treatment say, but it often clearly is in their interest to continue with the treatment in order to be relieved of their ailment.

It is certainly the business of medicine to promote a person's best interests, at least as far as their health is concerned. This may begin to sound at odds with the notion of respect for persons and to smack of the paternalism contemporary health care has attempted to reject, but this is not so. Indeed the idea of respect for persons requires that we respect a person's wishes, subject to the constraints of morality and the requirements of social living. The reason we think respect for persons requires respect for their wishes is that a person's wishes are an expression of their autonomy, and in respecting their wishes we respect their autonomy.

Generally speaking we take the view that the best way of respecting a person is to respect their wishes, even though their wishes may not be what is best for them. However, we also believe that there are circumstances when there are good reasons for overriding a person's wishes because their wishes would be seriously self-defeating or because there is a greater public interest at stake. Since it is the role of medicine to promote the objective interests of society as well as those of individuals, it may sometimes be necessary to do so at the expense of a person's wishes. Where this sacrifice of autonomy is not only in that person's interests broadly conceived, but in addition clearly in the public interest, the moral character of the imperative is manifest, although not of course established beyond doubt.

It should be clear, and must be emphasised, that we are not suggesting that patients or other people should be coerced into participating in medical research. Rather, our argument is that it ought to be expected that they would be willing to do so both in their own and in the public interest, and that this may require some sacrifice of personal freedom and comfort.

THE RESEARCHER'S DUTY OF CARE

Clearly the assumption of this level of public obligation in no way diminishes the researcher's duty of care. If anything, it requires the highest level of scientific and ethical scrutiny of research proposals, perhaps requiring a greater public involvement at all stages of the research process, together with improved methods for monitoring medical research activity.[3, 4]

In the context of medical research the potential for any harmful effects of the research must be minimised, although sometimes, as we shall see, research may of necessity entail morbidity, and even a risk of dying, from a new treatment in the course of its attempted verification. However, generally speaking, the benefits of medical research are very clear. We all benefit from living in a society, and, indeed, in a world in which medical research is carried out and which uses the benefits of past research. It is not too difficult to enumerate the benefits of research where a patient benefits directly. However, there are also indirect benefits, which derive, *inter alia*, from the knowledge that research is ongoing into diseases or conditions from which we do not currently suffer but to which we might succumb. Some research questions are of immediate and universal concern – for example the growing problem of antibiotic-resistant organisms that has begun to undermine the "magic bullet", which changed the face of twentieth-century medicine. The possibility of such a major reversal in the efficacy of medicine shakes our current, virtually assured, sense of safety, and increases our concern for the future safety of ourselves, our descendants, and others for whom we care.

Where we benefit from research but refuse to participate in it, we are clearly acting unfairly in some sense. To benefit from the contribution of others without even a gesture of reciprocity is to accept a free ride on the sacrifice of others. To volunteer to participate in medical research is to do what any reasonable, decent person should be willing to do if they wish and expect to receive the benefits of research, at least where the risks and dangers to research subjects are minimal. Where risks, dangers, or inconvenience of research is minimal, and the research well founded and likely to be for the benefit of one-self or others, then there is some, perhaps very modest, moral obligation to participate.

This seems to run contrary to the spirit of Helsinki. A moment's reflection reveals that there are many instances in which we recognise the legitimacy of placing some limitation on personal autonomy, and in some circumstances a severe restriction is justified where the interests of the community require this.[5] Compulsory military service where one is required to risk life and limb for one's country is perhaps the most extreme example, to say nothing of the plethora of safety regulations and legal restrictions that restrict out work, our leisure, and even our home life. All such restrictions involve some denial of autonomy and indicate that there are circumstances in which the interests of the individual are clearly *not* paramount. Let's take a moment to reflect on further examples where the public good is prior to the interests of the individual.

PARTICIPATION IN PUBLIC GOODS*

It is widely recognised that some restriction on personal autonomy is justified in the interests of the community and that this may even extend to the violation of bodily integrity.[5] Control of dangerous drugs, or control of road traffic, for example, both require limitations on personal freedom in the public interest. Vaccination is an interesting example of a public health programme in which people are strongly encouraged to participate in the public interest. Vaccination programmes are usually voluntary, although most societies regard a high compliance rate as essential and are not above using coercive measures just short of compulsory vaccination to ensure this. Although powers of compulsory vaccination are no longer used in the UK, compulsory treatment including vaccination is still possible in the case of children under provisions of the Children Act [1989]. Existing policies for immunisation programmes in the UK have been criticised as coercive to the point of compulsion.[6]

However, there are, of course, risks attendant on participation, and these are usually regarded as minimal, although some parents of children whom they believe to have been damaged by vaccines would dispute this. A parent, solely consulting her own and her child's best interests, when considering the issue

of measles, mumps and rubella (MMR) triple vaccine programmes, for example, would wish to be a free rider, exempting her child and hoping to benefit from the protection afforded by the fact that the overwhelming majority of other children would have been vaccinated. In such circumstances her child would be relatively well protected by the fact that other children were immune and would therefore neither contract nor pass on infection. Her child would benefit without running any risks attendant upon vaccination. If we think such behaviour wrong, we do so because we think that such free riding is unfair, and because we think that we all have an obligation to contribute to the safety of others and to the public interest. (It would probably also be self-defeating when others came to the same conclusion.) In the present example, the widespread success of the vaccination programme depends, of course, on a high level of public uptake, in order to achieve both "herd" and individual immunity.

Public health legislation[7] provides a good example of the existence of statutory powers where it is recognised that interference with a person's life and liberty is justified in the public interest. The Public Health (Control of Disease) Act 1984 gives the power to compulsorily exclude a person from work, allowing for compulsory medical examination and the compulsory removal of a person to hospital where they may be detained but not forcibly treated. It is also recognised that in the interests of public health it may be necessary to breach patient confidentiality and make public information about a person that is normally deemed private. Whilst the draconian measures possible under public health legislation would be tyrannical if extended to other areas of public interest, the example remains a useful illustration of the degree to which personal autonomy may be encroached upon in the public interest. By comparison our claim that participation in medical research ought to be regarded as a form of citizen's obligation, particularly where the risks to the individual are generally small and the gains to the public are potentially large, stands firm.

It could be argued that the measures made possible under public health legislation are only justified because they are necessary to *prevent* a serious harm occurring, but that it is a different story to suggest that similar obligations apply when attempting to do positive good. Whilst denying that there is an important difference between the "Janus faces" of our obligations here, we do not rely on this moral symmetry. Clearly we would not wish to argue that people be

---

*This term is used in a non-technical sense.

coerced into participating in medical research. We merely seek to point out some of the many examples which exist suggesting that a degree of self-sacrifice in the public interest is often expected and usually reasonable, and that participation in medical research ought to be regarded as one of these.

However, there are also examples where individuals and society as a whole are prepared voluntarily to sanction the sacrifice of personal autonomy in the interests of others. Where people find themselves in immediate and deadly peril, even when the danger is of their own making, then there is a common intuition and belief that every effort ought to be made to save them, even when the odds of success are small. So widely held is this feeling that society is willing to apply considerable public resources to this endeavour, supporting rescue organisations through charitable contributions in addition to supporting the statutory services through taxation. Such is the instinct to rescue those in danger that individuals are often willing to risk life and limb to save others. There are many senses in which participation in research involves features relevantly analogous to the examples we have discussed, as well as the many other examples of public duty or service, such as jury service and compulsory military service. All are important public goods for which citizens are called upon and, in the case of public health, required to make some sacrifice of autonomy and perhaps undergo some inconvenience or sacrifice of interests for the public good. It is this latter feature that is particularly important.

OBJECTIVE INTERESTS AND THE PUBLIC GOOD

Surely there is something mistaken in this view? Whilst it may be true to say that a person's interests are objective, it does not follow that everyone has the *same* objective interests. This seems most plausible where the type of research is concerned with a particular, say rare genetic condition, where it is possible to rule out the majority of people as potential beneficiaries. Even here, however, it is reasonable to claim that all people stand to benefit, if not directly, then indirectly from research of this type; and, if not from this type of research, then from the very institution of medical research itself. This seems to hold true of even the most challenging of circumstances, where the nature of the research requires that an experimental therapy is administered exclu-

sively to patients with a particular condition and where the nature of the research or the condition, or both, preclude a significant possibility of advantage to the individual patient.

Take for example a Phase I clinical trial of a new cancer drug. Here the principal aim of the trial is to observe the toxicity associated with the experimental therapy.[8] The inclusion criteria for such studies usually require that the patient's disease has relapsed following comprehensive use of established treatments, in effect, that patients have an incurable, and in the case of cancer, usually a terminal illness. In such trials the best that can be expected for particular participants is a partial remission. The most likely outcome, however, is that the patient's prognosis remains unchanged; quality of life may be worsened and in some cases, death may even be accelerated. What is certain in the case of research participants who have incurable cancer is that the patient will die of the disease within a relatively short time and will therefore be highly unlikely to benefit directly from the possible therapeutic application of the new drug.

However, many patients who volunteer for Phase I trials do so in the full recognition that the benefits of such research are precisely unlikely to be of benefit to them personally, yet they agree to participate for what are often described as altruistic reasons, for the benefit of others. Such gestures are perhaps in part due to the recognition that others have made similar sacrifices for the benefits they themselves have already enjoyed. They seem to recognise that they ought to make a similar sacrifice.

There is still a further sense in which such acts may be regarded as a benefit; namely in the objective sense already alluded to. In the class of interests a person may have, we can distinguish between at least two kinds of interest, *experiential* and *persisting*.[9, 10] In the course of our lives we all have the desire to have our various interests met. For some of our interests it matters whether they are fulfilled or not during our lifetime, since the degree to which such interests are satisfied is one of the ways in which we judge the goodness of our life. This is clearly the case for our experiential interests; since once our capacity for experience has ended, we can no longer have such interests. For most interests it is the person themselves who is the best judge of whether those interests have been met or not. We generally allow that the individual is therefore the best judge of the success of his or her own life. However, for *non-experiential* interests, it may as a matter of fact be true that a person is mistaken as to whether an important interest has been met. Take for example the view that the success of your life is entirely contingent upon the fulfilment of your ambition that your children grow into successful and happy adults.[11] Suppose that you are deceived into believing this to be the case, and you die happy in the belief that your life's ambition to be a successful parent has succeeded. Then it is not true of you that your life has been a success since your life has failed in this one defining interest. This remains true of you for as long as this state of affairs persists.

Now it is in the nature of interests that they can be either personal, impersonal or both, and a life may be judged a greater or lesser success in respect of the degree to which the impersonal interests of that life have been met. If it is true that after your death you leave this world better off than it would otherwise have been, then this fact is true of you irrespective of whether you were aware of this fact before your death. It is also true regardless of whether bettering the world was one of your acknowledged interests. The fact of this change to the world amounts to more than what Derek Parfit calls a mere "Cambridge-change", i.e. more than a mere change in the number of true sentences about an object.[11]

To leave the world a better place than it otherwise would have been, is what any decent person should wish to achieve. Arguably to do so is also in everyone's interests in the sense that acting honourably and morally always is, even where so doing may shorten one's life or cause pain and distress. Doing the right thing has seldom been cost free. Equally, to have contributed to the advance of medical knowledge by participating in medical research is to have made the world a better place. Each person has an interest in leaving the world a better place than they found it. If such an obligation holds for the very sick, even in circumstances where they are likely to experience direct harm from participating in research, then it holds *a fortiori* for others where the costs and risks are minimal.

It is important to be very clear about what we are here proposing. What we are saying is not to be mistaken as an argument for coercion into medical research. Coercion, as we have noted, can only be justified in extreme circumstances and should always be the very last resort. Nor is it an argument for the waiving of consent. Noting that there are circumstances where an important public good licenses the suspension or even the disregard for fully informed consent is not, of course, a recommendation that

consent should be abandoned. On the contrary, fully informed consent is the best guarantor of the interests of research subjects and is expressive of equal concern and respect for them as autonomous persons. However, such cases remind us that the principle of equality of concern and respect sometimes involves not only the balancing of competing claims, but also necessitates some respect being given to the difference in force, urgency, and moral weight of competing claims.

To note that coercion is justifiable is not to recommend coercion. If it were to be claimed that conscription into the military would be justifiable in cases of threats to national integrity, this might make more plausible and more palatable measures to recruit defence forces that fell short of conscription. In such a case a society would be unlikely to stress as paramount the right of all citizens to refuse to defend their country. In such a case we might, as a society, be justifiably content, for example, with obtaining "mere consent" to be recruited, rather than with an elaborate protocol of "informed consent".

INFORMED CONSENT AND THE PUBLIC INTEREST

There is no doubt that there is a pressing public interest in discovery and development of effective treatments for the major modern killers such as heart disease and cancers. Jeffrey Tobias argues that a real barrier to progress is the lack of consensus that exists over how to weigh different sorts of interest between "… those who insist that the individual patient in the consulting room should be the sole focus of concern for the doctor, and those who feel – and are prepared to say publicly – that they owe a duty not only to the patient sitting opposite but also to society at large which, with an equal passion, has charged us to get on in all haste and find that cure".[12] Here our sympathies, if not our final position with regard to consent, lie closer to those of Tobias. With regard to consent our position is more closely allied to that of Len Doyal who eloquently argues that informed consent should remain inviolate;[13] although consent *per se* adds nothing in terms of justification for a particular piece of research, it may well justify the involvement of the research subjects. This will be particularly true where the research, while well founded, is not of great urgency or while therapeutic is not of high priority, not life-prolonging for example.

We have argued that becoming a patient, like becoming a research participant, is not the sort of consideration that could possibly alter one's moral status. Tobias argues that the pressing public interest in cancer research might merit the waiving of informed consent where this requirement ultimately results in fewer patients being entered into clinical trials for which they are eligible. We have argued there are good moral reasons to accept some curtailment of individual autonomy where this serves an important public interest. However, whether or not it follows from this that the safeguard of consent should be altogether abandoned is a further and separate question to which we must now turn.

Whilst Jeffrey Tobias's motives are no doubt of the highest moral integrity, wholesale abandonment of informed consent would be incautious. One problem is that whilst there are such powerful commercial interests in the development of novel therapies, the moral and scientific integrity of the medical science community is not beyond reproach. An audit of clinical trials revealed that 88% of 226 sites where clinical trials were in progress had at least one error in compliance, which risked patient safety.[14] So long as careers and profits rest on the outcomes of clinical trials it is not inconceivable that conflicting interests may compromise the moral and scientific integrity of the researchers. Whilst informed consent is an imperfect palliative, it serves an important function in the scrutiny of the methods and motives of medical research.

Moreover, there are many things, which we would be morally justified in doing, that we should be very reluctant to do. There are powerful public policy considerations as to why coercion should always be a last resort in a democracy. It is always better to proceed by consent if at all possible. However, pointing out that the public good is sufficiently important to be secured by conscription may, as we have noted, demonstrate the justifiability of other measures to secure the desired and, by hypothesis, desirable outcome.

Establishing that conscription might be morally justified by the personal and public good it would secure shows that, *a fortiori*, less drastic or dramatic measures would be justified. These might include the provision of incentives to participate in research and the waiving of the requirement for consent, where concern for autonomy is not materially an issue, e.g. in the case of the research, use of stored archive samples from individuals now dead or where mechanisms are in place to secure anonymity and untraceability of the source of the sample. Both these suggestions are of course controversial and contravene many existing international protocols[1, 15] on research ethics. We do not have space here to examine or defend these suggestions further (but see refs. 16 and 17 for further discussion).

Conscription would also raise very difficult problems of selection of research subjects and of compliance. Are people to be dragged "kicking and screaming" into the laboratory or are they to be fined or imprisoned for non-compliance? Whilst problems of selection and enforcement are not insoluble, they make the likely acceptance of any such procedures in a democracy very remote. However, the arguments for conscription are worth rehearsing precisely because of the effect that they have on public education and on public consciousness. We need people to understand both the point and the urgency of research, and we need them to consider both the desirability of participation and its utility. If they also know that measures are in place to ensure that researchers are scrupulous in applying agreed protocols, that all research is rigorously assessed by competent and well-constructed ethics committees, and that the agreed protocols are also properly policed, then there is likely to be not only widespread acceptance of the idea of participation in research but more well-founded research. That this is not only in the individual but also in the public interest should be both sufficient motive and sufficient justification.

REFERENCES

1. The World Medical Association Declaration of Helsinki as amended by 48th General Assembly, Somerset West, Republic of South Africa, October 1996. Article 1, para 5.
2. Goodare H. The rights of patients in research. *BMJ* 1995; **310**: 1277–8.
3. Chalmers I. What do I want from health research and researchers when I am a patient? *BMJ* 1995; **310**: 1277–8.
4. Herxheimer A Clinical trials: two neglected ethical issues. *J Med Ethics* 1993; **19**(4): 211–18.
5. Harris J. Ethical issues in geriatric medicine. In: Tallis RC, Brockelhurst JC, Fillett H, eds. *Textbook of geriatric medicine and gerontology* 5th Edition. London: Churchill Livingstone, 1998.
6. Nicholson RH. U.K. moves towards compulsory vaccination. *Hastings Centre Rep* 1996; March–April: 4.
7. Public Health (Control of Disease) Act 1984 and Public Health (Infectious Diseases) Regulations 1988.

8. Souhami R, Tobias J. *Cancer and its management* 3rd edn. Oxford: Blackwell Science, 1998, pp. 85 ff.

9. Dworkin R. *Life's dominion*. London: HarperCollins, 1993, pp. 201 ff.

10. Harris J. *Wonderwoman and Superman*. Oxford: Oxford University Press, 1992, pp. 100 ff.

11. Parfit D. *Reasons and persons*. Oxford: Clarendon Press, 1991.

12. Tobias JS. *BMJ*'s present policy (sometimes approving research in which patients have not given fully informed consent) is wholly correct. *BMJ* 1997; **314**: 1111–14.

13. Doyal L. Informed consent in medical research: journals should not publish research to which patients have not given fully informed consent – with three exceptions. *BMJ* 1997; **314**: 1107–11.

14. Trial and error puts patients at risk. *Guardian* 1999; July 27, p. 8.

15. Council for International Organizations of Medical Sciences. *International ethical guidelines for biomedical research involving human subjects*. Geneva: CIOMS, 1993.

16. Harris J. Ethical genetic research. *Jurimetrics: J Law, Sci Policy*, 1999; **40**(1).

17. Research on human subjects, exploitation and global principles of ethics. In: Lewis Andrew DE, Freeman M, Harris J. eds. *Current Legal Issues 3: Law and Medicine*. Oxford: Oxford University Press (in press).

28 · Informed consent in medical research: the consumer's view

Naomi Pfeffer

Undoubtedly some readers' hackles will have risen on finding a chapter on consumers in a book on informed consent to medical research. Who are consumers? What, if anything, of medical research is 'consumed'? How can a medical research subject have anything in common with say, a viewer, of television programmes, who can select a programme from a number of different providers? There is no simple answer to these questions. A consumer sits at the centre of numerous current debates. Hence, there are many different types of consumer.

In considering how consumers' presence might be felt in relation to informed consent to medical research, this chapter examines three types: lay person, customer, and activist. Each type may question the frameworks and commitments of the medical research community, albeit in different ways. Each may draw attention to the unequal power relationship of, investigator and potential research subject, to their different rewards and disbenefits, which tend to be overlooked in debates about whether or not, how, and from whom, to seek informed consent.

CONSUMER AS LAYPERSON

The British medical research establishment's immunity to consumers was compromised in 1996 when The Standing Group on Consumers in NHS Research was set up. The Group believes consumers of the NHS have a right to participate in research that affects them. Consumers are defined as "patients, potential patients, carers, organisations representing consumers' interests, members of the public who are the targets of health promotion programmes and groups asking for research because they believe they have been exposed to potentially harmful circumstances, products or services."[1] In effect, consumer is a synonym for a lay person.

The Standing Group suggests seven reasons why investigators should involve consumers in research

and development such as: it will make research more relevant to patients, they can help recruit subjects, they can disseminate research findings, and consumer involvement is now on the political agenda.[2] The contribution consumers might make to the doctrine and practice of informed consent is not included, perhaps because lay people are constructed as the problem – not the solution – in debates about it. Should they and, if so, how can they, be made to understand the purpose and design of a clinical trial in which they are being asked to participate? The chances of them understanding what is involved appear slim. The term "lay" conjures up an image of people somehow disabled by illness and misunderstandings. "Lay" is taken to mean "inexpert."[3] People are lay because they lack specialist knowledge held by medical professionals whose status is based on the acquisition, through years of study and practice, of the complexities of biomedicine, the recondite principles of statistics and counterintuitive ethical imperatives such as equipoise. The distance separating doctors and lay people is widened by new discoveries of medical research; each finding added to the stock of knowledge makes more arduous the task of medical investigators seeking informed consent.

Ethical, legal, and regulatory requirements on informed consent to medical research insist investigators bridge the gap between themselves and potential research subjects with information. The task that confronts the investigator is designing and building what might be called, an information bridge. What route should it take, and out of what materials should it be constructed?

In medical research, information bridges are seen as the means for transporting the frameworks and commitments of investigators to potential research subjects. They are constructed out of materials found within medicine and, to a lesser extent, law. Undoubtedly, ensuring research subjects know what is in the protocol is crucial. For consent to be "real", subjects must understand what the research involves, why it is being carried out, by and for whom, its potential risks and benefits, and what their role entails.[4] Building information bridges is understood as a technical problem which, with occasional help from the legal profession, the medical research community can solve by itself. Plain English,[5] the use of narrative rather than description, translations into minority languages spoken in the local community, and diagrams are now recommended. How well different methods work is established by technical devices such as readability scores and experimental methods, including randomised controlled trials, which have even been brought together in a meta-analysis.[6] Success is measured by gathering evidence of research subjects' understanding and recall of the information on the information sheet.

Little interest has been shown in "consumer preference" in terms of media, for example, whether an interactive video is preferable to the printed word. Evaluations of effectiveness rarely take into account the difference context makes. Yet the quality of consent must differ if it is sought in an outpatient hospital clinic desperately trying to conform to Patient Charter standards, from a patient lying partially clothed on an examination couch in a cubicle separated from other patients by a curtain, from a patient the night before undergoing major surgery for cancer, or in a quiet room where, given ample time, the patient is able to ask the investigator for clarification of aspects of the research. These and other social factors are rarely considered. Yet we know that how potential research subjects are perceived influences investigators' willingness to seek informed consent. For example, Tobias admits to feeling differently about approaching a journalist and a street homeless person.[7] In turn, social distance influences, both positively and negatively, how people respond to investigators and their willingness to consent to research.

It is not surprising some investigators question the wisdom of confronting potential research subjects with stark and uncompromising details about clinical trials: information taken from lengthy protocols, however clearly written, rarely conveys a sense of concern or mutual respect for people. Information might be more readily accessible if it included what lay people might want or need to know about taking part in trials, not simply what investigators, sponsors, and regulators of research felt they ought to know. Availability of a car parking space, or a roof over one's head when the trial has ended, may be more crucial than number of blood tests in deciding whether or not to consent to research. The ethics of deliberately withholding information about things that are important to potential research subjects but which, from legal, regulatory, and investigators' points of view, are not obviously related to a trial, are never considered, perhaps because both law and ethics focus on protecting passive people rather than on engaging with active consumers of health care.

The "Deficit" Model of Lay Knowledge

How might investigators construct "consumer-friendly" information? Firstly, by acknowledging people have different commitments and frameworks to them. Secondly, by allowing consumer advocates to join the bridge-building team and, once there, recognising their capacity to make important contributions. This second step is difficult for investigators because it requires their abandoning what is sometimes called "the public ignorance" or "deficit" model of lay knowledge,[8] which buttresses the belief that lay people are wholly ignorant of medicine and medical research. According to the deficit model, the purpose of investigators' information is to fill an empty lay mind.

Some enthusiasts of the public ignorance model believe more people would consent to take part in medical research if they understood what it was about; the impression sometimes conveyed is of disobedient school children being forced, for their own good, to do homework. Others know from experience that it is possible fully to understand another person's point of view and still not agree with it. Some people may agree with another person but, for a host of reasons, decide not to be party to their project. The implications of people consenting to trials because they have not fully understood what they entail are rarely considered.

Support for the deficit model of lay knowledge is found in the significance of mental capacity in ethical and legal considerations of consent to medical research. However, competence and incompetence are medicolegal concepts. The term "incompetent" describes a cognitive barrier to informed consent such as age, mental illness, and unconsciousness; it serves as a caution to investigators considering research on vulnerable people. Different conceptual tools developed in anthropology and sociology are required to capture the complicated knowledge of and attitudes to research and medicine of the increasingly diverse population of Britain.[9, 10]

A moment's reflection reveals the absurdity of thinking that lay people having empty minds. They are filled with many different things, only some of which are concerned with their illness. Information about research has to engage with and is buffeted by these other concerns. Few people are completely ignorant about what is wrong with them. Nowadays everyone is swamped with information about health, medicine, and medical research, albeit presented in a different format to that of a trial protocol. As The Standing Group acknowledges, people with chronic conditions know a great deal about their disease (indeed, the Worldwide Web means some are better informed than their doctors about current research and new treatments).

Arguably, the failure to recognise that people's minds are not empty contributes to low recruitment rates. An illustration of this is a trial of the effectiveness of hydroxyurea in reducing the severity of sickle cell disease.[11] It followed an investigation in the USA of the benefits of urea which, in high doses, had been found to have toxic effects owing to dehydration. Many people with sickle cell living in the UK were aware of this finding. Yet because, in developing information about the hydroxyurea trial, investigators had sought to fill what they took to be empty minds, they had failed to grasp the importance of explaining crucial differences between the two substances. As a result, some highly motivated people with sickle cell refused to take part in the trial.

It is all too easy to assume that empty minds lead empty lives. It has been suggested that the burden of a trial – extra visits to a hospital or doctor's surgery and extra tests – are beneficial: people in trials benefit from more intense scrutiny than patients outside the trial receiving routine treatment.[12] However, this claim is based on clinical outcomes, not on process, which is crucial to many people. The trial burden can interfere with subjects' work, domestic arrangements, hobbies, and close relationships. For example, at the end of the investigation, a significant proportion of dying people who, for altruistic reasons, had consented to take part in Phase I and II trials of anticancer drugs, said they felt that they had been used by research rather than assisting it. Some complained that the information presented to them at the outset fulfilled legal obligations rather than expressed a concern for the quality of their remaining days.[13] Because, inevitably, experiences such as this one

are shared with others, they feed public attitudes towards medical research.

Another weakness has been identified in the public ignorance model of information bridge design: by focusing on investigations of new cures for cancer rather than, say, trials of new toothpaste formulations, medical research is represented as if it is always socially useful. Yet, almost daily, its credibility and validity is publicly threatened by attacks launched from both within and outside. In June 1998, Richard Smith, editor of the *BMJ*, was reported in *The Guardian* as having described most published research as "rubbish". He claimed only 5% of published articles reached minimum standards of scientific soundness and clinical relevance.[14] The quality of research that never sees the light of day is probably even lower. In considering why people should consent to take part in "rubbish" research, the research community and its sponsors, not lay people, become the problem.

CONSUMER AS CUSTOMER

Standing at just over 11% in 1993, the UK had the largest share of world biomedical publications of the G7 countries (UK, Canada, France, Germany, Italy, Japan, USA).[15]

If the UK research community is a major producer of medical research findings – admittedly, measured controversially, by number of publications – who then is the consumer? Probably the most common understanding of the word "consumer" is customer. Despite sounding out of place in debates about informed consent, thinking about who is the customer of medical research is an important undertaking: it reminds us that money frequently changes hands in medical research, albeit out of sight of research subjects. It also provides an explanation of why research subjects lack any direct influence over its topics and design, have no claim over its findings, and its topic is usually irrelevant to their situation.

The Triumph of Consumption

Unlike the lay person, the customer is always right! Indeed, customers have become a force to be reckoned with in postindustrial societies like Britain, where consumption now drives production. Until the recent past, consumption was considered the poor relation of production; producers determined both the substance and pace of consumption, paying scant regard to what consumers might prefer, and showing little interest in whether or not they were satisfied with what had been produced. Consumption was excluded from criteria used in the evaluation of production, which focused on conformity to standards set by "experts", docility of the workforce, size of dividends paid to shareholders, and wealth and influence of the owners of the means of production. Indeed, rejection of what was produced was interpreted as lack of judgement on the part of consumers, not a failure of producers.[16]

Nowadays, the richest markets are in postindustrial societies where consumers determine both pace and substance of production. Every act of consumption, every choice made, is monitored and analysed; information technology links cashpoints in shops in the UK to production lines in remote parts of the world. Technologies of surveillance are responsible for the omnipresence of consumers.[17]

The triumph of consumption over production explains why "consumer" is increasingly being used instead of patient: the word signals a reorientation of healthcare organisations away from professional/provider dominance towards a "patient-centred" ethos.

The change in terminology has been mistaken for a real transfer of power when none has taken place. The source of consumer/customer power is the contract, which acts as a control lever on the pace and substance of production. At present, in the UK, patients have no purchase on this lever. As research subjects, they still have almost no say in which topics are investigated and how they are researched. According to the Association of Medical Research Charities (AMRC), charities provide around 13% of the funding of medical research. Although many medical research charities rely on money donated by the general public, decisions on how funds should be spent are made mostly by scientific committees who often favour studies of no immediate practical application.[18] The Standing Group on Consumers in NHS Research is allowing lay people to select some topics for research and, in some NHS regions in England, it is mandatory that patient groups make comments on proposals for NHS-funded research. However, given the relatively small size of budget over which they may have some influence – around 10% of funds for research is found by the NHS and less than 3% by the Department of Health – they are unlikely to have much impact on the overall direction of research.

Findings of the main fields of research cannot be "bought" by patients in the same way as they can buy say, clothes or groceries. Bibliometric analysis puts research into oncology by UK investigators top of the list of publications, followed closely by genetics, cardiology, neurosciences, immunology, and histopathology. The successful "products" of research in these fields can be obtained by patients only through the agreement of a doctor who, in turn, recommends it only where an NHS healthcare purchaser is willing to pay for it.

Admittedly, consumption can involve more than payment with money; different kinds of things can be given and returned.[19] However, considerable energy is spent on preventing subjects from "consuming" medical research, and on making sure they are motivated only by altruism. Research ethics committees carefully weigh up "expenses" paid to healthy volunteers, ensuring any money offered is a "token of appreciation", not an inducement to consent. Information sheets on clinical research recognise and, sometimes, explicitly discourage, people's hope that virtue may be rewarded when a test substance or procedure proves to be a "miracle cure" of their disease. Patients are advised that any benefit emerging from a trial will be felt not by them but in the future, by people with the same illness. Other possible sources of satisfaction are denied to patients; they are usually the last to hear of results of trials in which they have taken part; and, at the end of a trial, they may find it impossible to obtain a treatment tested and found beneficial by them.[20]

Findings can also harm subjects. It is impossible to say how often this happens; episodes emerge in public only where there is conflict. A well-known example is the now infamous Bristol breast cancer survey, sponsored by the Cancer Research Charity: "findings" of higher rates of disease recurrence and lower survival in women who attended the Bristol Cancer Help Centre, subsequently proved erroneous, were widely publicised, causing great distress and anxiety amongst women who had taken part in the investigation, and who learnt that, statistically speaking, they would relapse.[21] Another more recent case is a clinical trial to assess the efficacy and safety of the oral chelating agent deferiprone for the prevention of iron overload in patients with transfusion-dependent forms of thalassaemia. The company sponsoring the trial attempted, and ultimately failed, to restrict investigators' freedom to tell patients and the scientific community about the concerns they had about deleterious effects of the drug being investigated.[22] The devil is in the detail of the contract which research subjects never see.

Sponsors are Customers

In the UK, according to the AMRC, in 1992–93, 56.3% of health research and development was funded by the pharmaceutical industry. Industry-funded research tends to have a more clinical profile; its more applied nature is directly connected to wealth creation. More than half of all clinical trials run in the UK are designed to test new drugs under development by pharmaceutical companies.

Most producers of pharmaceuticals are multinational corporations. The UK is an attractive market for their products because it is rich and a relatively large consumer of healthcare. It is also highly regulated.[23] Regulatory requirements compel commercial sponsors to be active consumers of medical research carried out in the UK: data from industry-sponsored clinical trials form the basis of the application to license a new drug so it can be introduced into clinical practice.

In discussions of industry-sponsored clinical trials, the term "sponsorship" might more appropriately be replaced by "customer". The relationship between industry and clinical investigators is a contractual one: industry contracts with investigators, who have direct contact with potential research subjects to carry out the research that it requires for regulatory purposes. From the patient's point of view, the research appears to emanate from their trusted and respected doctor, not a commercial organisation, although this is usually stated on information sheets. Yet clinical investigators are effectively providing a commercial service to industry. For a host of reasons, such as diminishing funds and pressure to carry out research, the dependence of clinical investigators on industry-sponsored research is increasing as they use it as a source of funds for "pet" projects.

The importance of industry support of medical research has been recognised by the FDA which, since February 1999, has insisted that doctors and scientists who conduct clinical trials in the UK of drugs, which may later be licensed in the USA, declare any financial interests. Spouses and dependant children of investigators are included in the arrangements to prevent financial interests being hidden within a family.[24]

A plethora of legal instruments safeguard the interests of customers.[25] In contrast, protecting the welfare of research subjects takes the form of a paper exercise. Research ethics committees issue "licences" to investigators to carry out studies described in protocols. The legal status of these committees is uncertain.[26] They are accountable not to patients but to health authorities who rarely monitor them. It is left to committees to decide whether or not to follow and how to interpret guidelines issued by the Department of Health and the various royal colleges. Anecdotal evidence suggests practice varies widely. Some committees are prepared to approve studies where informed consent is not sought and which, occasionally, are published with much soul searching in the *BMJ*. Meetings are held in secret. Accountability to research subjects takes the form of a published annual report, most of which are remarkable for their opacity.[27]

Gaining research ethics committee approval can be likened to passing a driving test. However, while the proficiency of drivers continues to be monitored by police and other forms of surveillance, and legal penalties can be incurred for breaking rules, no one is charged with monitoring whether and how investigators seek informed consent. Monitoring of the conduct of research might provide researchers with an added incentive not to cut ethical corners.[28]

Recently, a new "industry" devoted to safeguarding sponsors' interests has sprung up in response to the growing awareness of financial fraud and malpractice in the medical research community.[29] Yet, as the scandals in medical research described in Chapter 6 show, research subjects have a fight on their hands if they try and voice well-founded objections to the design and conduct of research. In the absence of a robust, transparent, open, and accountable system of regulation of clinical trials, informed consent is the only means of self-protection of medical research subjects.

CONSUMER AS ACTIVIST

The activists who have had the greatest impact on the medical research community are the people with HIV/AIDS in the USA, who exploited clinical trials for their own ends. In their desperation to obtain the active experimental drugs in placebo-controlled trials, they had their test medicines analysed. These subversive tactics persuaded the FDA to modify its procedures and standards for clinical efficacy of new drugs through innovations such as "fast-tracking" and "parallel track", intended to increase access to experimental drugs.[30]

The HIV/AIDS activists sought a direct benefit: a private form of consumption. Other patients are on the receiving end of the relaxation in regulations, an unintended consequence of their campaign. A softening of regulatory practice is also sought by right-wing liberals who demand individuals should be allowed the freedom to judge for themselves the risk/benefit ratio of everything including medical research. Reaching its zenith of popularity in the Reagan/Thatcher era, pro-market ideology seeks to undermine and eventually replace regulation by official, legal, and governmental methods with unfettered consumer choice, which, they claim, is the most efficient and effective method of disciplining producers. As yet, there is no sign of pro-market consumer activism challenging medical investigators in the UK, partly because the NHS militates against it. Another reason is difference in regulatory styles on the two sides of the Atlantic: in the USA, the consumers' voice is seen as making a legitimate contribution to the regulatory process, whereas, in the UK, it is regarded mostly as an irritant.[31]

Unmanageable Consumers

In the UK, a new way of containing the threat posed by the triumph of consumption was pioneered in the 1980s when what is sometimes called institutional consumerism was introduced into the public sector to a fanfare of consumerist-sounding, but non-enforceable rights. Many of these "rights" were not new but were recycled principles, such as the right to informed consent to medical research proclaimed in The Patient's Charter.[32] Institutional consumerism is a top-down form of consumer activism, described as fake because it creates the illusion of a coherent group enforcing its will when no such coherent group exists. In effect, institutional consumerism is a way of managing people. The only right they have is to choose, yet the choices they make are from a menu predetermined by others.[33] On the bright side, it has provided a foothold for consumer advocates from which they can draw the attention of professionals to patients' views.[34]

Another type of consumer activist is deliberately unmanageable.[35] Their platform draws on theories developed within what are sometimes referred to as new social movements – feminism, gay rights, disability rights, antiracism and "green" environmen-

talism – which have identified in the triumph of consumption a potential that can counter the power and interests of organized capital, the professions and management. It legitimises their ideas that healthcare, medical research, and the assumptions made by healthcare professionals, sponsors of research, and investigators should meet patients' interests as defined by patients.[36]

An illustration of "unmanageable" consumer activism in relation to medical research is *A charter for ethical research in maternity care* developed by The Association for Improvements in the Maternity Services and The National Childbirth Trust. Under the slogan "Research should be undertaken with women, not on women", it lists 23 issues research ethics committees and investigators should address when considering research on childbearing women.[37] Unfortunately, because endeavours such as this are rarely listed on databases such as Medline, they fail to reach the intended audience.

The process of "peer review" is but one of many barriers confronted by "unmanageable" consumer activists. Their groups are usually small and unstable because of limited funds: they are often suspicious of, or get into trouble if they accept funding tied to professional or commercial interests. They are sometimes confused with powerful political lobbies, usually backed by wealthy sponsors such as the pharmaceutical industry and leading clinicians. These groups are extremely influential: an audit of the US National Institutes of Health spending on research found that AIDS, breast cancer, diabetes mellitus, and dementia, all backed by vocal lobbies, received a disproportionately large share of federal spending in relation to their toll on public health. By comparison, depression, stroke, and emphysema were judged to be underfunded.[38]

A crucial difference between unmanageable consumer activists and powerful lobbies is how they understand the purpose of research. Not surprisingly, most powerful lobbies want more of the current research paradigm, which they helped shape. In contrast, unmanageable consumers seek to redirect research towards their own commitments and frameworks. They want it to find practical things, which may improve the quality of life of themselves and their carers. These goals are excluded by the current paradigm in part because many sponsors support clinical research for regulatory purposes, and in part because researchers do not usually live day-to-day with the condition that is the area of their research. Unmanageable consumer activists tend to think investigators have empty minds and the concepts and methods of the current research paradigm may do more harm than good.[39]

Both powerful lobbies and unmanageable consumer activists share a concern for a single issue. Consumers for Ethics in Research (CERES) takes a generalist approach, seeking to influence how medical research is designed and conducted for the benefit of the collective. Instead of "Research: what's in it for me?", the title given to a conference held in January 1988 by The Standing Advisory Group on Consumer Involvement in the NHS Research and Development Programme, the question it would ask is, "Research: what's in it for us?"

CONCLUSION

In fleshing out three different types of consumers, this chapter has demonstrated the importance of considering the implications of denying people the right of informed consent to medical research within the broadest possible framework, as well as thinking about it in the context of the immediate investigator/research subject encounter.

Denying people the right to informed consent to medical research is an easy but dangerous solution to an extremely complex problem posed by the current paradigm of research and the political economy in which it is undertaken. In speaking in favour of denial the problem and its context are ignored. In effect, arguments in favour of denial maintain the barrier between the wider and immediate context of the investigator/research encounter. Denial allows the different potential rewards and disbenefits of medical research to be disguised. Denial assumes methods of institutional protection afforded research subjects against the disproportionate power of the medical research community are adequate. Yet these are paper exercises performed by research ethics committees and journal editors who chose whether or not to publish the findings of unethical research. Denial condones the refusal of healthcare providers to acknowledge the complex often difficult social circumstances of patients and research subjects.

Looked at through the eyes of an unmanageable consumer, informed consent emerges as the only shield currently available to protect research subjects. However, it is important not to overstate its capacity to protect them. It is limited by the quality and substance of the information provided research subjects, and by the scant attention given to monitoring how, where, when, and by whom it is delivered.

REFERENCES

1. Hanley B. *Involvement works: the second report of the Standing Group on Consumers in NHS Research.* London: Department of Health, 1999.
2. Hanley B. *et al. Involving consumers in research and development in the NHS: briefing notes for researchers.* Winchester. The Help for Health Trust, 2000.
3. Williams R. *Keywords.* London: Fontana, 1985.
4. Doyal L. Informed consent in medical research: journals should not publish research to which patients have not given fully informed consent – with three exceptions *BMJ* 1997; **314**: 1107.
5. Consumers for Ethics in Research. *Spreading the word on research or patient information: how can we get it better?* London: CERES, 1994.
6. Edwards SJL, Lilford RJ, Thornton J, Hewison J. Informed consent for clinical trials: in search of the 'best' method. *Soc Sci Med* 1998; **47**: 1825–40.
7. Tobias JS. BMJ's present policy (sometimes approving research in which patients have not given fully informed consent) is wholly correct. *BMJ* 1997; **314**: 1111.
8. Irwin A, Wynne B eds. *Misunderstanding science? The public reconstruction of science and technology.* Cambridge: Cambridge University Press, 1996.
9. Ashcroft RE, Chadwick DW, Clark SRL, Edwards RHT, Frith L, Hutton JL. Implications of sociocultural contexts for the ethics of clinical trials. *Hlth Technol Assess* 1997; **1**(9).
10. Pfeffer N. Theories of ethnicity in health care and research. *BMJ* 1998; **317**: 1381–4.
11. Special issue on sickle cell and thalassaemia, *CERES News* 1995; **17**.
12. Stiller C. Survival of patients in clinical trials and at specialist centres. In: Williams CJ ed. *Introducing new treatment for cancer: ethical and legal problems.* London: John Wiley & Son, 1992.
13. Cox K. Investigating psychosocial aspects of participation in Phase I and Phase II anticancer drug trials (Unpublished PhD Thesis). Nottingham: University of Nottingham, 1999.
14. Boseley S. Medical studies 'rubbish'. *The Guardian*, 1998; June 24: 5.
15. The Wellcome Trust. *Mapping the landscape: national biomedical research outputs 1985–95.* London: The Wellcome Trust, 1998.
16. Pfeffer N, Coote A. *Is quality good for you? A critical review of quality assurance in welfare services.* London: Institute for Public Policy Research, 1992.
17. Mort F. The politics of consumption. In: Hall S, Jacques M, eds. *New times: the changing face of politics in the 1990s.* London: Lawrence & Wishart, 1989.

18. Hogg C. *Patients, power and politics: from patients to citizens*. London: Sage, 1999.

19. Douglas M, Isherwood B. *The world of goods: towards an anthropology of consumption*. London: Routledge, 1996.

20. Frardin JP. *Med Res CERES News* 1999; **27**: 1–2.

21. Goodare H, Smith R. The rights of patients in research. *BMJ* 1995; **310**: 1277–8.

22. Nathan DG, Weatherall DJ. Academia and industry: lessons from the unfortunate events in Toronto. *The Lancet* 1999; **353**: 771.

23. Abraham J. *Science, politics and the pharmaceutical industry: controversy and bias in drug regulation*. London: UCL Press, 1995.

24. Ferriman A. Drug trial investigators asked to declare financial interests. *BMJ* 1999; **318**: 831.

25. Ogus AI. *Regulation: legal form and economic theory*. Oxford: Clarendon Press, 1994.

26. Mander T. Legal standing of local research ethics committees. *Med Law Int* 1996; **2**: 149–68.

27. Nicholson R. What do they get up to? LREC annual reports. B*ull Med Eth* 1997; July: 13–24.

28. Smith T, Moore EJH, Tunstall-Pedoe H. Review by a local medical research ethics committee of the conduct of approved research projects, by examination of patients' case notes, consent forms, and research records any by interview. *BMJ* 1997; **317**: 1588–90.

29. Boseley S. Trial and error puts patients at risk. *The Guardian* 1999; July: 27–8.

30. Marks H. *The progress of experiment: science and therapeutic reform in the United States, 1900–1990*. Cambridge: Cambridge University Press, 1997.

31. Vogel D. *National styles of regulation*. Ithaca, New York: Cornell University Press, 1986.

32. Hambleton R, Hoggett P. Rethinking consumerism in public services. *Consumer Policy Rev* 1993; **3**: 103–111.

33. Ascherson N. Democracy means choosing what you're told. *The Independent on Sunday*, 1993; September 12: 21.

34. Williamson C. The rise of doctor-patient working groups, *BMJ* 1998; **317**: 1374–7.

35. Gabriel Y, Lang T. *The unmanageable consumer: contemporary consumption and its fragmentations*. London: Sage, 1995.

36. Williamson C. Reflections on health care consumerism: insights from feminism. *Health Expectations* 1999; **2**: 150–8.

37. Association for Improvements in Maternity Services. The National Childbirth Trust. *A charter for ethical research in maternity care*. London: Association for Improvements in Maternity Services.

38. Gottlieb S. US research funding depends on lobbying, not need. *BMJ* 1999; **318**: 17–15.

39. Oliver M. Changing the social relations of research production? *Disabil Handicap Soc* 1992; **7**: 101–14.

29 • The role of effective communication in obtaining informed consent

Angela Hall

THE ROLE OF EFFECTIVE COMMUNICATION IN OBTAINING INFORMED CONSENT

This chapter will argue that whatever information ethicists think patients *ought* to be given about their condition and their treatment is of little account if doctors do not have the communication skills necessary to transfer information successfully. Legally, the concept of informed consent requires only that doctors disclose information to patients. *Morally* valid consent, however, means that patients must understand the information that has been conveyed. Doctors need to ensure not only that their patients receive appropriate information but that they have heard and understood what they have been told, that they are competent to reason about alternative courses of action, and that they are acting voluntarily. Any agreement obtained through manipulation or coercion is not informed consent. In practice then, ensuring that all these requirements are met depends heavily on the communication skills of the person eliciting that consent.

IDENTIFYING THE PROBLEMS

In General Medical Settings

We know from countless reports in the media that there is considerable dissatisfaction with the doctor–patient relationship, with lack of understanding of the patient as a person who has individual concerns, viewpoints, and wishes. We know also from a very large number of research studies that there is a problem with the communication process in medicine. While it is beyond the scope of this chapter to include a comprehensive review of this literature, mention of the findings from some of the key studies indicates the breadth of the difficulties. For exam-ple, 54% of patients' complaints and 45% of their concerns were found not to have been elicited by physicians[1] and in 50% of visits, the patient and the doctor did not agree on the nature of the main presenting problem.[2] Another study found that doctors frequently interrupted their patients so soon after they began their opening statement (on average within 18 seconds) that they failed to disclose other significant concerns.[3] In a study of patients with cancer, one-third of those being treated palliatively believed that the therapeutic intention of the doctor was cure.[4] In a large study conducted in general practice, doctors rarely asked their patients to volunteer their ideas, often actually evaded these ideas and inhibited their expression.[5] There are consistent findings that between 10 and 90% (average 50%) of patients do not take their prescribed medication at all or take it incorrectly.[6] The majority of medicolegal complaints made by patients arise from failures and errors in communication.[7–9]

In Research Settings

There is no reason to think that the situation is any better in research settings. Talking with patients about the research element only introduces an additional layer of complexity. Legally speaking, there is a consensus that doctors have a stronger professional duty to communicate information about risks in the context of research than in the course of normal clinical care.[10] It is dismaying to find, therefore, that in the conclusion to a comprehensive review of the ethics of randomised clinical trials from the perspectives of patients, the public and healthcare professionals, Edwards *et al*. point out that " ... doctors seemed to have been aware that patients may not have fully understood what was going on. For many, informed consent seemed little more than a ritual."[11]

Support for this conclusion is found in a study by Titus and Keane, who studied 167 principal investigators applying to Midwestern review boards for approval for a range of research studies, including clinical trials, drug and device studies.[12] They were asked to say, in writing, how they would verbally describe components of their own process to gain consent from patients. The findings were disturbing. About one-third of the investigators gave a detailed description of the purpose and procedure of their study, but meaningful discussion of all other areas, including risks, benefits, and alternatives, was virtually non-existent; 80% demonstrated that they relied exclusively on asking closed-ended questions, precluding any form of dialogue with the patient; Few of the researchers seemed to have any appreciation of the need to assess potential subjects' understanding of what they had been told, which the authors perceived as "extremely troublesome" because it indicated how highly coercive the process remained.

Sutherland et al.[13] used interpretation of statements contained in a consent form about a hypothetical clinical trial as a surrogate for understanding in a sample of patients with cancer. Between 26 and 54% of patients were unable to interpret correctly the information given to them. The authors felt that the most striking misinterpretation, by 32% of the sample, was that the randomisation process would "select the best treatment for me" or would permit the doctor to decide "which treatment is the right one for me." Thus, although the consent form was explicit about the meaning of randomisation, a significant proportion of the sample was apparently unable to understand treatments being chosen on anything other than an individualised basis. Of particular interest in the context of this chapter was the finding that only 46% of patients correctly interpreted the statement "a particular type of cancer responds to radiation treatment in 10% of cases." This word "response" is part of the *lingua franca* of the oncology consultation but its meaning is ambiguous. Does it indicate that the tumour will shrink for a period of time and then grow again, or shrink and disappear? What are patients to make of this kind of information? This point is being emphasised because one of the most basic and important skills that doctors need is the ability to check that they and their patients share the same understanding of information.

Many other studies in a large variety of research settings have identified major problems in the communication of the most basic elements of the informed consent process. For instance, in a study investigating the effects of different drugs in 43 women with acute salpingitis,[14] five were not aware that a second laparoscopy was performed only for research purposes. Seven women reported that they had not been aware of the meaning of participating in the study and 17 women did not know that they could withdraw from the study whenever they wanted. The authors suggested that because of variations between centres, the providers of the information rather than the receivers were to blame for the low quality of perceived information. In another study of parents whose children were entered into a randomised trial, neither the need to assess safety as well as efficacy of the drug treatment, nor the right to withdraw from the study, was widely appreciated.[15] The great majority of the parents felt that drug trials carried low or no risks, suggesting, as the authors point out, an inordinate faith in the medical system to protect their children. A significant minority of the parents thought that informed consent was unnecessary anyway as they would trust the advice of their doctor. This study was interesting because although the design specified strict adherence to informed consent procedure, attitudinal and psychological barriers appeared to militate against full comprehension. Taking other research into account, these barriers include the inordinate trust in the medical system, the psychological need of some individuals to volunteer,[16] and the tendency to deny and downgrade the risks involved in participation in research.[17] Awareness of these barriers must be taken into account in the design of informed consent procedures. This reiterates the point made by Cassileth et al. in a study on informed consent from patients with cancer that, as patients become increasingly ill, their sense of personal control gives way to intensified dependence on their physicians.[18] This appeared to result in poorer attention to, interest in, and recall of information about consent. These barriers increase the potential for coercion and represent a big challenge to the communication abilities of clinicians, as does the clinical assessment of the patient's competence to reason about difficult or complex choices.

EVIDENCE THAT PROBLEMS CAN BE SOLVED THROUGH EFFECTIVE COMMUNICATION

Up to this point, the situation looks pretty dismal.

We need now to ask some important questions. First, is there evidence that effective communication skills can overcome these problems? It should be emphasised that clinical communication skill is now sufficiently grounded in theory and research to be accepted as a discipline in its own right, with its own subject matter and methods. As Kurtz *et al.*[19] have pointed out, "Knowing how to communicate in normal conversation is not the same as understanding the specific skills of communicating with patients. Communication in medicine is a professional skill that needs to be developed to a professional level." There is now widespread acceptance that communication is a core clinical skill, as important as clinical knowledge, competence in problem-solving, and physical examination. As a discipline it is able to draw on a very large body of research literature accumulated over the last 30 years to back its claims. This literature provides compelling evidence that effective skills in communication can overcome these problems and make a difference to patients as measured by outcomes. Increased patient satisfaction,[20–22] better recall and understanding of information,[23, 24] better adherence to treatment plans,[25, 26] and reduction in litigation[27] have all been shown to be associated with specific core interviewing skills. Importantly there is evidence that physical outcomes for patients are improved with more effective communication skills, such as symptom resolution in chronic headache,[28] better control of hypertension,[29] improved blood sugar control in diabetes,[30] and decreased need for analgesia after myocardial infarction.[31] Other studies have shown an improvement in psychological outcomes, such as reduction in patients' emotional distress, up to one year after skills have been used such as problem-defining, emotion-handling, and creating an atmosphere that encourages information exchange and questioning on the part of the patient.[32, 33]

EVIDENCE THAT COMMUNICATION SKILLS CAN BE LEARNED AND BE RETAINED

If effective skills can overcome problems in communication and improve patient outcomes, then the next question to ask is whether there is evidence that these skills can be learned and will persist? Before answering this question it may clarify matters to point out that the medical interview has been conceptualised as having three main functions,[34] which address the core objectives of the communication process between doctor and patient. The three functions of the model are:

- information gathering
- relationship building, and
- explanation and planning.

Skills specific to initiating and closing the interview have been incorporated into a similar model by Silverman *et al.*[35] Specific skills have been shown to be effective in achieving each functional goal. In practice, of course, these skills are inextricably related, but it is important to appreciate that the key to learning a complicated skill is to identify the *series* of skills that make up the whole and practice them separately before reintegrating them. There is a set of basic, fundamental, core communication skills that have been identified as "...the primary resource for dealing with all communication challenges; often all we need do to manage difficult communication issues is to apply these core skills carefully."[35]

One of the most influential series of studies demonstrating that interviewing skills can be learned was published by Maguire and colleagues between 1976 and 1986. They identified that senior medical students, trained in the traditional apprenticeship method, had serious deficiencies in their information-gathering skills. Few students managed to discover the patient's main problem or clarify its exact nature, let alone explore ambiguous statements, respond to cues, or cover personal topics. Most used closed, lengthy, multiple, and repetitive questions.[36] Importantly, students who underwent a training programme reported almost three times as much accurate and relevant information as the control group, who had received only the traditional learning methods.[37]

In a subsequent study, fourth-year medical students during their psychiatry clerkship were randomised either to a control group, who had clinical training alone (the traditional apprenticeship method), or to individual feedback by a tutor, who used either written ratings on performance, audiotape, or videotape.[38] There was no significant change in the ability of the control group to cover key areas in the history or in their use of skills. All three groups given systematic feedback were able to improve their ability to elicit accurate and relevant information, but only those given audio or videotaped feedback showed significant gains in key interviewing skills. The skills included clarification, the avoidance of jargon, repetition, complex and leading questions, response to verbal leads, facilitation, the ability to discuss more personal matters, and keeping control of the interview. Giving individual feedback is very time-consuming and hence expensive but a later study found that providing feedback within small groups of students was as effective as giving it to students on their own.[39] Students learning with a tutor who was familiar with the key points of the interview model, who allowed students to appreciate their strengths as well as their weaknesses, made more progress than students giving themselves feedback either individually or in small groups.

A subsample of these students was followed up five years later to see whether skills had persisted; interviews were conducted with patients who had physical as well as psychiatric illness.[40] Both groups had improved but the superiority in the skills associated with accurate diagnosis in the group given feedback was maintained. The only skills among the trained group that had deteriorated somewhat were the use of open questions and coverage of psychosocial problems; the control group was clinically inadequate in both of these respects and also in clarifying patients' statements.

Many studies conducted in different settings have now replicated these findings that skills can be learned. Evans *et al.* showed in addition that medical students who had learned key skills were diagnostically more efficient and effective than their control group counterparts and, significantly, took no more time to interview their medical and surgical patients.[41] Even brief training interventions have been shown to be effective. Innui *et al.* delivered a single session on compliance-aiding interviewing skills to physicians whose patients had hypertension.[26] These doctors subsequently spent more time than a control group in considering their patients' ideas and in patient education. Not only did the patients' understanding of their condition and adherence improve, they had better control of their hypertension, even six months after their doctors had been trained.

METHODS OF TEACHING COMMUNICATION SKILLS

These studies have been discussed in some detail because they highlight some very important points. They demonstrate that communication skills can be learned and will persist and they have also illumi-

nated our understanding about appropriate learning methods. The traditional apprenticeship model does not work for two reasons, according to Maguire. First there is a lack of a suitable framework making explicit what areas medical students should cover and what skills they should use. Secondly, it does not allow much, if any, opportunity for students to be given systematic feedback on how effectively they communicate with their patients. Evans *et al.* have demonstrated that didactic methods alone are not sufficient to bring about change in learners' skills.[41] There is a place for didactic or cognitive methods – in particular, introducing conceptual frameworks through which to view the medical interview and to stimulate interest and expand the understanding of learners. There is overwhelming evidence, however, that it is experiential methods of teaching that bring about lasting behavioural changes. These include direct observation of the learner interviewing a real or simulated patient, the provision of appropriate and constructive feedback, and enabling practice and rehearsal in a safe and supportive setting. We also know from these studies that the use of audio or video recording to guide feedback is particularly helpful. Videotape has the additional advantage of making it possible to give feedback on non-verbal as well as verbal behaviours.

COMMUNICATION SKILLS AND INFORMED CONSENT

Although the opening paragraph of this chapter identified the crucial importance of successful transfer of information in eliciting properly informed consent, little has been said up to this point about the specific skills involved. Information-giving is one of the components of the third function of the interview – the explanation and planning phase. In general it is known that doctors give relatively scanty information to their patients, with most patients wanting more information than they have been given.[35, 42–44] A Consumer Association survey identified a further difficulty for patients.[45] When asked reasons for patients not asking questions, nearly two-thirds of the sample said that they assumed the doctor had told them all that they needed to know. Indeed many people have made the point that it can be very difficult for them as patients to know *what* they need to know. The onus is on the doctor to provide what patients need in order to give fully informed consent.

REASONS FOR PROBLEMS WITH INFORMATION TRANSFER

Why should there be such a problem with information transfer?

Lack of Training for Medical Students

One reason is that undergraduate training programmes tend to concentrate on teaching the first two functions of the interview – information-gathering and relationship-building. There are good reasons for this. As Cushing has pointed out, the relationship between the components that constitute a communication skills curriculum and when and how they are taught is crucial.[46] Learning is based on doing, and the most effective learning occurs when the skills being taught are perceived by students to be relevant to what is expected of them on their clinical attachments. The fact is that medical students are not expected to give information nor make management plans with their patients before they qualify. Even if they are taught the skills necessary for effective information transfer, there is no opportunity for the practice that is essential to consolidate learning. The problem is that the point at which medical students qualify and need to use these skills coincides with the time when, for most, formal communication skills training ends. This third function of the medical interview – explanation and planning – has been described as the "Cinderella subject of communication skills teaching".[35] Sanson-Fisher et al.[47] has argued that training doctors in information transfer is the new challenge in communication skills teaching.

There is evidence to support these observations from Maguire et al.'s five-year follow-up study mentioned earlier.[40] The training that the undergraduates had received had not included anything on information-giving, although this was presumably a significant part of their job as these students were now senior house officers, registrars, or general practice trainees. The follow-up study required them not only to take a history but also to give designated information to their patients.[48] The findings make salutary reading. Although most gave simple information diagnosis and treatment, few mentioned aetiology, investigations, or prognosis; 70% made no attempt to discover the patient's views and expectations nor encourage questions; 90% did not categorise the information or attempt to negotiate with

their patients; 63% of these young doctors failed to repeat any advice given, and only 11 % made any attempt to check patients' understanding of what they had been told. These are all skills that have been identified by Ley[24] as fundamental to the informing process. The authors concluded that, "Some young doctors do discover for themselves how best to give patients information and advice, but most remain extremely incompetent."

Lack of Training for Senior Doctors

Medical students in fact have many opportunities to observe how their seniors manage information transfer and to reflect on the skills that are used. Some doctors will be excellent role models but, contrary to popular myth, there is no evidence that doctors' communication skills improve with experience alone. Doctors who qualified before1990 are unlikely to have received communication skills training, as was found in a study reporting training for 178 senior oncologists[49] which found that only 24% of the consultants in the sample had received any formal training at undergraduate level, this figure falling to 18% at postgraduate level. Senior registrars had fared better, as 60% had received undergraduate training. Only 20%, however, had received training as postgraduates and both groups of doctors said that this was usually delivered as part of a management course. Management courses are not the most appropriate setting for doctors to practise and be given feedback on how they transfer complex clinical information. Few regarded any of the methods used in their training (mainly lectures, seminars and/or observation) as effective; 75% of these doctors had some responsibility for teaching communication to their junior staff and students, despite having such little training themselves or indeed any education in how to teach. When asked to list their own communication difficulties, 51% explicitly mentioned the giving and pacing of complex information, including explaining clinical trials.

The Challenge to Professionals

Not surprisingly, given the problems that have been identified in the giving or exchanging of information, there has been much research endeavour aimed at identifying effective ways of improving the situation. The work of Ley mentioned above, identified important skills to help doctors give clearer information and improve patient recall.[24] However, improving recall does not necessarily guarantee an improvement in understanding. It was the work of Tuckett et al.[5] that has probably thrown most light on some of the necessary conditions for patients to understand information given to them. Ley had found in his review of studies on recall that 30–50% of information was forgotten by patients after the consultation, whereas the patients in the Tuckett et al. study (in a sample of 1302 consultations) only forgot 10% of information. Much of this difference is probably accounted for by differences in methodology. In the latter study, only recall of the key points made by the doctors was assessed, rather than every item of information, and the interviewers used probed recall to check understanding: 73% of the patients made sense of what they had been told. Consultations went wrong where there was an incongruity between the explanatory frameworks of the doctor and the patient. Skill is required to ascertain the correct type and amount of information that patients both want and need, to help patients understand and remember, and to achieve a shared understanding which incorporates the perspectives of both doctor and patient. Tuckett et al. point out that "It is, perhaps, asking a great deal of doctors to make what amounts to a fundamental alteration in the detailed way they think about and routinely conduct their task." They go on however, to make the point that, as a profession, doctors have been willing to be self-critical and evaluative. The challenge of involving patients more in decision-making is one to which professionals might be expected to respond with vigour.

CONCLUSION

During the last decade in the UK there has been increasing pressure from professional medical bodies to improve both the training and evaluation of doctors in communication skills. The GMC report *Tomorrow's doctors*[50] published in 1993 recommended that, among other things, communication skills teaching should be one of the core themes in the medical curriculum; all medical schools now include some curriculum training for undergraduates. What is essential now is that training is extended to postregistration doctors and into programmes of continuing medical education. This enables both the reviewing and reiteration of earlier learning and

the opportunity to move on and add new skills to meet the complex situations presented in daily practice. Barnard has pointed out that developments in the fields of medical ethics and communication skills have proceeded in relative isolation from each other and calls for concerted bridge-building between these disciplines and clinicians " ... lowering the barriers to collaboration and partnership".[51] Arnold calls for the discussion and teaching of ethical theory and communication skills together, pointing out that clinicians, both in practice and in training, would improve their performance in both areas simultaneously.[52] There is no doubt that collaboration between these three disciplines could do nothing but improve patient care. The eliciting of properly informed consent is one of the most demanding challenges that doctors face and they need all the help that they can get.

REFERENCES

1. Stewart M, McWhinney, Buck C. The doctor-patient relationship and its effect upon outcome. *J Roy Coll Gen Pract* 1979; **29**: 77–82.
2. Starfield B, Wray C, Hess K. The influence of patient-practitioner agreement on outcome of care. *Am J Public Health* 1981; **71**: 127–31.
3. Beckman H and Frankel R. The effect of physician behaviour on the collection of data. *Ann Int Med* 1984; **101**: 692–6.
4. Mackillop W, Stewart W, Ginsburg A, Stewart S. Cancer patients' perceptions of their disease and its treatment. *Br J Cancer* 1988; **58**: 355–8.
5. Tuckett D, Boulton M, Olson C, Williams A. *Meetings between experts: an approach to sharing ideas in medical consultations*. London: Tavistock, 1985.
6. Butler C, Rollnick S, Stott N. The practitioner, the patient and resistance to change: recent ideas on compliance. *Can Med Assoc* 1996; **154**: 1357–62.
7. Vincent C, Young M, Phillips A. Why do people sue doctors? A study of patients and relatives taking legal action. *Lancet* 1994; **343**: 1609–13.
8. Shapiro R, Simpson D, Lawrence S, Talsky A, Sobocinski K, Schiedermmayer D. A survey of sued and non sued physicians and suing patients. *Arch Intern Med* 1989; **149**: 1290–6.
9. Beckman H, Makarkis K, Suchman A, Frankel R. The doctor-patient relationship and malpractice: lessons from plaintiff depositions. *Arch Int Med.* 1994; **154**: 1365–70.
10. Doyal L. Informed consent in medical research. *BMJ* 1997; **314**: 1107–11.
11. Edwards S, Lilford R, Hewison J. The ethics of randomised controlled trials from the perspectives of

patients, the public and healthcare professionals. *BMJ* 1998; **317**: 1209–12.

12. Titus S, Keane M. Do you understand? An ethical assessment of researchers' description of the consenting process. *J Clin Ethics* 1996; **7**: 60–8.

13. Sutherland H, Lockwood G, Till J. Are we getting informed consent from patients with cancer? *J Roy Soc Med* 1990; **83**: 439–43.

14. Lynoe N, Sandlund M, Dahlqvist G, Jacobsson L. Informed consent: study of quality of information given to participants in a clinical trial. *BMJ* 1991; **303**: 610–13.

15. Harth S, Thong Y. Parental perceptions and attitudes about informed consent in clinical research involving children. *Soc Sci Med* 1995; **41**: 1647–51.

16. Harth S, Johnstone R, Thong Y. The psychological profile of parents who volunteer their children for clinical research: a controlled study. *J Med Ethics* 1992; **18**: 86.

17. Woodward W. Informed consent of volunteers: a direct measurement of comprehension and retention of information. *J Clin Res* 1979; **27**: 248.

18. Cassileth B, Zupkis R, Sutton-Smith, March V. Informed consent-why are its goals imperfectly realised? *New Engl J Med* 1980; **302**: 896–900.

19. Kurtz S, Silverman J, Draper J. *Teaching and learning communication skills in medicine*. Oxford: Radcliffe Medical Press, 1998.

20. Stewart M. What is a successful doctor-patient interview? A study of interactions and outcomes. *Soc Sci Med* 1984; **19**: 167–75.

21. Eisenthal S, Koopman C, Stoekle J. The nature of patients' requests for physicians' help. *Acad Med* 1990; **65**: 401–5.

22. Hall J, Roter D, Katz N. Meta-analysis of correlates of provider behaviour in medical encounters. *Med Care* 1988; **26**: 657–75.

23. Bertakis K, Takayama J, Phibbs C *et al.* The communication of information from physician to patient: a method for increasing patient retention and satisfaction. *J Fam Pract* 1977; **5**: 217–22.

24. Ley P. *Communication with patients: improving satisfaction and compliance*. London: Croom Helm, 1988.

25. Schulman B. Active patient orientation and outcomes in hypertensive treatment. *Med Care* 1979; **17**: 267–81.

26. Innui T, Yourtee E, Williamson J. Improved outcomes in hypertension after physician tutorials. *Ann Intern Med* 1976; **84**: 646–51.

27. Levinson W. Physician-patient communication: a key to malpractice prevention. *JAMA* 1994; **272**: 1619–20.

28. Headache Study Group of Western Ontario, 1986. Details in Silverman J, Kurtz S, Draper J. *Skills for communication with patients*. Oxford: Radcliffe Medical Press, 1998.

29. Orth J, Stiles W, Scherwitz L *et al.* Patient exposition and provider explanation in routine interviews and hypertensive patients' blood pressure control. *Health Psychol* 1987; **6**: 29–42.

30. Rost K, Flavin K, Cole K. Change in metabolic control and functional status after hospitalisation. *Diab Care* 1991; **14**: 881–9.

31. Mumford E, Schlesinger H, Glass G. The effects of psychological intervention on recovery from surgery and heart attacks: an analysis of the literature. *Amer J Public Hlth* 1982; **72**: 141–51.

32. Roter D, Hall J, Kern D *et al.* Improving physicians' interviewing skills and reducing patients' emotional distress. *Arch Intern Med* 1995; **155**: 1877–84.

33. Fallowfield L, Hall A, Maguire P, Baum M. Psychological outcomes of different treatment policies in women with early breast cancer outside a clinical trial. *BMJ* 1990; **301**: 575–80.

34. Bird J, Cohen-Cole S. The three-function model of the medical interview: an educational device. In: Hale M, ed. *Models of consultation liason psychiatry*. Basil: S Karger, 1990.

35. Silverman J, Kurtz S, Draper J. *Skills for communication with patients*. Oxford: Radcliffe Medical Press, 1998.

36. Maguire P, Rutter D. History taking for medical students. 1. Deficiencies in performance. *Lancet* 1976; **2**: 556–8.

37. Rutter D, Maguire P. History taking for medical students. 2. Valuation of a training programme. *Lancet* 1976; **2**: 558–60.

38. Maguire P, Roe P, Goldberg D, Jones S, Hyde C, O'Dowd T. The value of feedback in teaching interviewing skills to medical students. *Psychol Med* 1978; **8**: 695–704.

39. Roe P. *Teaching interviewing skills to medical students*. MSc Thesis, 1980, Manchester University.

40. Maguire P, Fairbairn S, Fletcher C. Consultation skills of young doctors. 1. Benefits of feedback training in interviewing as students persist. *BMJ* 1986; **292**: 1573–6.

41. Evans B, Stanley R, Mestrovic R *et al.* Effects of communication skills training on students' diagnostic efficiency. *Med Educ* 1991; **25**: 517–26.

42. Waitzkin H. Information giving in medical care. *J Health Soc Behav* 1985; **26**: 81–101.

43. Beisecker A, Beisecker T. Patient information-seeking behaviours when communicating with doctors. *Med Care* 1990; **28**: 19–28.

44. Pinder R. *The management of chronic disease: patient and doctor perspectives on Parkinson's disease*. London: Macmillan Press, 1990.

45. Consumer Association. 1990.

46. Cushing A. Editorial: Communication skills. *Med Educ* 1996; **30**: 316–18.

47. Sanson-Fisher R, Redman S, Walsh R *et al.* Training

medical practitioners in information transfer skills: the new challenge. *Med Educ* 1991; **25**: 322–33.

48. Maguire P, Fairbairn S, Fletcher C. Consultation skills of young doctors. 2.Most young doctors are bad at giving information. *BMJ* 1986; **292**: 1576–9.

49. Fallowfield L, Lipkin M, Hall A. Teaching senior oncologists communication skills: results from Phase 1 of a comprehensive longitudinal program in the United Kingdom. *J Clin Oncol* 1998; **16**: 1961–8.

50. General Medical Council. *Tomorrow's doctors*. London: GMC, 1993.

51. Barnard D. Communication skills and moral principles in health care: aspects of their relationship and implications for professional education. *Patient Educ Counsel* 1986; **8**: 349–58.

52. Arnold R, Forrow L, Barker L. Medical ethics and doctor–patient communication. In: Lipkin M, Putnam S, Lazare A, eds. *The medical interview*. New York: Springer, 1994.

30 · Informed consent and medical education

Chris Ward

HISTORICAL BACKGROUND

In the early 1900s medical students were prepared for life as a doctor through didactic teaching based on rigid scientific methodology and a submissive clinical apprenticeship to hospital staff, who worked occasionally and voluntarily in so-called "teaching" hospitals. Overwhelming paternalism ruled in relation to both patient and student. In 1925 Abraham Flexner described the medical curricula in America and Europe[1] where, in the index of this classical text, there is no mention of any patient behavioural themes or topics, such as sociology, psychology, communication skills, or the doctor/patient relationship. Medical ethics was nowhere to be seen or taught. Flexner was unable to resist comment:

> Scientific medicine is today sadly deficient in cultural and philosophic background … there is a vast difference between local chauvinism, holding to things as they are, and an enlightened spirit, seeking stimulus and suggestions, wherever they are to be found. It is upon the latter that progress largely depends. Thus, gradually, men become aware of the extent to which chance has determined development, and of the extent to which intelligent effort may reconstruct educational institutions.

Sadly Flexner's analysis and recommendations went unheeded but, astonishingly, so did the powerful emphasis made on patients' rights that emerged through the Nuremberg Code and Declaration of Helsinki. It beggars belief that in the background of the unspeakable part that doctors played in the pseudoscience of racial hygienics and in the chilling exploitation of so-called inferior human beings in "research", the recognition of patients' rights in the clinical and educational context in the United Kingdom should be so underplayed. The General Medical Council responsible for standards in undergraduate education also failed to address

this subject in recommendations made to the Government and expressed in the Medical Acts of 1958 and 1967.

This was all too obvious to the author as a clinical student in the early 1960s, when ward rounds were conducted in an entourage of students, houseman and registrars, led by a consultant with no training in teaching or communication skills. A discussion of a "case" would take place around the bed with scant respect for privacy, confidentiality, or the patient's own views. After this parade of consultant power it was the job of the houseman and the ward sister to later carry out a secondary ward round in an effort to console patients, and to try to explain and clarify the intended investigations and treatment. The patient-centred approach was never discussed or encouraged, as dramatically witnessed in the undergraduate teaching in the VD Clinic (now called the genitourinary clinic), where clinic "skills" were learned from the examination of the affected parts only, while the top half of the patients was concealed by a blanket. The impression was given to us, as clinical apprentices, that their fate was somehow divine retribution for human frailty. Heaven knows what the patient thought of the whole humiliating process, and no student was given the chance to find out.

A more enlightened approach to medical education came from the Education Committee of the General Medical Council in 1980[2] based on the Medical Act of 1978, where a plea was made to "reduce congestion and overcrowding in the medical curriculum by instructing less and educating more." Among many teaching objectives it was stated that the student should acquire a knowledge and understanding of the ethical standards and legal responsibilities of the medical profession, although the expected ingredients of these standards and responsibilities were not identified. The response in medical schools was poor and patchy and, in the battle for curricular time, the traditional and bullish academic departments dominated and were not prepared to give way to "minor" topics such as medical ethics. The Pond Report of 1987[3] on the teaching of medical ethics had limited impact among deans of medical schools, so that the subject remained largely marginalised and surfaced for the attention of medical students only through the enterprise and energy of a few enthusiasts.

It needed the more prescriptive approach of *Tomorrow's doctors*,[4] which strongly insisted that today's medical students should all be initiated into an integrated course, whereby the notion of education rather than instruction is once again emphasised. In drafting this document, the Education Committee of the General Medical Council have taken into account the high calibre of successful entrants to medical school, by encouraging further enterprise and curiosity through greater emphasis on small-group teaching and the facilitation of self-directed learning. The goal is to produce medical graduates with a broadly based education to equip them to take the necessary steps towards differentiation in the appropriate career of their choice. Among the general educational aims to which the GMC have given priority are attitudes of mind and behaviour that befit a reflective and sensitive doctor. These include understanding the importance of respect for patients in ways that encompass, without prejudice, their diversity of cultural background. Of equal importance is the recognition by students of patients' rights in all aspects, particularly those pertaining to confidentiality and informed consent. A further recommendation is the development of the ability to analyse ethical problems including recognition that good medical practice depends on a partnership between the doctor and the patient based on mutual understanding and trust. The doctor may give advice and recommend treatment, but the patient must decide whether or not to accept it. Finally, under curriculum themes comes "Finding out: research and experiment" with emphasis on an understanding of the scientific method and the pivotal role of the fully informed patient within it.

Thus within the core curriculum of medical education there should be an unequivocal focus on the fundamental right of patients to determine their own therapeutic destiny and how this is achieved, through a relationship of trust based on truthful dialogue that does not withhold or distort any relevant facts. The practical expression of this special rela-

tionship is informed consent, which is a process that cannot be morally or legally denied to any patient of "sound mind".[5] The essence of this relationship is best expressed in the following statement:

> The primary goal of healthcare in general is to maximise each patient's well-being. However, merely acting in a patient's best interests without recognising the views of the individual as the pivotal decision-maker, would fail to respect each person's interest and self-determination .... When the conflicts that arise between a competent patient's self-determination and his or her apparent well-being remain unresolved after adequate deliberation, a competent patient's self-determination is or usually should be given greater weight than other people's views on that individual's well-being.
>
> Respect for the self-determination of competent patients is of special importance. The patient should have the final authority to decide.[6]

However, having established the notion of informed consent as such an essential ingredient of the core curriculum, how and when should the concept be introduced? How should it be taught? Who should teach it? How should the students' knowledge and attitudes in relation to consent be assessed? How should the teachers be taught and what mechanisms are there for insuring that the teaching of both theory and practice of informed consent is of a high standard?

EARLY AWARENESS OF INFORMED CONSENT

As one of the many criteria necessary to convince prospective medical students as well as student selection committees that they wish to be admitted to medical school, some sort of experience of healthcare is searched for either through past observation or "hands-on" activities. At one time such experience was easy to acquire simply through a 'phone call to a local hospital or GP surgery. However, as patients, managers, and doctors themselves have become increasingly aware of the potential harm in breaching confidentiality, particularly in a community where a school sixth-former wanting work experience lived, the conditions for gaining such experience are now more constrained. Thus patients should give permission for fledging medical students to be present. At the age of 17 or so, a sixth former (11th-year student) should become acutely aware of the theme of consent by understanding that it would be unreasonable for their own mother, say, to be seen in a GP surgery, outpatient clinic, or in an unconscious state in the operating room, by one of their school friends, unless she had been prepared for the event and given permission to be present. This notion is extrapolated to medical practice, where they should witness a doctor giving information about a possible investigation or treatment, to a level that they would expect if that patient were a close relative or friend.

Some hospitals or practices prefer not to be involved in offering work experience and close their doors to sixth-formers. This blocks essential experience for future medical students as an insight into practical clinical medicine and an understanding of confidentiality and informed consent. But, recognising that work observation is a helpful and practical way for students to get information about a medical career, whilst also being sensitive to the ethical issues, the British Medical Association has published a helpful booklet: *Guidelines for work observation*[7] outlines basic safeguards for both sixth-formers and medical staff in respecting the confidentiality, privacy, and autonomy of patients. The guidelines emphasise both the importance of the doctors explaining the concept of confidentiality to young observers, and also the fact that they can only attend patients who have given their permission. It also strongly recommends that work observation should take place outside the observer's immediate locality.

Should a prospective student be called for interview at the medical school, it is standard practice to include questions relating to medical ethics when the interviewer turns to the personal statement in the UCAS form. For example, questions about work experience naturally offers a chance to evaluate the sensitivity of the students about the issues of confidentiality or informed consent. It is possible that they may already have been prepared for this moment by interview rehearsals at school or by day release or immersion residential course. For example, the Medlink course at Nottingham University consists of lectures and seminars on all aspects of "being a doctor", and includes presentations on medical law in relation to negligence and the common areas within medical ethics (informed consent is acknowledged to be a common strand). By these means both the knowledge base and discursive skills may be so enriched that, by the time any well-prepared student is accepted for a place in medical school, he or she should already have a reasonable introduction to the principles of consent.

INTRODUCTORY YEARS AT MEDICAL SCHOOL

Within the information pack posted to the homes of students prior to registration and in the course of the welcome addresses, freshers' week, and the foundation course, there will be a range of introductions and guides both written and oral. These include how to behave with patients who, within the first term of the now integrated curricula, will be an integral part of experience and learning. The common theme is the importance of respecting the sensitivity and vulnerability of patients who have agreed to physical and emotional exposure for the benefit of the students. It is made clear to those students that they must now respond in kind by keeping the event in confidence and by personally asking the permission of the patient to proceed with the consultation. If patients change their minds and decide not to participate in early contact teaching, they know that they must accede to this request. These actions and related attitudes are comparable to the practical courtesies that should be intrinsic to the attitude of any healthcare worker to a patient in routine activities, but how should medical ethics and law be taught to medical students?

One extremely positive response to the educational recommendations of the General Medical Council in respect of ethics and law has been a series of meetings convened by teachers of the subjects in order to negotiate a consensus on a model for such teaching within the core curriculum.[8] The core topics in the box relating to consent are extracted from that consensus statement.

Informed consent and refusal of treatment

- Significance of autonomy: respect for persons and bodily integrity
- Competence to consent: conceptual, ethical and legal aspects
- Further conditions for ethically acceptable consent: adequate information and comprehension, non-coercion
- Treatment without consent and proxy consent: when and why morally and legally justifiable
- Assault, battery, negligence and legal standards for disclosure of information
- Problems of communicating information about diagnosis, treatment and risks: the importance of empathy

Specific consent issues are raised under a variety of the subsequent list of core topics

- The clinical relationship – truthfulness, trust and good communications
- Confidentiality and good clinical practice
- Medical research
- Human reproduction
- New genetics
- Children
- Mental disorders and disabilities
- Life, death, dying and killing
- Vulnerabilities created by the duties of doctors and medical students
- Resource allocation
- Rights

However the teachers, who submitted the consensus statement, recognised that identifying the content of the core was not enough and that suggestions should also be made for the organisation of teaching of ethics and law. So it was recommended that the teaching should be overseen and coordinated by at least one full-time senior academic in ethics and law, and that the subject should be introduced systematically and at an early stage of the course before being fully integrated within the curriculum. As for any other core subject, both the topics and those teaching the topics should be formally assessed. To expedite this goal, courses and workshops should be provided for the teachers, while sufficient time and human and financial resources should be set aside for the teaching. Within the clinical setting, where there are rich opportunities for debating ethics, especially consent issues, students should be encouraged to present moral problems that they have encountered as a feature of their overall clinical analyses of patients. In this regard case presentations are particularly valuable.

It was emphasised that the standards embodied within the core curriculum in ethics and law applied to medicine should be regarded as minimal requirements towards helping students to become doctors who engage in good professional practice.

TEACHING AND LEARNING OPPORTUNITIES

Small group learning, promoted in the new curriculum, is an ideal format within which to air and debate relevant topics. Problem-based learning sessions, in particular, have been described as the most important development since the move of professional training into educational institutions,[9] and are proving to be popular with students and tutors.[10] They can be designed so as to place informed consent within case scenarios in such a way as to become either a main or secondary study objective. Clinicians teaching in the small group environment or early patient contact sessions have comparable opportunities. Important as small group teaching is, however, students also need a more formal and structured style of teaching to give them the necessary conceptual and practical skills as regards the moral theory, legal principles, and clinical relevance of informed consent. Here the lecture format complemented with all appropriate teaching aids and backed up with focused seminar groups is also worth incorporating into the curriculum, especially around the time that students are learning basic clinical skills with patients. By these means students should be well equipped to continue into the curriculum where clinical experience is a more dominant component. By including such academic ingredients within the second and third year teaching, some students would hopefully become sufficiently intrigued and provoked to study the subject in greater depth either within the study module of a BSc or as a BSc in healthcare ethics and law, both of which are now in existence or being developed within UK medical schools. So, in the later years of the course, when clinical experience and patient involvement form a major part of undergraduate education, both students and their clinical teachers should be ideally placed to explore the more pragmatic and practical implications of consent.

In every year of their training, medical students are not only learning from patients but also from each other, for example by measuring the effect of pharmacological agents in teaching laboratories, or by playing the role of a patient, both for learning clinical skills or for examination purposes within the Objective Structured Clinical Examination (OSCE). In this role they are likely to become more aware of their own vulnerabilities and need for privacy and confidentiality of information, and transpose these experiences to the circumstances of the patient. Should they, as students, be approached to participate in medical experiments, their minds are compelled to focus more precisely on consent themes through apprehension of the unknown. In this area they will be assisted through the guidelines of the National Union of Students for Participation in Medical Experiments, where it is stated that students must be provided with full information about any study, both in oral and written form, and that their consent should always be obtained in writing and independently witnessed, while a copy should be retained for the student's own reference. The paragraph that captures the spirit of consent in terms of self-determination within the context of research, reads: "At any time, students should be able to free themselves from a previously agreed series of experiments. This is a basic human right and must be stated clearly on the volunteer information sheet and consent form."[11]

CONSENT AND THE STUDENT/PATIENT RELATIONSHIP

The General Medical Council pamphlet *Seeking patient consent: the ethical considerations* is provided within the student introductory pack. Although it is a useful teaching aid and outlines good professional practice, it contains only one sentence concerning students in training whereby doctors should inform the patients of "the extent to which students may be involved in an investigation or treatment".[12] The British Medical Association is more expansive and does not assume that a patient, by seeking treatment in a teaching hospital, is implicitly consenting to the various measures commonly associated with teaching. Rather, it is regarded as important to inform patients about such measures, to allow them to have a genuine option in the matter, and when they agree to participate to record their explicit consent.[13] The same process of obtaining consent applies to all other sources of teaching, such as patient records, photographs, video films, or clinical teaching via linked TV cable systems. In hospitals where students are taught it should be standard practice to describe the teaching function of the institution in the leaflets relating to outpatient and inpatient attendance, as well as within the consent form. This extract from one used at the Charing Cross Hospital in London is an example:

> Student doctors and nurses cannot learn all they need to know from textbooks or lectures. Teaching students is an important part of the work in this hospital and we need your assistance with this. During the period of treatment you may well be asked to have students present. We would be grateful if you would co-operate with us but you have the right to refuse. A refusal will not affect your standard of care.

However, a patient going through the hospital admission process is unlikely to take on board all written information and there is no substitute for one-to-one discussion and explanation. In that exchange the purpose of the presence of students and the identity of students must be clarified and not obscured through reference to "young doctors" or "assistants". In a survey by questionnaire within teaching hospitals, 41% of patients had on one or more occasions participated in some undergraduate clinical teaching without being informed; 80% felt aggrieved if they were not informed although, on average, 88% were in principle positive to participating of which a majority group of elderly patients were prepared to be involved without preparation.[14] Within the community setting where clinical teaching is rapidly expanding, 75% of surveyed patients preferred to know in advance whether students would be present when they attended their general practitioner; 37% did not wish the student to see all their medical notes and 18% were worried that the student might discuss their case outside the surgery.[15]

It is a considerable privilege for a medical student to be able to benefit from the generosity of patients admitted to hospital or attending the GP surgery, and it follows that as a moral obligation, apart from a basic courtesy, students should clearly explain that their association is primarily for educational purposes and to obtain explicit verbal consent to take histories or undertake a physical examination. Potentially embarrassing examinations should only be performed with the permission of the clinical teacher and in the presence of a chaperone, unless the patient explicitly agrees otherwise. In the event of student involvement with the unconscious anaesthetised patient, such as intubation, pelvic examination or suturing, that activity must be specifically agreed by the patient through written consent. This procedure is endorsed for medical students in relation to gynaecology and obstetrics, where it is insisted that written consent for a pelvic examination under general anaesthetic should be given for a named rather than a generic medical student. "Such practice is perceived to have other educational advantages in that by the students personally obtaining consent they come to recognise not just the intrinsic importance of the act but inculcate a life-long respect for the autonomy of patients."[16]

By following such practice there are other long-term benefits in terms of the fiduciary relationship as understood by patients who are more likely to trust the "system", while students come to acknowledge and enjoy the rapport of friendship and trust that is so essential in promoting the well-being of any patient.

CONSENT AND THE CLINICAL TEACHER/STUDENT RELATIONSHIP

Students educated by the methods described so far are likely to have a better understanding and greater skills in relation to the theory and practice of informed consent compared to those who qualified under the previous system of undergraduate or postgraduate teaching and who now teach them. This is an ideal situation in which to develop a partnership in learning between the student and teacher, which increasingly permeates the new integrated curriculum. The teacher has the experience, expertise, and clinical knowledge of the circumstances in which consent is demanded, but not necessarily the moral and legal understanding of the contemporary boundaries of good professional practice.

However, the standards of teaching will vary from effective and sensitive implementation of respect for self-determination through the consent process to, extremely rarely, an atavistic degree of paternalism. In such an important stage of preparation for more independent clinical practice, one could argue that the education departments of medical schools could be creatively interventionist in identifying and promoting the teaching activities of those clinicians who take a particular interest in all aspects of student flourishing, while encouraging constructive change by feedback and education of those whose teaching falls below the expected standard. In other words, those who teach well and conscientiously should continue to teach and be correspondingly rewarded; those who are bad teachers and who refuse to accept offers to make them better ones, or remain bad teachers even after accepting the offer, should, in the interests of students, not teach and should have any funds allocated for teaching withdrawn. Certain medical schools have now expressed their firm intention to carry forward these processes.

However desirable the partnership in learning might be, the awe in which some students still hold teaching clinicians does not always lead to a balanced relationship. It is the author's personal experience in the course of using the unconsented pelvic examination under general anaesthetic in case-based

teaching that all students recognise the moral and legal issues in terms of assault and battery and breach of autonomy. However, if ordered by the consultant to carry out the unconsented examination (as is extremely unlikely), about 20% would not challenge that decision, for fear of jeopardising their future, and be prepared to carry it out. Such an example emphasises the importance of additional student support within the clinical teaching environment, so that personal tutors and directors of clinical studies are empowered to act as mentors and advocates to the students in such a way as to implement the teaching process, and to reassure students that any information that they would wish to share, such as perceived abuse of patients, would be treated and acted on in strict confidence.

INFORMED CONSENT: ASSESSMENT OF THEORY AND PRACTICE

"The balanced, sustained, academically rigorous and clinically relevant presentation on both ethics and law in medicine," as proposed in the Consensus Statement,[8] can only become a reality if it is formally assessed and examined to the same standard of all other subjects within the curriculum. There are opportunities for formative and summative assessment of the theory and practice of informed consent at each stage of the course. These include small group teaching, MCQs, OSCEs, traditional or modified essay questions, role-playing, presentations and posters, BSc modules, and clinical attachments. By these means one is able to assess the relevant knowledge and reasoning skills, but this is not enough; in order to achieve a consistently and uniformly high standard of relevant teaching, the teachers must be taught how to teach and the qualitative assessment process must be in place. Other means of self-assessment for long-term outcomes are also required, such as the effect teaching and learning has on the eventual clinical behaviour of medical graduates, and an assurance that the investment of scarce educational resources will result in a satisfactory and measurable dividend.[17]

By knitting together the academic, educational, and quality assessment strands that are recommended by the GMC to form the fabric of the undergraduate curriculum, the goal can be achieved of "maintaining attitudes and conduct appropriate to a high level of professional practice."[18] Educational committees and quality assurance agencies might be satisfied; but of still greater relevance is the proper implementation of the consent process as a natural and normal activity within clinical practice and clinical research, so that the public receive maximum benefit both directly and indirectly through today's students becoming not only the empathetic doctors and clinical investigators of tomorrow but the effective teachers of tomorrow's students.

CONCLUSION

It is now seven years since the recommendations of the most radical restructuring of undergraduate medical education in the last 70 years. Medical ethics and medical law have received strong backing as important and continuous educational themes, within which the recognition and respect for the rights of patients in determining their therapeutic destiny dominates. All aspects of healthcare incorporate the notion of autonomy and the inextricably linked practice of informed consent, whether they involve beginning or end-of-life issues, or in-between in the form of teaching, training, research and innovation, and day-to-day practice at the clinical coalface, or Government health policy as the greatest influence on all these functions.

However, it is only two years since the publication of the Consensus Statement by teachers of medical ethics in the UK medical schools as to the list of core topics. Furthermore, the impact of the new integrated curriculum on the quality of medical graduates is yet to be realised. This raises questions as to how and when should such an appraisal be made. Also, while it is quite reasonable to assume that a greater emphasis in teaching on medical ethics and law in general, and on the theory and practice of informed consent in particular, will help to generate higher and more uniform standards of professional care, one will need the evidence to prove the case. There is much, much more work to be done.

REFERENCES

1. Flexner A. *Medical education: a comparative study.* New York: MacMillan, 1925.

2. General Medical Council. *Recommendations on basic medical education.* London: GMC Education Committee, February 1980.

3. Pond D. *Report of a working party in the teaching of medical ethics.* London: IMF Publications, 1987.

4. General Medical Council. *Tomorrow's doctors: recommendations on undergraduate medical education.* London: GMC, 1993.

5. *Schloendorf* v. *Society of New York Hospital* (1914) 105 NE 92.

6. Presidents Commission for the Study of Ethical Problems and Biomedical Behavioural Research (1983). *Deciding to forego treatment.* Washington DC: US Government Printing Office, 1990; **44**: 26–7.

7. British Medical Association Career Progress of Doctors Committee. *Guidelines for work observation.* London: BMA, 1999.

8. Consensus statement by teachers of medical ethics and law in UK Medical Schools: Teaching medical ethics and law in the undergraduate curriculum. *J Med Eth* 1998; **24**: 188–92.

9. David MH, Harden RM. Problem based learning: a practical guide. *Med Teacher* 1999; **21**: 131–40.

10. Maudsley G. Roles and responsibilities of the problem based learning tutor in the undergraduate medical curriculum. *BMJ* 1998; **318**: 657–61.

11. Foster C. *Guidelines for student participation in medical experiments.* Manual for Research Ethics Committees. London: Kings College, 1994.

12. General Medical Council. *Seeking patients consent: the ethical considerations.* London: GMC, 1999.

13. British Medical Association. *Medical ethics today: its practice and philosophy.* London: BMJ Publishing Group, 1993; p. 19.

14. Lynoë N, Sanderlund M, Westberg K, Duckeh M. Informed consent in clinical training – patient experiences and motives for participating. *Med Educ* 1998; **32**: 65–71.

15. O'Flynn N, Spencer J, Jones R. Consent and confidentiality in teaching in general practice: survey of patients' views on presence of students. *BMJ*, 1997; **315**: 1142.

16. The Royal College of Obstetricians and Gynaecologists. *Intimate examination: report of a working party.* London: RCOG Press, 1997.

17. Mitchell K, Myser C, Kerridge I. Assessing the clinical ethical competence of undergraduate medical students. *J Med Eth*, 1993; **19**: 230–6.

18. Hope T. Ethics and law for medical students: *J Med Eth*, 1998; **24**: 147–53.

Part 5

Conclusion

31 · The moral importance of informed consent in medical research: concluding reflections

Len Doyal

My original *BMJ* paper defended the right of competent adults to consent to participate in all medical research involving clinical interventions. I argued that their choice should be informed by accurate information about aims, methods and potential risks. There is no need to repeat the arguments which I marshalled to justify this conclusion. Suffice it to say, they were based on the close links between respect for individual autonomy and respect for human dignity. Most of the new contributions to this volume appear to support this position or at least something like it.

Much as I support the importance of informed consent in medical research, however, my *BMJ* paper did not argue for a total ban on medical research without consent. It should be allowed in some cases where the subject is incompetent (e.g. children with the consent of parents, trauma cases with an appropriate risk–benefit ratio). Some research involving competent adults should be exempted from the requirement to obtain informed consent (e.g. epidemiological research where there is no intention to make further contact with participants). While morally complex, the reasons for such exemptions concern the potential importance of the research to the public good and its irrelevance to the immediate objective interests of unknowing participants.

Thus I accepted in my paper that for some forms of medical research, violations of individual autonomy can be morally justified. Yet the exceptions which I endorsed would not apply to the vast majority of medical research involving competent adults. Again, there appears to be a broad consensus in this book that these sorts of exceptions are acceptable, though do note arguments in the contrary in the chapter by Bennett.

More specifically, Part 1 of the book examines the harmful and unreasonable things that have been done to individuals in the name of medical progress and the public interest. If we have learned anything from this unfortunate history it is that medical researchers cannot be trusted to regulate the ethical and legal acceptability of their work. This applies just as much to their moral intuitions about what constitutes a reasonable standard of informed consent as it does to other aspects of research ethics – applying an acceptable risk–benefit ratio, for example.

As the chapter by McNeill and Pfeffer makes clear, there is little point in focusing blame for such moral myopia entirely on individual clinical researchers. Enthusiasm and a desire to get the job done are necessary to maintain the personal momentum which most medical research demands. Because of their need to achieve good results, research institutions in both the public and the private sectors may place insufficient emphasis on the rights and safety of research participants. Such unintentional moral blindness can confront potential research participants with unanticipated risks, over and above those associated with ordinary care. The fact that the production of this book has been accompanied by several new scandals about research and informed consent in the UK and elsewhere, underlines the importance of continuing to maintain strict discipline among researchers about this issue.[1-5] This is no matter how benign researchers regard experimental interventions or how difficult or distressing they anticipate that the process of obtaining informed consent will be.

Bringing the reader up to date, Part 3 builds on arguments and issues explored in the papers and correspondence published in the *BMJ* and making up Part 2. It also underlines the degree to which legal regulations and professional guidelines continue to demand a high standard of disclosure of information to potential participants in medical research. Most chapters do not question this imperative, although it is true that several do outline both theoretical (McLean, Chadwick, Fennell) and practical (Johnson, Farsides/Draper, Hurwitz) reasons why it may be difficult to achieve. Indeed, the chapters on current international regulation (Foster, Meslin, Nicholson) demonstrate the wide recognition of the moral importance of informed consent in medical research, while also noting agreement about the circumstances where this requirement might be waived. For the most part, these repeat the proposals in my *BMJ* paper.

There are some fascinating contributions to the book which still very much engage with specific arguments in my paper and on which I have not had an opportunity to comment. Equally, some other chapters raise new and important questions which also warrant further analysis. All of these are excellent in their own right. However, to take the debate further, I will use the opportunity of this conclusion to respond to some of the interesting points that they raise. I am aware that this may appear to give me, at least for the moment, the last word on the matter. In one sense, this is inevitable. However, it is not my intent. On the one hand, there is no doubt that the debate about informed consent in medical research will – and should – continue and I do not regard any of my comments on these chapters as without the potential for counterargument by the authors involved. I simply wish to try to make the issues that require further debate as clear as possible. On the other hand, the *BMJ* is very keen for the debate to continue where it started – on its pages – and will welcome related contributions for potential publication.

FURTHER REFLECTIONS ON PAPERS PUBLISHED IN THE *BMJ*

The first group of papers for which further comment seems appropriate were printed in the same issue as the *BMJ* as my "response to recent [earlier] correspondence". Three are of particular interest:

- Lindley (pp. 133–6) argues that were my emphasis on informed consent to be adopted universally then some medical research important to the public interest would become impossible. This is because it entails more than minimum risk and requires the participation of incompetent patients.

- David and Solomon Benatar (pp. 137–8) maintain that I am in breach of the very moral standards I defend in my paper. This is because of the exceptions to the rule of consent which I there outline.
- Warnock (pp. 129–30) rejects my argument that with some exceptions, journals should only publish the results of research where informed consent was obtained.

I will assess each of these responses in turn.

Richard Lindley's View

Here, a powerful defence is mounted for the importance of some clinical research entailing substantial risks for incompetent patients. Lindley convincingly shows that there are some circumstances where participation in such research must be in the interests of patients who cannot give their informed consent. He takes me to task for suggesting otherwise. Contrary to Lindley's suggestion, however, my paper argues that such research can be acceptable. I argue that when it is, the risks should be deemed minimal when compared to those associated with the standard available treatment or when there is none, with no treatment. Yet it follows that if the risks of using the best available treatment are high – however one wishes to define the word "high" – then those of a promising new treatment may be considered minimal if they are believed on reasonable evidence to be no higher. I go on in my paper to make it clear that waivers of informed consent in such circumstances must be interpreted in practice by research ethics committees which may exercise some latitude in their decisions.

Note that I do not, as Lindley suggests, offer any advice in my paper about how such committees should interpret the relative importance of a small chance of a patient's *death* through the administration of a new treatment when compared with a larger chance of *permanent and severe mental disability without* this treatment. On the one hand, Lindley is quite right to raise this issue. It is neglected in the literature on the acceptability of risks in medical research and there should be further debate about it, especially in the face of disability so severe as potentially to make life no longer worth living. But I suspect that a significant proportion of members of a research ethics committee would be most concerned about Lindley's favourable comparison of apparent prospect of improvement of disability by approximately 100 plus per 1000 survivors with a definite risk of approximately 9 plus extra deaths per 1000 – at least without much more information than he provides about the level of potential disability for those who survive (p. 134). Morally, I would argue that research ethics committees should always err on the side of caution when the lives of incompetent patients are at stake and where the potential benefits of risking life are not abundantly clear. To argue as much is not to advocate a strait-jacket on the types of research involving incompetent patients that Lindley and I both wish to promote. It is to suggest that we need to be very careful about our evaluation of risk–benefit ratios for those who cannot do so for themselves.

Finally, I am happy to endorse Lindley's suggestion for more public education about why risky research with incompetent adults may be in their best interests.

Significantly, the FDA have made such local education a prerequisite for granting waivers of informed consent in such research. If Lindley and others with the same beliefs are serious however, then they should also endorse such education as a precondition of relevant research in the UK, very much along the lines outlined by Pfeffer in her chapter on consumer participation. What they should not suggest – as Lindley appears to – is that it might be appropriate to allow the public to determine the acceptability of research without consent. This should remain the province of an independent committee with the specialist expertise required for an accurate evaluation of risk–benefit ratios and their moral consequences.

David and Solomon Benatar's View

With both force and clarity, the Benatars explicitly endorse my argument that informed consent should always be obtained from competent adult participants in any research involving an experimental intervention. They also agree with some of the exceptions which I outline to the duty to obtain such consent (e.g. anonymised testing of blood where the link has been irrevocably broken with the identity of the source) and provide other interesting arguments about how this can be morally justified. However, the Benatars go on to maintain that I have not maintained sufficient consistency with my own moral arguments because I accept the moral appropriateness of some uses of medical records without informed consent.

They reason that one of the studies which I argue should not have taken place because of lack of informed consent – that on HIV and admission to surgical care in Natal – actually conforms to my criteria for allowing some epidemiological studies to proceed without consent. Readers should check these criteria in my paper (pp. 89–90). The Benatars rightly point out that the study in question involved taking blood without consent for the purposes of HIV testing and the patients involved were later told that this had been done. They correctly maintain that the results of these tests were (a) not forced upon patients without consent, (b) were essential for the purposes of the research and (c) were anonymised as regards public scrutiny (i.e. some of my criteria). Most importantly, they refer to another criterion – "that it is not anticipated that contact will be made with the patients as the result of research findings" and argue "that merely informing patients that they had been subject to an HIV test as part of a study does not constitute contact with patients as a result of research findings" (p. 137). Therefore, they argue the Natal study is permissible on my terms. While their criticism of the Natal study itself is excellent and more detailed than my own, there are two flaws in the Benatars' reasoning about my own work.

First, in my discussion of medical records, I specifically state that they should only be used without consent "if no further consequences follow for such patients" (p. 89). The HIV study obviously violates this principle. Patients were rightly told after the study that they had been tested for HIV and offered post-test counselling. The investigation would have been even more unethical were this not so. Consequently, from the beginning of the study the researchers knew that further consequences *would* follow for the patients – being asked to choose whether or not to be given potentially traumatic information about the results of a test for a life-threatening disease to which they had not agreed. Therefore, the study remains unethical for the reasons which I originally cited.

Second, I am grateful to the Benatars for pointing out what might be seen as an ambiguity in one of my criteria for allowing epidemiological research without consent. I state that consent must always be obtained for such studies "where contact will be made with patients as a result of research findings" (p. 89). The Benatars observe that "merely informing patients that they had been subject to an HIV test as part of a study does not constitute contact with patients as a result of research findings" (p. 137) and argue that this means that the HIV study conforms to my criteria for not obtaining informed consent. The problem with this argument is that I never suggest in my paper that this criterion should be applied to studies involving *clinical* interventions. Again, as regards this type of research, I argue that informed consent should always be obtained unless findings can be strictly anonymised and future contact with patients thus made impossible. The criterion concerning "research findings" to which the Benatars call attention was developed only in relation to epidemiological studies, precisely because they involve no clinical intervention. In such studies, the *only* bases for any future contact with patients are their findings, though readers should consult the fuller arguments by the Benatars in the longer version of their paper published on the *BMJ* website.

Finally, the Benatars powerfully argue that many of the problems with the Natal study would have been obviated by the strict anonymisation of the blood tests made without obtaining informed consent. Once such anonymisation occurs, no further consequences can follow for any patients involved. Indeed, the Benatars point out that I give a similar argument in my paper for the use of human tissue without consent. Yet they remain curiously silent about the difficult implications of their own strong endorsement of the principle of informed consent for epidemiological research. This places them on the horns of a dilemma. If the Benatars want to be consistent in rejecting my exceptions to the principle of informed consent for epidemiological research, they must also rule out all such research which is not strictly anonymised. It is commonly accepted that this would bring a great deal of important epidemiological research to a halt, research that I would allow. The debate of what types of epidemiological research to allow without consent will clearly continue. For further details, readers should again consult the chapter by Hurwitz.

Mary Warnock's View

This contribution addresses the question of how prescriptive we should be in constraining editorial discretion about the publication of the results of research obtained without informed consent. Warnock begins by providing a fine exposition of the Kantian background to the principle of informed consent in research, one consistent with that in my *BMJ* paper. She stresses that since clinical research always has an instrumental aim over and above any good that it might provide for participants then the "evil" of compulsion is removed if "people offer their services voluntarily" (p. 129). Thus she interestingly argues for a principle of "non-exploitation", indicating that this means much the same as the principle of respect for autonomy which I evoked in my paper. She outlines why this principle – her formulation of which will be an important contribution to future debates about informed consent – is so important in medical research, referring to notorious abuses of the past and their potential future occurrence. Finally, she endorses two familiar exceptions to the rule – "the use of anonymous data, collected for a particular study ..." and "... the use ... of discarded or unwanted tissue ..." (also presumably strictly anonymised) (p. 130). So far, so good.

What then occurs is surprising. Warnock concludes by apparently advocating blanket editorial discretion in publishing research findings where consent has not been obtained. This is because "any other policy seems to me to rely on a dogma – that there are no other principles worth considering in the ethics of research except the principle of non-exploitation – and to rely on an exceptionally wide and unrealistic view of what counts as exploitation" (p. 130). So after providing good arguments for respecting the autonomy of adult and competent research participants, she appears to open the door to other competing principles to which any editor might be attracted. We know that there are such competing principles – the public interest, for example. But if it is acceptable to publish for this or other reasons, what are we to make of the force of her own argument that "to make use of people, especially when they are not aware of what is going on, is generally agreed to be wrong"? (p. 129).

Warnock cannot have it both ways. She wants editors "to distinguish things that differ" and suggests that in doing so they will have to rely on moral principles. If these principles are to be consistent with the moral emphasis she herself gives to the importance of obtaining informed consent in much clinical research then this same emphasis will inevitably place constraints on editorial discretion to publish research where consent has not been obtained. Thus she says that: "It seems to me a misuse of words to suggest that not obtaining informed consent in itself constitutes a harm; sometimes it amounts to exploitation, sometimes it does not" (p. 130). Yet the only exceptions to the rule to which she actually refers and presumably condones are ones that I also elaborate in my *BMJ* paper – research anonymised so that results cannot be linked back to patients. Indeed, because I am willing to allow some epidemiological research which is not anonymised without consent, Warnock appears to advocate even more potentially stringent constraints than my own.

Yet the primary debate in Part 2 of this book is about editorial discretion to publish research which extends beyond such constraints. Many contributors argue that such discretion should be exercised even for the publication of some research involving *clinical interventions* on competent adults who have neither been anonymised nor consulted. If Warnock wants to broaden editorial discretion to encompass research of this kind too then she should come clean and say so, along with providing appropriate moral justifications. To do otherwise is to embrace an unconstrained form of discredited moral intuitionism. Since I cannot believe that this is Warnock's intent, I conclude that in reality her position about editorial discretion is substantially the same as my own – that it should be confined to specific exceptions to the general rule of informed consent.

COMMENTS ON SOME COMMISSIONED CHAPTERS

Most of the commissioned chapters in this book do explicitly endorse my emphasis on the moral and legal importance of informed consent in medical research. However, three fascinating and innovative chapters in Part 4 raise possible exceptions.

- Gillon argues that "full" informed consent is impossible in most medical research. Further, he insists that what he calls "extensive informed consent" can itself be immoral through violating the right of some participants not to receive unwanted information about their experimental care.
- Chalmers and Lindley attack "ethicists" who have implicitly reinforced a "double standard" of informed consent in clinical care through emphasising the unknown risks of participating in experimental care while remaining silent about the often greater risks of non-experimental care.
- Harris and Woods ultimately endorse the importance of obtaining informed consent for participation in medical research but place even more emphasis on the competing moral importance of the duty of patients to participate in the public good.

Let us now examine each of these contributions in turn.

Raanan Gillon's View

In my *BMJ* paper, I argue that researchers have a duty to obtain "fully informed consent" from all competent adult patients who are subject to any form of clinical intervention. In a chapter full of profound clinical insight and experience, Gillon strongly rejects this view for two reasons. First, he rightly argues that if by "full information" one means – "all of the information which might be given with no principle of selectivity applied" – then this becomes impossible. On the one hand, one can always find yet more information to give to potential research participants. On the other hand, providing too much information can be self-defeating because no one would be able to understand it all. Much better, Gillon argues, to use the phrase "extensively informed consent" to cover the sorts of cases where he agrees that what I call fully informed consent should be obtained (e.g. all cases of non-therapeutic research).

To be sure, a limit does have to be put on the amount of information that researchers can practically give participants in research and Gillon powerfully argues why. They will only have so much time available for understanding, so much intellectual capacity to understand, so much energy to try to understand – and so on. But who would not agree? I know of no contributor to the extensive literature on informed consent in medical research who does not accept such limitations, many of whom also use the phrase "fully informed consent". We do so to indicate that agreement to participate in such research has been obtained through the disclosure of appropriate information in *each* of the different *categories* of information that are required by the Helsinki Declaration. These are the: "aims, methods, anticipated benefits and potential hazards of the study and the discomfort it may entail" (p. 5). Patients should also be given information about alternative standard and experimental treatments, if any. Understood in this way, there is nothing impractical or incoherent about the principle of fully informed consent. It refers to the importance of information being provided in all of these categories, while recognising that clinical researchers must have some discretion in how much they provide in each.

Gillon goes on to develop his second argument

against my view that researchers should always obtain fully informed consent – now understood by him to mean "extensively informed consent" – for participation by competent adults in any research involving clinical intervention. In a deeply textured and subtle argument to which I cannot do justice here, he refers to the conduct of two types of research to make his case. On the one hand, some research compares two or more standard treatments for the first time. On the other hand, research might compare a standard treatment with a promising new treatment where the relative ineffectiveness of the former leads researchers to believe that participation in a trial of the latter will be in the patient's best interest. To the degree that the intentions of clinicians involved in both types of research embody what Gillon calls the "Hippocratic commitment", he suggests that the interests of patients will be protected (p. 258). In the presence of such commitment, therefore, Gillon reasons that the "extensive" informed consent from patients that he concedes it is necessary to obtain for non-therapeutic trials should not be a requirement for trials from which the patient might clinically benefit. He argues that what he calls "adequate" informed consent will do instead, even if it means not providing patients with appropriate information in each of the Helsinki categories.

Thus, in therapeutic research clinical researchers should have the discretion to evaluate the desire of patients for information about the research in which they are being asked to participate. Like Jeffrey S Tobias, Gillon argues that clinical researchers should not force unwanted and potentially distressing information on patients already made vulnerable by the impact of their illnesses. In circumstances where patients are being experimentally treated for illness, they should be able to fall back on their trust of the medical profession, without fear that they will be told something that they would rather not hear or read.

Gillon's argument is based on the premise that patients have just as much right to refuse information about their participation in therapeutic research, as they do to demand it. The difficulty with this argument is that patients may have objective interests in information about the process and outcome of such research. It would presumably not be acceptable for them to waive their rights to it on the basis of arbitrary whim fuelled by ignorance. For example, patients may have personal plans of which researchers know nothing. These plans may be inconsistent with the schedule of activities demanded by participation in the research or may be impeded or made impossible by some of its potential side effects. Thus for the refusal of information by a patient to be adequately informed, some basic information must be provided about the research to which they are agreeing.

Gillon accepts this point when he states that irrespective of patients' wishes, some information should be disclosed in the case of the comparison of two standard treatments. This includes "likely side effects plus an indication that the treatment could itself could be risky", along with further information about the fact that the clinical researcher does not know which is the best treatment and that the patient will be randomised to try to find out (p. 261). Where he apparently wants to draw the line as regards disclosure is information about the distressing details of side effects and information about poor prognosis altogether. This is puzzling. Patients may be just as fearful of potentially distressing news which Gillon agrees that they must be given before participating in research (e.g. likely side effects and the fact that doctor does not know which treatment is best) as they may be worried about other sorts of information which he argues that researchers should have the discretion not to disclose.

The fact is that despite their commitment to Hippocratic values, clinical researchers cannot be sure that keeping patients in ignorance will serve their objective interests. These interests may not necessarily be understood by patients to be linked to their participation in a clinical trial. Patients – especially those with cancer (Gillon's paradigm case) – may be confused about their illness because they have been only minimally informed in other therapeutic contexts where doctors thought that this was their preference. To allow them to participate in a clinical trial without full informed consent – as per the categories of Helsinki – might well lead them to disappointment and disillusionment. For example, the new treatment may fail without patients being warned that this is a possibility or it may lead to side effects which conflict with what they perceive as an acceptable quality of life or with important life plans which they had not anticipated would be hampered. At this point, such patients will hardly thank the clinical researcher who reminds them that it was they who said that they did not want to know about the detail of such possibilities. Patients may rightly believe that by honouring their poorly informed preferences for incomplete information the clinical researcher responsible for their care acted against their objective interest and in breach of their Hippocratic commitment.

At the end of the day, and in a spirit of partnership in care, patients need to be helped to protect their own interests. In my view, Gillon places too much faith in clinical researchers to do this job for them. As he well knows, doctors make mistakes and the history of clinical research is riddled with well-meaning intentions which were not in the interests of the patients involved. The fact that clinical researchers may strongly believe that participation in their trials is their patient's best option provides no guarantee that this is so. Patients need to understand this, even if it is distressing. The issue which demands yet further discussion and debate is whether or not it is morally better to distress patients in the short term than to undermine what might be their objective interests in the long term. Future debate should move in this direction and I have no doubt that my good friend Raanan Gillon will be a significant contributor to it.

Iain Chalmers and Richard Lindleys' View

This chapter highlights another problem with Gillon's argument. With great panache, Chalmers and Lindley argue that too much of the discussion about the ethics of medical research has overly emphasised its risks at the expense of playing down the risks of standard therapy. They demonstrate that such therapy is often without a rigorous scientific base and that it may well pose greater risks. Further, they marshal convincing evidence to show that participation in trials may reduce risks and provides more benefit than relying on standard, unassessed therapies. Consequently, a more balanced ethical analysis of informed consent in medical research would make these points. I completely concur with this view and hope that it will have the significant impact on future debates that it deserves to. I will take the authors' arguments more into account in my own writing on the subject in the future.

However, with Gillon in mind, what I find perplexing in Chalmers and Lindley's analysis is a refusal to address explicitly the issue at hand: the moral importance of informed consent in medical research. They do seem to embrace this, citing, for example, Lantos' criticism of standard treatment because "consent may be obtained in a manner governed only by the risk of malpractice litigation" and need not meet up to the scrutiny of a research ethics committee (p. 268). No room for clinical discretion about information based on nothing more than the "Hippocratic commitment" here! Chalmers and Lindley are scathing about the arbitrariness of standards sometimes found in non-experimental clinical care, whatever the feelings of professional duty of those who practise it. Such doctors may dangerously overrely on clinical intuition. The same danger of arbitrariness presumably follows about moral intuition concerning informed consent. One would have thought, therefore – contra Gillon – that Chalmers and Lindley's rejection of what they call the "double standard" of consent between non-experimental and experimental care would demand that patients be both properly informed about the risk of participating in both.

Unfortunately, this is not how Chalmers and Lindley conclude their chapter where they appear to wash their hands of the entire issue of the standard of consent which should be appropriate to both standard and experimental care. They argue: "to have discussed the lack of a single standard on informed consent ... would have served only to distract attention from ... the double standard ... on the requirements for consent to treatment in well-controlled treatment experiments ... and consent to treatment in the poorly-controlled experiments of routine clinical practice ...." (p. 271). Either this means that – as per the above – they believe that routine practice should aspire to the standard of consent to be found in medical research or that the latter should be dumbed down to the level of routine practice, the very level which they so successfully criticise on other grounds. Since I cannot believe that they would advocate the latter, I will continue to interpret them as arguing for the former. In either case, they cannot escape from the necessity to establish the best moral standards for consent to both research and standard care. An optimal moral basis for medical care and research is just as significant as the optimal evidence base which they have both done so much of importance to promote.

John Harris and Simon Woods' View

One of the most important moral tensions in debates about informed consent in medical research is the conflict between the right of competent adults to choose to opt out of participation and the moral duty which they can also be argued to have to participate. Harris and Woods provide a range of interesting and effective arguments from which it follows that we all have a duty to so participate – both in the public interest and also in our own. As regards the public interest, not to participate entails accepting a free ride in the form of optimal medical care and public safety. This is derived from the previous participation of others in medical research and is unfair. Concerning our own interest, they agree that to the degree that these interests are objective and not dependent upon our experience then to "leave the world a better place than it otherwise would have been, is what any decent person should wish to achieve" (p. 280). It is suggested that such arguments are also behind other examples of compulsion which are tolerated in our society to serve the public good (e.g. jury service).

Harris and Woods go on to reason that the fact that we have a moral duty to participate in medical research does not entail that we should be forced to do so: "On the contrary, fully informed consent is the best guarantor of the interests of research subjects and is expressive of equal concern and respect for them as autonomous persons" (p. 280). Yet the authors also argue that the primary reason for not introducing compulsion to participate in research concerns public policy rather than substantive moral principle. On the one hand, they claim current regulation of research is at present insufficient to protect the safety of participants and "whilst informed consent is an imperfect palliative, it serves an important function in the scrutiny of the methods and motives of medical research" (p. 281). On the other hand, they suggest there may be less intrusive ways of encouraging participation in research deemed to be in the public interest (e.g. better education and incentives). However, to argue in this way, envisages circumstances where compulsion would be tolerated (e.g. the guarantee of effective regulation and the failure of alternative methods of encouragement). Here, the force of Harris and Woods' argument must lead to their endorsing compulsion, remembering – as they indicate themselves – that other commentators about medical research are already close to doing so.

There is no space to develop a rival view here, especially in light of the fine quality of the arguments in question. Suffice it to say that Harris and Woods agree with my analysis of informed consent in practice. Indeed, their arguments concerning the poor regulation of some medical research at present and the potential risks which this represents to participants add to the strength of my argument and pose

serious problems for Gillon's confidence in the effectiveness of the Hippocratic commitment. Yet an argument can be developed which rejects the moral primacy of the principle of the duty of individuals to protect the public good over that of the duty of others to respect individual autonomy. Rather than placing priority on the former, one might reason that both principles have equal moral standing. Seen in this way, the sacrifice of either principle always leads to moral harm. The issue then becomes how in specific circumstances to minimise such harm, much as I reasoned in my *BMJ* paper in trying to justify some epidemiological research without informed consent. Such an approach seems to me to be consistent with many of Harris and Woods' practical conclusions about public policy. To place too much moral emphasis on the public good risks too much harm to the public, as indicated by many of the horrors perpetuated in its name in the last century, including some of the notorious medical research outlined in this book.

CONCLUSION

Since the dark days of Nuremberg, we have come a long way in our understanding of the moral importance of informed consent in medical research. When one compares the conduct of research now with that of the time of Beecher and Pappworth, there is much to be pleased about. Because of the regulatory frameworks documented in this book, participants in research can now be much more confident that they will be not exposed to potential harm to which they have not explicitly agreed. They can equally be assured that decisions about the amount and quality of information they require in order to make an educated choice will be independently reviewed and not left to the discretion of researchers themselves. There can be no doubt that as a result of such review, some potential research has been modified or stopped which would have otherwise kept patients in ignorance of significant risks, denying them their right to self-protection. The fact that the conduct of conventional medical care raises similar problems about risks and educated choice does no more than underline the importance of similar vigilance there.

Yet it should also be remembered that progress concerning the rights of participants in research has been hard won. Success has sometimes evolved in the face of continued insistence that limits should be placed on such rights. This is made all the more worrying by the growing threat to human rights posed by probable trends in medical research. For example, research involving the use of human tissue is becoming increasingly diversified, especially in the field of genetics. Progress will demand the creation of tissue banks from which appropriate experimental material can be drawn without the necessity to extract it each time from donors. Providing that, among other things, such tissue is strictly anonymised and has not been taken for the sole purpose of future research, it is widely agreed that the issue of consent does not arise. Yet there will be many circumstances where anonymisation is impossible because future contact with donors (and possibly their relatives) will be necessary.

Here, enormous pressure may be exerted to relax the rules of consent in the name of medical progress. Thus researchers may wish to ask patients to donate tissue for future studies without specifying what type of research this will be or what provision will be made for the feedback of information to them. For all of the reasons which have been argued by so many in this book, such desires should be resisted. To the degree that patients can be seen to have a potentially objective interest in the results of research involving themselves or their tissue then ways should be found for their informed consent to be sought.

Further, as Hall and Ward argue in their chapters, there is no point in stressing the moral and legal importance of a high standard of informed consent in medical research without also underlining the importance of providing the necessary education and resources for this standard to be a realistic possibility. Attempting to convey complex technical information to patients who may be vulnerable and frightened by the choices that confront them can be a demanding task. It may require specialised training, as well as appropriate levels of time, staffing and other resources. In this context, "ought" is constrained by "can" and those responsible for the finance and organisation of medical research and medical education at whatever level should remember this in their decision making. If we cannot afford to conduct medical research so that the autonomy of participants really is respected then the research should not be done. Otherwise, we risk pretending that informed consent has been obtained because certain rituals which gesture in this direction have been performed (e.g. the signing of a piece of paper). To rest content with such gestures – to equate them with an acceptable level of informed consent

in either research or non-experimental therapy – remains a breach of human rights and an offence against human dignity.

Finally, let us conclude by returning to the issue of whether or not journals should publish research inconsistent with an acceptable standard of informed consent. Perhaps unsurprisingly, I can still see no reason for doing so and would speculate that most – but by no means all – of the contributors to this book would agree. What is beyond doubt is that there is nothing new about this problem and no reason to believe that moral standards have only just evolved to the point where a clear conclusion might be reached. We have seen that in his famous paper of 1966, Beecher endorsed the principle of informed consent in medical research. He also wrote (p. 36):

> In the view of the British Medical Research Council it is not enough to ensure that all investigation is carried out in an ethical manner: it must be made unmistakably clear in the publications that the proprieties have been observed. This implies editorial responsibility in addition to the investigator's. The question rises, then, about valuable data that have been improperly obtained. ... Even though suppression of such data ... would constitute a loss to medicine ... this loss ... would be less important than the far reaching moral loss to medicine if the data thus obtained were to be published.

Writing three decades later, I continue to believe that this eloquent statement should still be our guide in thinking about the matter of editorial discretion concerning medical research where informed consent has not been appropriately obtained.

REFERENCES

1. Bristol Royal Infirmary Inquiry. Interim report: removal and retention of human material. Bristol Inquiry Unit, May 10, 2000.
2. Nicholson R. Retaining organs after post-mortems. *Bull Med Ethics* 2000; **157**: 3.
3. Nicholson R. Evidence to the independent inquiry into clinical trials in North Staffordshire. *Bull Med Ethics* 2000; **158**: 13–24.
4. Charatan F. US halts University of Oklahoma clinical research. *BMJ* 2000; **321**: 195.
5. Farham B, Bradbury J. Suspicions raised over breast-therapy trial. *Lancet* 2000; **355**: 553.

32 · Contemporary challenges in clinical research: paying lip service to informed consent, or a genuine shift of gear?

Jeffrey S Tobias

WHAT DOES "INFORMING THE PATIENT" REALLY MEAN?

Like the rest of us, the clinical trialist learns from bitter experience – or at least he thinks he (or she) does, only to make the same errors time and again. Those engaged in the frustrating, laborious but essential task of pursuing clinical trials, with the aim of providing better evidence for medical judgments, know that patient preference for background information varies to an almost bewildering degree. The first might require a lengthy exposition of options, choices, opinions; the next rejects any such discussion out of hand. As a doctor and committed clinical trialist, I doubt (perhaps somewhat arrogantly) that other professional groups recognise this extreme variability so clearly, since patients who make contact, for example with consumer or self-help groups, are of course self-selected; far more are broadly satisfied by the doctor's attention and explanation, and look no further for additional advice. For some patients, an hour's discussion – possibly followed by another, all tape-recorded – may be insufficient, though a more frequent complaint nowadays (at least in my judgment) is that *too much* information is presented for many patients to assimilate. It is as if the radically altered culture of information and consumer selection has in recent years engendered in the doctor an unwelcome sense (unwelcome to the patient, that is) of his (or her) being there simply to lay out the choices somewhat like a market trader at a country fair. The medical profession, stunned by repeated complaints of paternalism, high-mindedness and over-hasty treatment has reacted far too sharply, rejecting its proper twinned role of providing information but also expressing a well thought-out opin-ion based on medical experience and judgment. How often over the past few years have I heard a patient complain in despair: "after I was given the diagnosis of breast cancer I was told I could have a lumpectomy with breast preservation and radiation therapy, or a mastectomy – but the choice was up to me". Many doctors will both recognise and react to this example; few will believe themselves guilty – but in the final reckoning, it's what the patient takes away from the consultation that really matters; the doctor may fail to recognise that the expression of a well-argued preference is just as important as going through the various options – a key component of good medicine rather than unwished-for paternalism.

I feel by now I recognise what "consent" is, but I'm not so sure about "informed". It is the doctor's duty, of course, to give as full and frank an explanation as he or she feels the patient requires – most doctors recognising instinctively that some patients express little interest or need, others a great deal. At each encounter we need sensitivity, humanity and the ability to communicate effectively, with well- or ill-educated, anxious and sometimes incapacitated patients. Even the best informed of them – sometimes doctors themselves, of course – find it difficult to make or even participate in personal decisions under these adverse circumstances. Many now come armed with information from books, magazine articles or the internet, perhaps scarcely recognising that none of these sources can substitute for the doctor's wider understanding of what needs to be done. One sharp distinction to be drawn between present-day communication and the patient–doctor relationship of shall we say five years ago (hardly the olden days!) is the much enhanced level of information now available to patients – a change which I naturally applaud, whilst recognising its inherent dangers. So "informed" is inevitably a relative rather than an absolute term, with the degree of completeness resting on so many variables including of course, the nature and reliability of the source. Those of us who see cancer patients arriving in clinic armed with weighty volumes (often best-sellers) on curing cancer by diet or lifestyle change will know what I mean. In the end, one of the toughest tasks for an informed, intelligent and inquisitive patient, normally fully in control of their life, is to recognise and place trust in the skill and goodwill of their chosen medical adviser – a task made still more difficult in an era of highly specialist medicine in which few patients requiring hospital treatment can still enjoy the luxury of a single doctor able to take charge competently of all aspects of their case. The problem may in principle be as acute for all patients (not just the intelligent, inquisitive, etc.) yet the plight of the relatively well-informed often strikes me as particularly poignant as they embark on their difficult and painful medical journey, with its many attendant indignities and inevitable loss of control.

WHEN DOES "RESEARCH" BECOME "TREATMENT"?

These introductory remarks placed within a closing statement in a volume on informed consent seem to me as much related to "treatment" as to "research" so I deliberately illustrate the enduring medical dilemma (how much discussion? how little?) in the context of a "typical" doctor–patient interaction over medical management as I do not see a moral distinction between the two. Traditionally, perhaps, there might have been "established treatment" (radical mastectomy, for instance) and "research" (a newer type of treatment, often vigorously advocated by one or two passionate believers yet rejected by the majority) such as lumpectomy with radiation, preservation of the breast, but no mastectomy. Yesterday's orthodoxy becomes today's standard practice, sometimes almost overnight, as for example with the immediate adoption a decade ago of clotbusting treatment with aspirin and streptokinase for heart attacks. The public at large – and many who sit on ethics committees, I should think – have little conception that these two apparently separate aspects of medical activity are in fact tightly enmeshed or, perhaps more accurately, joined at the

hip. Many of today's fully accepted treatments, hallowed by tradition and historical precedent, have little evidence base to support them, including widely practised procedures such as tonsillectomy, prolonged bed rest for back pain, vitamin supplementation, use of cough suppressants for "chestiness" – an almost endless list. Whereas "research" – now that's another matter! All of us feel entitled to the best available treatment (better than the best, if possible) dimly recognising perhaps the concept of clinical research trials as a means to discovering which novel treatment is genuinely better. Many of course (patients and doctors alike) habitually confuse "novel" with "progress".

Nonetheless, remarkable medical advances have been made over the past thirty years since I qualified in medicine, every one of them underpinned by research activity, often initiated by lone mavericks or a few brave souls dissatisfied with current treatment. Doubtless some have moved too hastily from laboratory science to the clinical arena, though in recent years, local and national research ethics committees have played an important moderating role, guiding the hand of overzealous researchers. Inevitably, in some cases, such committees are clearly at odds with similar ones elsewhere, who might judge the same piece of research ethically acceptable in one part of the country, but not, say, in a neighbouring health region. To some extent, the development of MRECs (multicentre research ethics committees) have solved this unacceptable restriction though voices have been raised in protest including that of the President of the Royal College of Physicians. In a recent editorial entitled "Multi-centre Research Ethics Committees: has the Cure been Worse than the Disease?", he pointed out that since the development of MRECs, established in 1997, "frustrated research workers have regularly told me that the new system is a disaster".[1] Professor Alberti also referred to two articles in the same edition of the *BMJ* as his editorial, both tracking the record of multicentre research submissions. In the larger of these, by Tully and colleagues from the Institute of Child Health, London,[2] 125 local research ethics committees' activities were addressed; although the development of multicentre committees had shortened the process of dealing with applications, their study protocol had still not been approved by nine of the committees, as far out as six months after submission of the application! The median time of response was just under six weeks, a reasonable enough period one might think, though half of the committees had asked for amendments, and two-thirds of these concerned non-local issues – expressly (as Alberti pointed out) *against the guidance* from the Department of Health. In a further article of an even simpler trial design, Larcombe and Mott were frustrated in their study of lifestyle health behaviour in young adult survivors of childhood cancer – essentially a straightforward questionnaire-and-interview protocol, hardly rocket science – by endless red tape from both local and multicentre research committees.[3] The quickest responses (all by Chairman's action) had been under a fortnight, the slowest $4^{1}/_{2}$ months, for a study which had already received ethical approval from a multi-centre committee! Many researchers faced by such difficulties become understandably dispirited, taking the view that the game is simply not worth the candle.

To give one recent example of the fine line between research and treatment, the use of post-operative pelvic radiotherapy following hysterecto-my for uterine cancer – hardly any longer a research question at all, you might say – was assessed in a large-scale randomised study from Hol-land in which all but one of that nation's cancer cen-tres participated, itself a remarkable enough achievement.[4] Specific lessons were learnt about which type of patient might benefit and which not, but the important point within the present discus-sion is that even a relatively standard "treatment" should be regarded as fair game whenever necessary, to a renewed scrutiny which can only be described as "research". The line of division is so faint as to be better removed entirely, a move in the right direc-tion which would engender a far greater sense of co-operation and partnership between patient and doctor: a welcome and more grown-up attitude by society at large to the need both for continuous research effort, and for querying established approaches.

The most important lessson I learnt during my year as a postgrad at Harvard Medical School was encapsulated in their proud slogan "Clinical research is an obligation, not an option" emblazoned in lecture halls and seminars across the campus. I certainly thought of that when reading the recent startling news reports[5] about a comparative trial of an experimental neonatal ventilator, the CNEP device (continuous negative extra-thoracic pressure), which expanded babies' lungs to help them breathe without the need for intubation – an extremely worthwhile line of research since intubation of an infant requires such remarkable skill, not always

available for a difficult obstetric delivery during the small hours. It makes sense to assess whether a type of ventilation without intubation but with a sophis-ticated face-mask type of support might be benefi-cial. In the event, sadly, the comparative study performed in North Staffs, UK, showed no benefit; indeed, a possible slight disadvantage. Between 1989 and 1993, 122 babies were put on the CNEP machine; of these 43 died or were brain damaged compared to 32 in the control group placed in a con-ventional ventilator. Statistically, the outcome was not significantly different, but the main outrage causing such public disquiet was the alleged lack of parental consent and, worse still, a claim that in some cases, their signatures on the permission (consent) forms might have been forged. These points were made by an NHS panel who found that "experiments have taken place at the hospital without safeguards to ensure that the parents of babies who took part in random trials knew what was happening and agreed to it". It seems clear that whilst statistically significant results are always required before the medical profession takes serious notice of a new treat-ment, the public's view is understandably different, and the message from both the panel report and the media frenzy was that 11 of these babies died or were serious damaged unnecessarily. Regardless of the sci-entific outcome, the real source of understandable anger and bitterness was once again the consent issue, far more than the arguably inferior 'medical' result.

ALTERNATIVES TO THE CONTROLLED RANDOMISED TRIAL?

All this makes the concept of "informed consent" still more complex since those who insist upon following a (preferably written) line should recognise that the spotlight needs to be focused not only on the rela-tive minority of committed researchers, who for the most part genuinely recognise that questioning orthodoxy with a well-constructed trial protocol should be applauded rather than viewed as a threat; but also on those who recommend "treatment" which may have little if any firm evidence base. As the writer and journalist Carolyn Faulder pointed out in her book *Whose body is it? The troubling issue of informed consent*,[6] (p. 2)

> informed consent is *the* ethical issue in medicine today, and unless we sort out our views and determine what we really mean when we talk about the patient's right

to give informed consent, we are imperilling our ability to make wise and humane decisions about all the other bioethical problems now facing us. I say this, well aware that many people, including even some of the ethicists and doctors who are most concerned about the prevailing lack of informed consent, particularly in clinical trials, will think I am over-stating the case.

Personally, I don't. Not much has changed in the 15 years since Faulder published her book, though multicentre research ethics committees have certainly imposed a greater degree of conformity. Perhaps we can claim to have moved closer to an increased understanding both by doctors and patients of the need for research generally, and also – at least arguably – the moral issues relating to the patient's decision whether or not to participate in a clinical trial. The quality of clinical research has generally improved with an increasing recognition that single-centre studies with small numbers of patients are usually meaninglesss and that statistical number-crunching is an essential part of the game. Meta-analyses allow proper and reliable conclusions to be drawn from large-scale studies where bias is effectively removed, with the patient groups sufficiently large for treatment, rather than chance, to be the determining factor in measuring outcomes. As Faulder points out, there may be alternatives to randomised controlled trials but like most clinical researchers, I am greatly concerned that other approaches, for example the careful observation of a concurrent control series treated differently from the "novel treatment" group, are fraught with difficulty and likely to include biases which even (especially!) the researcher may fail to recognise. A treatment recommendation based on weaker evidence than that obtained from a randomised clinical trial is like a recommendation based on a mere hunch or an idiosyncratic preference.[7, 8]

This issue was recently addressed by two "special articles" in the *New England Journal of Medicine* together with an editorial,[9, 10] the two articles essentially supporting the use of 'observational' (i.e. non-randomised) studies but the editorial taking a quite different view, reminding us that "only randomised treatment assignment can provide a reliably unbiased estimate of treatment effects" – a position with which I wholeheartedly agree. It may be a matter of some conjecture but my personal view is that the conceptual development of the randomised controlled trial is probably the greatest medical advance of the last century. Since improvements in medical treatment are hardly ever self-evident, clinical trials of one type or another are invariably required to confirm or

refute that a novel approach is genuinely better, and have played a central part in the development of an evidence-based medical culture. However, both for doctors and much more importantly for society at large, it is important for the distinction between conventional treatment and research to be recognised as frequently artificial; what should follow is a clearer recognition by all parties that there is little in medicine that is written in tablets of stone. Just as today's cutting edge research technology becomes tomorrow's standard practice, an established methodology, so vigorously practised and defended within the profession, may prove unnecessary. Participation in research is surely the best way of keeping doctors on their toes. Earlier in this volume, Chalmers and Lindley eloquently argue the case that double standards – with the often foolish and unwarranted distinction between treatment and research – remain all too common, with the unacceptable moral conclusion that informed consent is somehow seen as crucial in the one situation, but, curiously, unnecessary in the other. In my view, this irritating distinction is profoundly damaging for the proper pursuit of research trials aimed both at the definition of better new treatments, and the rejection of outmoded or unnecessarily damaging traditional practice.

WHAT IS "ETHICAL" ANYWAY?

It might seem somewhat disingenuous at this late stage to pose such a contentious, even impertinent question, but the continuing bioethical debate confirms this fundamental query as a live issue – and with continuing debate comes conceptual development. My own view is that we can be less certain of "absolutes" in medical ethics than in most spheres of moral philosophy. Just as treatments shift and (hopefully) improve, so the limits of what society regards as "ethical" are not perhaps as fixed as we might fondly imagine. Take, for example, the celebrated case of Mrs Diane Blood, in which assisted conception to achieve fertilisation using her late husband's semen was denied her on ethical grounds, since her husband had died before formal consent to usage of his sperm had been obtained – even though the technology for fertilisation was of course in place. The legal judgment in the UK was that such *in vitro* fertilisation should be denied her, at least within these shores, but that no legal impediment could be brought to bear, should she decide to seek medical help elsewhere – which, of course, is just what she did, taking her dead husband's sperm sample with her.

My own view about this sorry affair was that we had let Mrs Blood down, by an unnecessarily purist and narrow-minded interpretation of current ethical and legal opinion. By what *moral* authority could even the highest court in the land deny access, given what seemed to me at the time (and still does) an entirely common-sense view that Mrs Blood's late husband's consent could implicitly and most reasonably have been assumed, since they were man and wife living harmoniously together at the time of his death. Certainly there was no issue of consent on the part of Mrs Blood! And her husband, no longer alive, was unable either to give consent – *or to withhold it*. Technology nowadays certainly drives ethics (think for example of the huge moral questions thrown up by the virtual completion of the Human Genome Project). To the great relief of Mrs Blood, what was felt unethical in the UK was rightly accepted as perfectly acceptable in Belgium, where successful fertilisation was achieved. Or take the example of cloning – unlike the Blood case, currently unresolved but clearly a technology capable of offering powerful opportunities for medical advance. How many members of the public realise that the whipping up of fears about Frankenstein-type monsters seriously hinders the cooler and more clear-headed debate which we so badly need, in order to look more carefully at the clear potential benefits, for instance in patients suffering severe burns – often of course children – for whom additional supplies of cloned human skin could literally make the difference between life and death. The technology is there: will the ethics keep up? And with waning authority from religious and other leaders of society, whom will we choose to oversee such decisions? After all, in an increasingly consumer-oriented society, where the customer increasingly calls the tune, should we not argue for more democratic means of deciding how far to exploit the benefits that modern biotechnology now routinely offers?

Even within the narrower issue of informed consent in clinical trials, one might reasonably argue the ethics of provoking anxiety in the many (by over-explicit explanation of highly unlikely side effects, for example) for the benefit of the few, i.e. those who do develop the side effect – a common enough problem in clinical medicine, but especially acute in the research setting. I am not here suggesting that only those who engage actively at the coal face of clinical research have the right to debate these issues, far

from it; but I do feel, however, that doctors and healthcare professionals in general are perhaps more keenly aware of the practical difficulties to which an insistence on "the ethical approach" can sometimes lead, particularly with vulnerable patients who are often more than willing to participate in clinical research, but less concerned about the niceties or conundrums of ethics and consent. I accept of course that a fine line exists between trust and exploitation; but will it really be to society's and the individual's advantage if we were to recommend more in the way of "ethical policing" of the medical profession, or would it simply act more frequently to stifle essential research? If trust between doctor and patient is not enough, then what should replace it? A serious question, not just conceptually but perhaps even more important, in terms of practicality. At present, at least in the research setting, a common solution to this formidable problem is the use and involvement of other professionals than doctors (often trial co-ordinators, research nurses and so on), who witness the discussion between doctor and patient, and often at a later stage enlarge on what the doctor had to say. "Witness" implies less than active participation, which may seem an affront to the concept of the fully integrated research nurse – though on ethical grounds, this key professional would inevitably become less independent if viewed more fully as a clinical researcher him- or herself. My own view is that nothing inspires confidence in the patient so much as a clear explanation by the doctor of what is wrong, what needs to be done, and whether there is a clinical trial available which might be appropriate or potentially beneficial to the individual concerned.

INFORMED CONSENT AND OUR GENOMIC FUTURE

As recently pointed out in a *Lancet* editorial, demand for trial participants has never been so high – partly of course because more drugs are currently in development than ever before.[11] In 1995, for example, 2585 drugs were in pre-clinical animal testing in the USA; three years later that number had increased to 3278. In the decade up to 1990, the average number of individuals included within new-drug-application trials had more than tripled to over 4000. Increasing developmental costs put considerable pressure on the pharmaceutical companies to bring new drugs to the market place in as short a time as possible.

These powerful commercial trends have stimulated a report by the US Department of Health and Human Services Office of Inspector General [*Recruiting human subjects: pressures in industry-sponsored clinical research*] which criticised many recruiters in the USA for adopting practices that seemed to compromise patient confidentiality, abuse the doctor–patient relationship, and ignore basic requirements for informed consent. Doctors, for example, are often paid substantial fees to get their patients to enrol in trials, raising serious questions about a potential conflict of interest. The report also found that on occasion, recruiters appeal directly to the public, with misleading advertisements giving the impression that an unproven experimental drug could be an effective new treatment or encouraging news stories in the media, to suggest that the investigational drug is more promising than the facts strictly allow. One industrial press article quoted by the OIG (and also by the *Lancet* editorial) noted: "Done correctly, publicity can look like an endorsement by your well-respected newspaper reporter or TV news anchor. It can be an excellent way to generate phone calls needed to fill studies". What's more, the report also noted a worrying trend to undertake more trials in developing countries such as China where research costs are lower, and it is much easier to find participants who have never received treatment for their particular condition – once again reminding us (as in the Diane Blood case) of the wide international variable standard of ethical acceptability within the whole bioethical research arena.

A further recent event of considerable significance to the research community in the USA has been the suspension of testing of a cancer vaccine under study at the University of Oklahoma.[12] Federal regulators from the newly constituted Federal Office for Human Research Protections have insisted that the research be halted for a number of reasons including the criticism that "the informed-consent form given to volunteers overstated the possible benefits of the experiment and understated the risks", a charge closely analogous to those made by Beecher and Pappworth over 30 years ago. This highly publicised decision affected around 75 studies on the campus at the University of Oklahoma Health Sciences Center in Tulsa, the suspension occurring, it seems, largely because of the auditors' concern that "adequate precautions to protect the safety of patients [had] not been taken".

They certainly do things differently in Iceland! In 1998 a commercial organisation, deCODE genetics, were given the exclusive rights to incorporate the medical records of all Icelandic citizens into a database which would also contain genetic information on those who agreed voluntarily to donate a DNA sample to the company. Iceland's relative isolation, small population (270 000), and extensive population-based record system make it an ideal location for genetic research, and by correlating the medical and genetic data, deCODE hopes to discover medically useful knowledge with – of course – considerable commercial opportunity.[13] According to the law, the centralised database, termed the Icelandic Healthcare Database (IHD), with information from the entire healthcare system, would be collected under the assumption of "presumed consent". This might be regarded as a somewhat nebulous concept, but in the context of the project the authors of the *New England Journal of Medicine* sounding board article regarded it as "the consent of society to the use of health care information according to the norms of [that] society. These norms may vary from one society to another and may change with time ...".[14]

Some would doubtless argue that presumed consent is inconsistent with the right of individuals to decide for themselves, amounting to a new and ground-breaking standard for research and healthcare data produced in the process of delivering medical services. However, the authors state robustly "It is not certain that we would have health care as we know it today if explicit consent had [previously] been a pre-requisite for the use of medical data". On the other hand, as pointed out by the author of the sounding board article (himself from the Boston University School of Medicine and Public Health), "Although a community can approve a research project, it cannot legally or ethically require individual members of the community to participate." In recognising the many benefits from "group participation", I rather like the concept described here of "community consultation" rather than "community consent". Perhaps the answer, as Annas suggests, is to propose that individual consent should not be necessary for research if the DNA in this project were to be stripped of its identifiers, so that it could not be traced back to the individual person, providing research with non-linkable data (sometimes termed "anonymous" research) with its protection of individual privacy.

These are weighty issues indeed. DNA molecules are entirely separate from medical records, though in the future, it is likely that the DNA molecule and the medical record could merge when it becomes possible to sequence an individual's entire genome and put the information on a computer chip or disk – and that moment has very nearly arrived! Ownership of such information would then be a matter for authoritative ethical bodies to consider, but they would have many nettles to grasp. Who would take ownership of such information? Should special consideration be given to highly sensitive medical information relating to psychiatric or drug-dependency data? What about the status of children and minors? Should patients be encouraged to have their entire genome scanned without knowledge of the thousands of genetic tests which could be run, akin to consent to a battery of tests during annual physical examinations of healthy subjects? – and so on.

One thing is for sure: with these rapid developments in electronic information transfer and genetic biotechnology, advances in science and medicine will take off at an ever-accelerating pace over the next decade.[15] Despite attacks by those believing in alternative approaches to gathering reliable data, the randomised trial remains of paramount importance even though I accept as a serious ethical difficulty (as Truog and colleagues pointed out) that "studies have shown that patients rarely demonstrate an adequate understanding of consent forms and often do not understand the meaning or implications of randomisation".[16] In the end we will all have to rely (as these same authors recommend) on the "reasonable-person standard" to determine whether persons should be informed about becoming subjects in a randomised, controlled trial – a standard which would require informing prospective subjects whenever enrolment in the study could lead to additional testing, clinic visits or other inconveniences beyond those associated with ordinary treatment or, as one correspondent pointed out,[17] "if the investigators plan to collect and maintain records of confidential information apart from the standard medical record". This same correspondent recommended using the legal analogy of a standard interpreted by a jury of one's peers, in judging whether or not consent should be regarded as essential before enrolment within a clinical trial.

In concluding this brief survey of contemporary and future issues within the current debate on consent, I feel strongly that, as pointed out by Dresser and Truog, there is a pressing need for greater community involvement in decision-making with respect to clinical trial proposals – a concept already "up and running" in the UK, with increasing input from such bodies as the Consumers' Advisory Group for Clinical Trials which has already helped to shape some of our important prospective trial programmes. Only when the community at large wakes up to its responsibility as genuine partners in clinical research will we make real progress in this contentious, labyrinthine and highly charged debate.

REFERENCES

1. Alberti KGM. Multicentre research ethics committees: has the cure been worse than the disease? *Br Med J* 2000; **320**: 1157–8.
2. Tully J, Minis N, Booy R, Viner R. The new system of review by multicentre research ethics committees: prospective study. *Br Med J* 2000; **320**: 1179–82.
3. Larcombe I, Mott M. Multicentre research ethics committees: have they helped? *J Roy Soc Med* 1999; **92**: 500–1.
4. Creutzberg CL, Van Putten WLJ, Koper PCM *et al*. Surgery and postoperative radiotherapy vs surgery alone for patients with stage-l endometrial carcinoma: multicentre randomised trial. *Lancet* 2000; **355**: 1404–11.
5. Boseley S. NHS on trial over secret baby tests. *The Guardian*, May 9, 2000.
6. Faulder C. *Whose body is it? The troubling issue of informed consent*. London: Virago Books, 1985. Benson K, Hartz AJ. A comparison of observational studies and randomised, controlled trials. *New Engl J Med* 2000; **342**: 1878–86.
7. Marquis D. How to resolve an ethical dilemma concerning randomized clinical trials. *New Engl J Med* 1999; **341**: 691–2.
8. Freedman B. Equipoise and the ethics of clinical research. *New Engl J Med* 1987; **317**: 141–5.
9. Concato J, Shah N, Horwitz RI. Randomised, controlled trials, observational studies, and the hierarchy of research designs. *New Engl J Med* 2000; **342**: 1887–92.
10. Pocock SJ, Elbourne DR. Randomized trials or observational tribulations? *New Engl J Med* 2000; **342**: 1907–9.
11. Anon. Safeguarding participants in clinical trials. *Lancet* 2000; **355**: 2177.
12. Weiss R, Nelson D. US halts testing on cancer patients. *Internationl Herald Tribune*. 12 July, 2000.
13. Gulcher JR, Stefansson K. The Icelandic healthcare database and informed consent. *New Engl J Med* 2000; **342**: 1827–30.
14. Annas GJ. Rules for research on human genetic variation – lessons from Iceland. *New Engl J Med* 2000; **342**: 1830–3.

15. Meek J. New age of cloning for health care. *The Guardian*, June 29, 2000.
16. Truog RD, Robinson WW, Randolph A, Maurice A. Is informed consent always necessary for randomised, controlled trials? *New Engl J Med* 1999; **340**: 804–7

and **341**: 450 (correspondence, August 5, 1999).
17. Dresser R. Is informed consent always necessary for randomised, controlled trials? [correspondence] *New Engl J Med* 1999; **341**: 449.

Index